AF437252

ANNALS OF
THE NEW YORK ACADEMY
OF SCIENCES

Volume 730

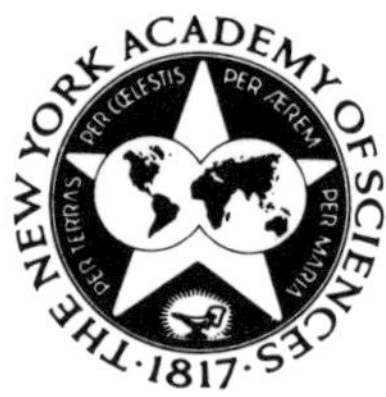

EDITORIAL STAFF

Executive Editor
BILL M. BOLAND

Managing Editor
JUSTINE CULLINAN

Associate Editor
ANGELA C. FINK

The New York Academy of Sciences
2 East 63rd Street
New York, New York 10021

MICROBIAL PATHOGENESIS
AND
IMMUNE RESPONSE

ANNALS OF THE NEW YORK ACADEMY OF SCIENCES
Volume 730

MICROBIAL PATHOGENESIS
AND
IMMUNE RESPONSE

Edited by Edwin W. Ades, Richard F. Rest, and Stephen A. Morse

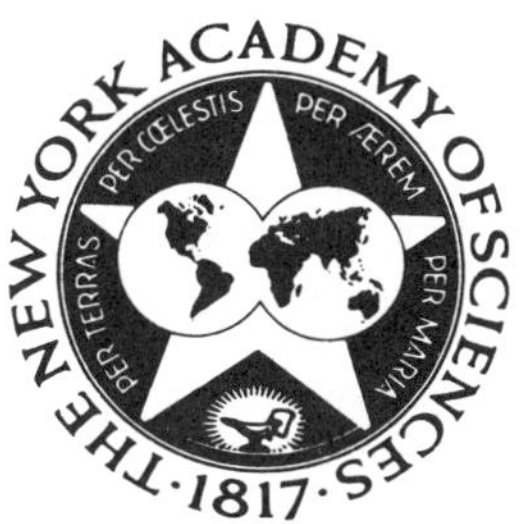

The New York Academy of Sciences
New York, New York
1994

Library of Congress Cataloging-in-Publication Data

Microbial pathogenesis and immune response / edited by Edwin W. Ades, Richard F. Rest and Stephen A. Morse.

    p. cm. — (Annals of the New York Academy of Sciences, ISSN 0077-8923 ; v. 730)

    Includes bibliographical references and index.

    ISBN 0-89766-895-2 (alk. paper : cloth). — ISBN 0-89766-896-0 (alk. paper : paper)

    1. Pathogenic microorganisms—Congresses. 2. Infection—Immunological aspects—Congresses. I. Ades, Edwin W. II. Rest, Richard F. III. Morse, Stephen A. IV. Series.

    [DNLM: 1. Bacteria—pathogenicity—congresses. 2. Bacterial Infections—immunology—congresses. 3. Infection—immunology—congresses. 4. Infection—microbiology—congresses. W1 AN626YL v. 730 1994 / QZ 65 M626 1994]

Q11.N5 vol. 730

[QR175]

500 s—dc20

[616'.014]

DNLM/DLC

for Library of Congress

94-25683

CIP

PCP

Printed in the United States of America

ISBN 0-89766-895-2 (cloth)

ISBN 0-89766-896-0 (paper)

ISSN 0077-8923

ANNALS OF THE NEW YORK ACADEMY OF SCIENCES

Volume 730
August 15, 1994

MICROBIAL PATHOGENESIS AND IMMUNE RESPONSE [a]

Editors and Conference Organizers
EDWIN W. ADES, RICHARD F. REST, AND STEPHEN A. MORSE

CONTENTS

[a] This volume is the result of a conference entitled **Microbial Pathogenesis and Immune Response**, which was sponsored by the New York Academy of Sciences and held on September 8–11, 1993 in Lake Buena Vista, Florida.

Financial assistance was received from:

Supporter
- CENTERS FOR DISEASE CONTROL AND PREVENTION

Contributors
- ABBOTT LABORATORIES
- AMGEN INC.
- IMMUNEX RESEARCH AND DEVELOPMENT CORP.
- THE R. W. JOHNSON PHARMACEUTICAL RESEARCH INSTITUTE
- SMITHKLINE BEECHAM PHARMACEUTICALS
- SYNTEX DISCOVERY RESEARCH, DIVISION OF SYNTEX (USA) INC.

Preface

EDWIN W. ADES

Centers for Disease Control and Prevention
Atlanta, Georgia 30333

This is the record of the conference on "Microbial Pathogenesis and Immune Response" which took place in Orlando, Florida, September 8–11, 1993. Our rationale for this meeting was that most researchers interested in infection and immunity focus on either microbial pathogenesis or immunology and immunity, rarely on both. Thus, the objective of this meeting was to bring together an international group of basic and clinical researchers from government, academia, and industry who, individually, were interested either in the molecular mechanisms of microbial pathogenesis or in human immune response. Our focus was to use the information exchanged at this meeting to formulate clearer approaches to immune regulation of and vaccine development for various human pathogens.

We knew that many of the invited speakers have never heard each others' presentations and were anxious to agree to speak. Certainly, those attending the meeting found an exciting, stimulating mix of molecular pathogenesis and host immune response. Indeed, the mix of cytokines and microbial pathogenesis was unique to this meeting, which focused on developments applicable to or promising as therapeutic modalities. The scientific themes included experimental and clinical data and the latest molecular, cellular, and genetic approaches in areas of intense research activity in microbial pathogenesis. Presentations (oral and poster) covered *in vitro* studies, experiments in animal models, and pre-clinical and clinical epidemiologic relationships between infection and disease. The overall emphasis was to identify effective and efficient strategies for harnessing immunologic approaches to infectious disease.

The meeting ended with a discussion and summary of the talks by two world renowned researchers, Dr. Fred Murphy, Dean, School of Veterinary Medicine, University of California, Davis, and Dr. Stephen Morse, Director, Division of Sexually Transmitted Diseases, National Center for Infectious Diseases, Centers for Disease Control and Prevention.

We have been encouraged about this meeting by the positive remarks heard when formulating the speakers' rostrum. We hope that the interactions fostered between individuals will stimulate new ideas and new approaches.

The organizers wish to thank the New York Academy of Sciences and those companies and government agencies that helped to fund this meeting.

Structure and Function of the Parasitophorous Vacuole Membrane Surrounding *Toxoplasma gondii*

K. A. JOINER,[a] C. J. M. BECKERS, D. BERMUDES,
P. N. OSSORIO, J. C. SCHWAB, AND
J. F. DUBREMETZ

Yale University School of Medicine
New Haven, Connecticut 06510-8056
and
U42 Inserm
Villenueve d'Ascq, France

Toxoplasma gondii is growing in popularity as a model for studying intracellular parasitism.[1] The parasite has also gained more attention recently as the most common cause of focal central nervous system infections in patients with the acquired immunodeficiency syndrome,[2] and it continues to cause more than 3,000 cases per year of congenital birth defects in the United States alone.

T. gondii infects nearly all animals and most birds and is one of the most widely distributed of all intracellular parasites. *In vitro,* tachyzoites of *T. gondii* can invade and replicate within essentially all nucleated cells, an unusual feat for any intracellular organism. The intracellular tachyzoites reside within a vacuole that is incapable of acidifying or fusing with any membrane-bound organelle within the host cell endocytic system[3-6] and as such is effectively hidden from the host, yet the parasite replicates rapidly. The fusion incompetence of the vacuole is established at the time of cell entry and does not depend on secretion by the parasite of a soluble inhibitor of the fusion or acidification events. On the basis of these findings and in conjunction with the known morphology of the newly formed parasitophorous vacuole membrane (PVM), we hypothesized that fusion incompetence results from the absence of protein signals for vesicular fusion events. Nonetheless, the PVM surrounding *T. gondii* serves a critical additional function which is likely to depend on proteins, by allowing access of necessary nutrients from and exchange of metabolites with the host cell. A second potential function for the PVM, binding of host cell mitochondria and endoplasmic reticulum,[7] is also likely to be protein dependent. We believe that proteins that provide or contribute to these additional functions for the PVM are likely to be derived from parasite secretory organelles, but little direct data exist to support this hypothesis.

[a] Address for correspondence: K. A. Joiner, LCI 808, Section of Infectious Diseases, Yale University School of Medicine, 333 Cedar Street, New Haven, CT 06510-8056.

Our laboratories have been identifying and characterizing parasite proteins that associate with the PVM and that are likely to contribute to the functions just described. In particular, we have focused on proteins derived from a characteristic set of secretory organelles common to Apicomplexan parasites (such as Toxoplasma, Plasmodia, Cryptosporidia, Babesia, Theileria, and Eimeria), the rhoptries and dense granules[8] which discharge at selected times during and after cell invasion. The rhoptries are large, club-shaped anterior structures which are connected by thin ducts to the apical end of the parasite. During cell invasion only, rhoptries discharge their lumenal contents[7] through the duct into the forming vacuolar space. In contrast, the dense granules exocytose their contents into the vacuolar space after invasion is complete.[9–12] At least 10 rhoptry proteins (ROP1-9 and PO56) and 5 dense granule proteins (GRA1-5) have been identified in *T. gondii* using monoclonal antibodies.

DENSE GRANULE PROTEINS AND THE PVM

The major *T. gondii* dense granule proteins associated with the PVM are the 30-kD protein GRA3[13,14] and the 21-kD protein GRA5.[15] Our studies have focused on GRA3. Discharge of GRA3 into the vacuolar space is observed within 10 minutes after parasite invasion and increases in amount as the vacuole matures. The kinetics of GRA5 association with the PVM are not yet defined. Dense granule proteins GRA1, 2, and 4 are confined to the vacuolar space.[11,14,16] The function of GRA3 or of other dense granule proteins is not yet known.

GRA3 undergoes a conformational change after exocytosis; GRA3 liberated from parasite dense granules is a soluble monomeric protein, whereas GRA3 is inserted into the PVM as an amphiphilic homo-oligomer.[17] Soluble globular proteins which polymerize in association with transition to an amphiphilic form generally express epitopes specific for the polymerized form and lose epitopes specific for the monomeric form (reviewed in ref. 18). GRA3 undergoes such a conformational change during polymerization and PVM association. A monoclonal antibody that immunoprecipitates monomeric GRA3 does not immunoprecipitate the polymeric form of the molecule.

The deduced amino acid sequence for GRA3 predicts a protein with a long NH_2-terminal signal sequence which is cleaved from the protein during *in vitro* translation in the presence of dog pancreatic microsomes (Bermudes, Dubremetz, and Joiner, in preparation). Four additional short hydrophobic stretches in the protein may participate in PVM association. The mechanism and functional consequences of GRA3 association with the PVM is an active area of study in our laboratories.

RHOPTRY PROTEINS AND THE PVM

Immediately following invasion, the rhoptry protein ROP1 is associated with the PVM.[19] However, within 16 hours after invasion, ROP1 is no longer detectable.[14] In contrast, the rhoptry proteins ROP2, 3, 4, and PO56 are stably associated with the PVM.[20] Using permeabilized cell systems, we have shown that ROP2, 3, 4, and PO56 are exposed on the cytoplasmic side of the PVM. These molecules behave as transmembrane proteins in the PVM, based on salt elution studies and labeling with the photoactivatable membrane probe TID. The deduced amino acid sequence for full-length ROP2[20–22] encodes a protein with a signal sequence and a potential transmembrane domain near the COOH-terminus of the molecule. Topology studies using antibodies recognizing short fusion peptides from the protein show that the amino terminus of ROP2 is cytoplasmically exposed.[20]

Rhoptries are unusual organelles biochemically[23] and morphologically. The appearance within the lumen of rhoptries of membranous whorls[24] analogous to the surfactant-containing lamellar bodies of Type II pulmonary alveolar cells suggests that pre-formed membranes exist within the rhoptry. Discharge of these pre-formed membranes might then contribute to PVM formation. Direct confirmation of this hypothesis has been difficult (reviewed in ref. 25).

As mentioned above, ROP2, 3, 4, and PO56 behave as integral membrane proteins in the PVM. The mechanism for membrane insertion of these proteins is not yet clear, and no analogous data are available for any other coccidian parasite. Most eukaryotic membrane proteins are stably inserted into membranes cotranslationally (reviewed in ref. 26). In contrast, toxins and other pore-forming molecules are synthesized as soluble precursors which are secreted in soluble form and later inserted into membranes (reviewed in ref. 27). In this context, there are three potential explanations for the cytoplasmic exposure of ROP2, 3, 4, and PO56 epitopes in the PVM: (1) The proteins are packaged in a lipid bilayer in the rhoptries which contributes to formation of the PVM[7,28,29]; (2) the proteins are inserted into or through the PVM during or after invasion; or (3) the proteins are not inserted into the PVM but are bound by hydrophobic interactions to both sides of the PVM. Experiments are underway to distinguish between these possibilities.

PERMEABILITY OF THE PVM

The PVM functions as a molecular sieve, allowing the passive diffusion of charged and uncharged molecules of less than 1,400 daltons bidirectionally between host cell cytoplasm and the vacuolar space. This conclusion is based on microinjection of variously sized flourescent tracers into the cytoplasm of *T. gondii*-infected cells.[30] This result is most consistent with a proteinaceous pore in the PVM, which we hypothesize is of parasitic origin. An analogous structure was recently identified in the PVM surrounding *Plasmodium falciparum*.[31]

The presence of a pore across the PVM provides a simple yet elegant mechanism for exchange of nutrients and metabolites between the parasite and the host cell. The presence of a PVM pore of sufficient diameter to allow the diffusion of amino acids, monosaccharides, and purine nucleosides into the vacuolar space eliminates the need to have specific transporters for each of these components within the PVM. Instead, transporters within the otherwise impermeable parasite plasma membrane provide the specificity for nutrient uptake. Conversely, metabolic byproducts of the organism (such as pyruvate) do not accumulate within the vacuole space; they immediately diffuse across the PVM.

Most likely, the pore across the PVM is a proteinaceous channel of parasitic origin. Alternatively, the pore could be a proteinaceous channel of host cell origin or a combination of host and parasite molecules. One of our long-term goals is to understand the structure of the PVM pore and its role in the intracellular survival and replication of *T. gondii.*

ORGANELLE ASSOCIATION WITH THE PVM

Host cell endoplasmic reticulum (ER) and mitochondria localize to the PVM during and immediately after invasion,[32] suggesting a specific recognition event. The ER and mitochondrial membranes are tightly apposed to the PVM. Using mitochondria-specific dyes at the light microscopic level, we found that the association of mitochondria with the PVM does not depend on host cell microtubules or microfilaments, is maintained even when parasites are killed after invasion, and does not depend on mitochondrial membrane potential or mitochondrial DNA (Ossorio and Joiner, in preparation). Although the mechanism for the association is not yet known, the foregoing results are most consistent with a specific ligand-receptor interaction between the PVM and the mitochondrial outer membrane. In addition to defining the components of this interaction, we ultimately hope to determine the function that PVM-associated host cell mitochondria and ER play in the intracellular survival and replication of *T. gondii.*

CONCLUSION

Rhoptry and dense granule proteins associated with the PVM are certain to have important roles in the intracellular survival of *T. gondii.* Defining the role of these or other parasite proteins in PVM-associated functions such as transport, permeability, and organelle recruitment will facilitate an understanding of intracellular parasitism in general and coccidian parasites in particular.

REFERENCES

1. McLeod, R., D. Mack & C. Brown. 1991. *Toxoplasma gondii:* New advances in cellular and molecular biology. Exp. Parsitol. **72:** 109–121.
2. Luft, B. F. & J. S. Remington. 1992. Toxoplasmic encephalitis in AIDS. Clin. Infect. Dis. **15:** 211–222.
3. Jones, T. C., S. Veh & J. G. Hirsch. 1972. The interaction between *Toxoplasma gondii* and mammalian cells. I. Mechanism of entry and intracellular fate of the parasite. J. Exp. Med. **136:** 1157–1172.
4. Jones, T. C. & J. G. Hirsch. 1972. The interaction between *Toxoplasma gondii* and mammalian cells. II. The absence of lysosomal fusion with phagocytic vacuoles containing living parasites. J. Exp. Med. **136:** 1173.
5. Joiner, K. A., S. A. Fuhrman, H. Mietinnen, L. L. Kasper & I. Mellman. 1990. *Toxoplasma gondii:* Fusion competence of parasitophorous vacuoles in Fc receptor transfected fibroblasts. Science **249:** 641–646.
6. Sibley, L. D., E. Weidner & J. L. Krahenbuhl. 1985. Phagosome acidification blocked by intracellular *Toxoplasma gondii.* Nature **315:** 416–419.
7. Porchet-Hennere, E. & G. Nicolas. 1983. Are rhoptries of coccidia really extrusosomes? J. Ultrastruct. Res. **84:** 194–203.

8. CHOBOTAR, B. & E. SCHOTYSECK. 1982. *In* The Biology of the Coccidia. P. L. Long, ed. University Park Press. Baltimore, MD.

9. CHARIF, H., F. DARCY, G. TORPIER, M. F. CESBRON-DELAUW & A. CAPRON. 1990. Characterization and localization of antigens secreted from tachyzoites. Exp. Parasitol. **71:** 114–124.

10. LERICHE, M. A. & J. F. DUBREMETZ. 1991. Characterization of the protein contents of rhoptries and dense granules of *Toxoplasma gondii* tachyzoites by subcellular fractionation and monoclonal antibodies. Mol. Biochem. Parasitol. **45:** 249–260.

11. SIBLEY, L. D. & J. L. KRAHENBUHL. 1988. Modification of host cell phagosomes by *Toxoplasma gondii* involves redistribution of surface proteins and secretion of a 32 kDa protein. Eur. J. Cell Biol. **47:** 81–87.

12. ENTZEROTH, R., J. F. DUBREMETZ, D. HODICK & E. FERREIRA. 1986. Immunoelectronmicroscopic demonstration of the exocytosis of dense granule contents into the secondary parasitophorous vacuole of *Sarcocystis muris* (Protozoa, Apicomplexa). Eur. J. Cell Biol. **41:** 182–188.

13. ACHBAROU, A., O. MERCEREAU-PUIJALON, A. SADAK, B. FORTIER, J. A. LERICHE, D. CAMUS & J. F. DUBREMETZ. 1991. Differential targetting of dense granule proteins in the parasitophorous vacuole of *Toxoplasma gondii*. Parasitology **103:** 321–329.

14. DUBREMETZ, J. F., D. BERMUDES, A. ACHBAROU & K. A. JOINER. 1993. Kinetics of apical organelle exocytosis during *Toxoplasma gondii* host cell interaction. Parasitol. Res. **79:** 402–408.

15. LECORDIER, L., C. MERCIER, G. TORPIER, B. TOURVIEILLE, F. DARCY, J. L. LIU, P. MAES, A. TARTAR, A. CAPRON & M.-F. CESBRON-DELAUW. 1993. Molecular structure of a *Toxoplasma gondii* dense granule antigen (GRA 5) associated with the parasitophorous vacuole membrane. Mol. Biochem. Parasitol. **59:** 143–154.

16. MERCIER, C., L. LECORDIER, F. DARCY, D. DESLEE, A. MURRAY, B. TOURVIEILLE, P. MAES, A. CAPRON & M.-F. CESBRON-DELAUW. 1993. Molecular characterization of a dense granule antigen (GRA2) associated with the network of the parasitophorous vacuole in *Toxoplasma gondii*. Mol. Biochem. Parasitol. **58:** 71–82.

17. OSSORIO, P. N., J. F. DUBREMETZ & K. A. JOINER. 1993. A soluble secretory protein of the intracellular parasite *Toxoplasma gondii* associates with the parasitophorous vacuole membrane through hydrophobic interactions. J. Biol. Chem., in press.

18. YOUNG, J. D.-E., S. A. COHN & E. R. PODACK. 1986. The ninth component of complement and the pore-forming protein (perforin 1) from cytotoxic T cells: Structural, immunological and functional similarities. Science **233:** 184.

19. SAFFER, L. D., O. MERCEREAU-PUIJALON, J. F. DUBREMETZ & J. SCHWARTZMAN. 1992. Localization of a *Toxoplasma gondii* rhoptry protein by immunoelectron microscopy during and after host cell penetration. J. Protozool. **39:** 526–530.

20. BECKERS, C. J. M., J. F. DUBREMETZ, O. MERCEREAU-PUIJALON & K. A. JOINER. 1994. The *Toxoplasma gondii* protein ROP2 is associated with the parasitophorous vacuole membrane, surrounding intracellular stages, and is exposed to the host cell cytoplasm. J. Cell Biol., in press.

21. MERCEREAU-PUIJALON, O., M.-N. FOURMAUX & J. F. DUBREMETZ. 1993. Expression of apical organelle antigens by a *Toxoplasma gondii* genomic library. *In* Toxoplasmosis. J. E. Smith, Ed. **78:** 19–31. NATO ASI Series.

22. SAAVEDRA, R., F. D. MEUTER, J.-L. DECOURT & P. HERION. 1991. Human T cell clone identifies a potentially protective 54-kDa protein antigen of *Toxoplasma gondii* cloned and expressed in *Escherichia coli*. J. Immunol. **147:** 1975–1982.

23. FOUSSARD, F., M. A. LERICHE & J. F. DUBREMETZ. 1991. Characterization of the lipid content of *Toxoplasma gondii* rhoptries. Parasitology **102:** 367–370.

24. BANNISTER, L. H., G. H. MITCHELL, G. A. BUTCHER & E. D. DENNIS. 1986. Lamellar membranes associated with rhoptries in erythrocyte merozoites of *Plasmodium knowlesi:* A clue to the mechanism of invasion. Parasitology **92:** 291–303.

25. JOINER, K. A. 1991. Rhoptry lipids and parasitophorous vacuole formation: A slippery issue. Parasitol. Today **7:** 226–227.

26. SINGER, S. J. 1990. The structure and insertion of integral proteins in membranes. Annu. Rev. Cell Biol. **6:** 247–296.

27. OJCIUS, D. M. & J. D.-E. YOUNG. 1991. Cytolytic pore-forming proteins and peptides: Is there a common structural motif? TIBS **16:**

28. NICHOLS, B. A., M. L. CHIAPPINO & G. R. O'CONNOR. 1983. Secretion from the rhoptries of *Toxoplasma gondii* during host-cell invasion. J. Ultrastruct. Res. **83:** 85–98.

29. MIKKELSEN, R. B., M. KAMBER, K. S. WADKA, P. S. LIN & R. SCHMIDT-ULLRICH. 1988. The role of lipids in *Plasmodium falciparum* invasion of erythrocytes: A coordinated biochemical and microscopic analysis. Proc. Natl. Acad. Sci. USA **85:** 5956.

30. SCHWAB, J. C., C. J. M. BECKERS & K. A. JOINER. 1994. The parasitophorous vacuole membrane surrounding intracellular *Toxoplasma gondii* functions as a molecular sieve. Proc. Natl. Acad. Sci. USA. **91:** 509–513.

31. DESAI, S. A., D. J. KROGSTAD & E. W. McCLESKEY. 1993. A nutrient-permeable channel on the intraerythrocytic malaria parasite. Nature **362:** 643–646.

32. PORCHET-HENNERE, E. & G. TORPIER. 1983. Relations entre *Toxoplasma* et sa cellule-hote. Protistologica **19:** 357–370.

Serum Resistance of *Neisseria gonorrhoeae*

Does It Thwart the Inflammatory Response and Facilitate the Transmission of Infection?[a]

PETER A. RICE,[b] DANIEL P. McQUILLEN,[b]
SUNITA GULATI,[b] DARSHANA B. JANI,[b]
LEE M. WETZLER,[b,c] MILAN S. BLAKE,[c] AND
EMIL C. GOTSCHLICH[c]

[b]*The Maxwell Finland Laboratory for Infectious Diseases*
Boston City Hospital
Boston University School of Medicine
Boston, Massachusetts 02118

[c]*The Laboratory of Bacterial Pathogenesis and Immunology*
Rockefeller University
New York, New York 10021

The differences in local inflammation associated with serum-sensitive (SS) strains and strains of *Neisseria gonorrhoeae* that manifest phenotypically stable serum-resistance (SR) have been linked to the ability of SS strains to generate greater amounts of the complement-derived chemotactic peptide C5a.[1] We have shown that stable SR strains bind quantitatively more iC3b *in vitro* and *in vivo* than do SS strains regardless of sialylation (which converts SS strains to an unstable SR phenotype). This suggests that stable SR strains may inactivate C3b and thereby prevent effective C5 convertase formation.[2]

To further validate these observations and investigate differences in the molecular form of C3 bound to the different phenotypes, gonococci were opsonized in pooled normal human serum (PNHS) containing tracer amounts of ^{125}I-C3 followed by treatment with methylamine to release ester-linked C3b and C3b cleavage fragments that were then analyzed by SDS-PAGE. Surprisingly, more of the ester-linked α'_1 (68-kD) fragment of iC3b was released from the SS strain and the sialylated SS strain (converting it to unstable SR) compared to the stable SR strain. However, additional bands whose molecular weights did not correlate with known C3 cleavage fragments were present in lanes from the SR strain, suggesting the presence of C3α' fragments bound to gonococcal outer membrane components through methylamine-resistant (presumably amide) linkages. Similarly, immunoblot analysis using a mono-

[a]This work was supported by National Institutes of Health grants AI 15633, AI 32725, AI24760 (PAR), AI 18637 (M.S.B.), and AI 10615 (E.C.G.) and Physician Scientist Awards AI 01061 (D.P.M.) and AI 00680 (L.M.W.) from the National Institute of Allergy and Infectious Diseases.

clonal antibody (mAb) directed against an iC3b neoantigen indicated increased binding to high molecular weight acceptors on the stable SR strain with similar amounts of the α'_1 fragment of iC3b released from all three phenotypes. Low concentrations of trypsin cleave the α-chain of iC3b releasing an intact C3c molecule, whereas C3b is relatively resistant to trypsin proteolysis.[3] Limited trypsin digestion released significantly more C3c from the SR strain than the SS strain or the sialylated SS strain. Therefore, the previously described differences in total iC3b bound to these phenotypes appear to result from increased amide-linked iC3b on the surface of stable SR strains. The interplay between the amounts of ester and amide-linked C3b fragments may influence the inflammatory potential of the phenotypes. Using a liposomal membrane construct containing lipooligosaccharide (LOS) antigens purified from SS and stable SR gonococci and the anti-iC3b mAb, we also demonstrated that the SR LOS was more effective in inactivating C3b to iC3b when incubated in serum.

A second mechanism of stable serum resistance is the effect of blocking antibody that sterically inhibits the binding of bactericidal antibodies to the relevant reactive epitopes, which reside largely on LOS[4] and porin molecules.[5] It has been shown that IgG antibody in normal human serum, which specifically recognizes a common gonococcal membrane antigen called the reduction modifiable protein (Rmp) or Protein III (PIII), blocks killing of *N. gonorrhoeae* by human immune serum.[6] Rmp is an antigenically conserved outer membrane structure present on all strains of *N. gonorrhoeae* and is a potent immunogen in humans. Recently, we reported that a small amount of contamination with Rmp in a candidate porin vaccine preparation gave rise to an Rmp blocking antibody response when administered to humans.[7] Rmp has 75% homology with the carboxyl terminal portion of enterobacterial OmpA protein. Twenty-five percent of Rmp protein that is located upstream of the OmpA shared portion is unrelated to OmpA.[8]

We showed previously that OmpA-specific normal IgG blocks killing of *N. gonorrhoeae*, indicating that blocking antibody in normal human serum is directed against the OmpA-shared Rmp sequences.[9] To characterize the immunogenicity of Rmp and the specificity of the antibody response to Rmp in natural infection, we hypothesized that an Rmp antibody response may be directed against the unique portion of Rmp (not shared with OmpA). To evaluate the development of blocking Rmp antibodies after gonococcal infection, we used Rmp genetic constructs of *N. gonorrhoeae* that were deleted of specific Rmp sequences that harbored the putative epitopes recognized by blocking antibodies, and then we tested disseminated gonococcal infection (DGI) immune serum for blocking against these mutants. Two of the mutants had specific deletions in Rmp protein outside the OmpA shared domains. The first mutant (deficient between two cysteine residues upstream of the OmpA shared portion) was 16-fold more serum sensitive to the DGI serum than to either the wild-type or the second mutant (constructed to have a deletion downstream of the OmpA shared portion). A third mutant (control) lacking Rmp altogether was fourfold more sensitive to the DGI serum than was the first mutant, whose upstream disulfide loop had been deleted.

These experiments differentiate the presence of two sites that are targets for Rmp blocking antibody: the OmpA site and the upstream disulfide loop. We showed that development of Rmp blocking antibody in immune serum is directed at the upstream disulfide loop of Rmp and is superimposed on a background of blocking antibody directed at OmpA shared determinants in *N. gonorrhoeae.*

To examine a possible role for blocking antibody in facilitating transmission of gonorrhea from men to women, we measured antibody concentrations to Rmp and two other major outer membrane antigens present on gonococci, Por (porin protein [PI]) and LOS in women exposed to men infected with *N. gonorrhoeae.* We then correlated the amount of Rmp antibody present with the likelihood of having become infected. Antibodies to LOS and Por have been shown to be bactericidal[4,5] and might, therefore, be considered *a priori* to have an "opposing" effect compared to that of Rmp antibody. We found that women who became infected had higher levels of Rmp antibody and lower levels of LOS and Por antibodies. This suggests that the net bactericidal function as reflected in serum might be important in protecting against gonorrhea.

METHODS AND RESULTS

C3 Binding Assay. Binding of C3 to gonococci incubated in PNHS was measured. An SS pelvic inflammatory disease isolate (strain 24-1; PorIB) and a stable SR isolate from asymptomatic cervical infection (strain 252; PorIB) were used in these experiments. Strain 24-1 (SS) was also grown with 80 μg/ml of CMP-*N*-acetyl-neuraminic acid, with resultant conversion of this strain to unstable SR. Transparent, nonpiliated organisms were grown to mid-log phase, washed in HBSS^{2+} − 0.1% gelatin (HBSS^{2+} gel), and resuspended at 1×10^8 organisms/ml. Organisms were suspended at a final concentration of 0.5×10^8 ml in HBSS^{2+} gel containing 5% PNHS to which was added trace amounts of ^{125}I-C3, or 20% PNHS in Western blot experiments. The reaction mixtures were placed in a shaking water bath at 37°C and duplicate 200-μl aliquots removed at various times up to 60 minutes. Aliquots were layered over ice-cold HBSS^{2+} gel and centrifuged followed by removal of the supernatant, resuspension, and repeat centrifugation to remove noncovalently associated C3.

Molecular Form of C3 Ester-Linked to the Surface of N. gonorrhoeae. Initial experiments employed ^{125}I-C3. Half of the pellets were solubilized by boiling for 10 minutes in 1% SDS, followed by the addition of 200 mM methylamine (final concentration 40 mM) in carbonate buffer (pH 11) and incubation for 60 minutes at 37°C to release ester-linked C3 fragments. Methylamine release of ester-linked fragments indicted that more iC3b (released as a 68-kD α'_1 band on SDS-PAGE) was bound to the SS organism and the sialylated SS organism (unstable SR) than to the stable SR organism, in contrast to our prior observations of total iC3b bound.[2] However, additional labeled bands present in the stable SR strain lanes suggested the possibility that additional C3 might be amide linked to this phenotype. We therefore repeated the C3 binding/methylamine release experiments using 20% PNHS followed by Western blot analysis with HRP-conjugated anti-iC3b neoantigen mAb. Although binding of anti-iC3b neoantigen mAb to the α'_1 fragment of iC3b released from both strains was equivalent, binding to high molecular weight bands (>150 kD) was noted only in lanes from the stable SR strain. Taken together, these results suggested the presence of additional iC3b that was amide bound to gonococcal surface acceptors and thus was resistant to release by nucleophilic attack by methylamine.

Quantitation and Analysis of Amide-Bound C3. To determine the percentage of iC3b and C3b bound covalently through amide linkages to the organism surface we used a modification of a previously described method,[10] which was based on the observation that low concentrations of trypsin cleave surface-bound iC3b but not C3b,[3] releasing the intact C3c fragment into the supernatant. Washed, PNHS-incubated organisms (100 μl) were added to an equal volume of various dilutions of TPCK trypsin (Sigma) and incubated at 30 °C for 10 minutes. Soybean trypsin inhibitor (30 μg/tube) was added immediately, followed by centrifugation through 400 μl of ice cold HBSS^{2+} and aspiration of the supernatants. Both pellets and supernatants were then gamma counted, and the percentage of ^{125}I-C3 released into the supernatants was determined. Pellets were immediately solubilized in SDS sample buffer, while supernatants were precipitated in absolute methanol at 4 °C overnight before solubilization and SDS-PAGE autoradiography. Release of C3c from each of the three strains reached a plateau between 0.016 and 0.062 μg/ml of trypsin and did not increase at higher concentrations. Of the total C3 bound covalently to the three strains, approximately twice as much was bound to the stable SR strain in the form of amide-linked iC3b, compared to the SS strain or the sialylated SS strain (unstable SR). This difference accounts for the previously observed differences in total iC3b binding to the different phenotypes.[2]

iC3b Binding to Liposomes Sensitized Solely with Lipooligosaccharide (LOS). Unilamellar liposomes containing LOS (purified from SS strain 24-1[1] or SR strain 71H[4] by hot phenol water extraction and alkaline hydrolysis) were prepared as described[2] except that no enzymes were encapsulated in their internal aqueous space. Trace amounts of ^{3}H-cholesterol were added to the liposome preparations to permit normalization of liposome number. Liposomes were then incubated with either 5% PNHS or 5% C3-depleted NHS (Cappel) for 60 minutes at 37°C, washed, incubated with horseradish peroxidase-conjugated anti-human iC3b neoantigen mAb (Quidel) for 60 minutes at room temperature, washed, and developed with TMB substrate. Liposomes containing SR (strain 71H) LOS bound twice as much iC3b as did those containing SS (strain 24-1) LOS after PNHS incubation. These results suggest that LOS phenotype alone may account for the observed differences in iC3b binding.

Development of Antibody Directed against Reduction Modifiable Protein (Rmp) after Disseminated Gonococcal Infection (DGI). To examine the role of an alternative antigen, Rmp (or PIII), in serum resistance of gonococci we measured Rmp and OmpA blocking antibodies in a patient with DGI for approximately 3 weeks after the onset of symptoms. In the first 2 weeks, there was a threefold rise in Rmp antibody that persisted thereafter. OmpA antibody levels remained constant throughout the convalescent period. More than three quarters of baseline levels of Rmp antibody were directed at OmpA.

Subspecificity of Rmp Antibodies. To examine the possibility that blocking antibodies in DGI serum, as in normal serum, were directed against Rmp sequences that are shared with OmpA, we measured the amount of Rmp antibody in DGI immune serum and DGI serum depleted of OmpA antibody. Sixty percent of Rmp antibody was removed from the immune serum by immunoabsorption with OmpA. More than half the Rmp antibody was cross-reactive with OmpA. The residual Rmp antibody was directed against Rmp determinants that were not shared with OmpA.

Blocking Activity in DGI Immune Serum Fractions. We next examined the relative role of blocking by OmpA antibody in DGI immune serum by comparing resistance to killing of *N. gonorrhoeae* in intact DGI immune serum *versus* DGI serum depleted of OmpA antibody; each serum was tested against a strain used subsequently to create Rmp deletional mutants (see below). Depletion of OmpA antibody from DGI serum enhanced its ability to kill fourfold.[9] As in normal human serum, OmpA antibody contributes to blocking activity in immune human serum.

Construction of Rmp Mutants. To identify other non-OmpA shared Rmp target sites for blocking, we utilized three Rmp mutants of *N. gonorrhoeae*. The first Rmp mutant lacked Rmp altogether and was created by insertional inactivation of the Rmp gene.[11] Transformants were isolated on ampicillin-containing medium and were shown to be deficient in Rmp as a result of interruption of the Rmp open reading frame. On SDS-PAGE gel and Western blot of the parent strain (UUIP-Tr) and the resultant Rmp-deficient mutant (UUIX-5), the Rmp band was absent in the mutant; in addition, Rmp monoclonal antibody 2E6[12] failed to bind to the mutant.

A second Rmp mutant (PIIISS$^-_{cat}$) was created lacking the amino acids between the 2 cysteine residues upstream of the OmpA shared portion of the molecule (the disulfide loop between residues 47 and 64[8]). This resulted in a mutant that contains Rmp which is approximately 2,000 MW smaller than intact Rmp.

The third mutant (PIIIpT$_{cat}$) has a deletion downstream of the OmpA-shared portion. A translation stop codon was inserted near the carboxyl end which caused premature termination about four amino acids before the carboxyl terminus and removed a region that contained three histidines. A chloramphenicol transacetylase cartridge (*cat* gene) used for selection was inserted just before the transcription terminator (at a *Cla*I site) and well after the reading frame of the Rmp gene.

Loss of Blocking Activity Directed against Rmp Mutants. We used the Rmp mutants and the parent strain to test blocking by the DGI immune serum obtained 25 days after the onset of symptoms. DGI immune serum tested with the disulfide loop deficient Rmp mutant (PIIISS$^-_{cat}$) showed 75% loss of blocking compared to the loss seen using the strain that was totally deficient in Rmp (UUIX-5). *Cat* gene insertion after the structural portion of the gene (PIII$_{cat}$) had no effect. Immune serum tested with the mutant PIIIpT$_{cat}$ showed only minimal loss of blocking activity.

Do Gonococcal Antibodies Influence Transmission of Gonorrhea? To evaluate the possible influence of gonococcal blocking antibodies in facilitating transmission of gonorrhea, we measured antibody concentrations to gonococcal Rmp (PIII) in serum samples of women who were the definite or probable sexual contacts of men with gonococcal urethritis. Rmp was purified from strain UUIP-Tr by cation exchange chromatography[13] and was used to determine the amount of specific antibodies in sera by quantitative ELISA.[6]

To normalize antibody values in infected patients for the influence of acute infection, we took two serum samples (at enrollment and 14 days later) from a subset of infected women. Rising antibody levels to Rmp were measured at each time point, and the slope of the rise regressed back to the point during the male's spread period where the exposure occurred. The average slope for all such determinations was used to calculate the predicted level of antibodies at the time of first exposure for each infected woman.

In the group of women who became infected after exposure, the mean level of antibody (IgG) to Rmp protein was approximately threefold higher, corrected back from the time of enrollment, than that of exposed patients who did not develop infection. Logistic regression, holding the number of sexual exposures to the infected male partners as an independent variable, showed a significant association between Rmp antibody level and transmission ($p < 0.01$).

We performed a similar analysis using Por and LOS antigens to assess the likelihood of transmission as a function of the antibody levels to these antigens. To include the effect of serovar (or type) specificity of Por or LOS, antigens were prepared from each strain and antibody levels in women determined specifically against the antigens contained in the strains to which they had been exposed. Por was prepared by recovering the separated protein directly from SDS-PAGE gels of supernatants prepared from whole cells extracted with sodium acetate buffer.[14] Purity of the Por proteins was assessed by repeat SDS-PAGE of recovered Por proteins and showed single bands in all cases. Rmp contamination of these preparations was assessed by probing dot blots with monoclonal antibody 2E6.[6] All the preparations were free of Rmp. In separate pilot experiments, to assess antigenicity of these preparations, we compared antibody concentrations in three female sera using counterpart Por proteins purified by anion-exchange chromatography.[14] The results indicated no difference in measurements of antibody concentrations when Por prepared by either method was used.

In the group of women who became infected after exposure, the mean level of antibody (IgG) to Por was approximately threefold lower and the level to LOS was not significantly different (both levels corrected back from the time of infection) from that of those exposed patients who did not develop infection. However, IgG antibody levels to LOSs that were isolated from serum-sensitive (SS) gonococci *vs* serum-resistant (stable SR) gonococci were significantly higher in women exposed to but uninfected by these strains.

We considered the likelihood of gonococcal transmission as a function of antibody status to the composite of all three antigens, and applied a formula that we previously showed to predict the level of bactericidal activity present in serum.[6]

$$\frac{[\text{Por} + \text{LOS}]\ \text{antibody}}{[\text{Rmp}]\ \text{antibody}}$$

Application of this composite formula to the uninfected and infected groups resulted in the determination of a ''protective'' factor that exceeded by more than twofold the ratio of the antibody levels in these two groups against each antigen considered separately.

DISCUSSION

The liposome data presented herein may implicate LOS as an acceptor for iC3b (presumably through binding to amino groups on heptose residues in the basal oligosaccharide or attached to other oligosaccharides). Alternatively, C3 has been shown to bind to bactericidal IgG[15]; thus, anti-LOS IgG that remained associated with the liposomes may actually be the C3 acceptor. Additionally, protein antigens including Por and Rmp might also serve as acceptors. The acceptor molecule(s) to which amide-linked iC3b is bound on stable SR strains remains to be determined. C3b bound through amide linkages to acceptor molecules is generally more biochemically stable against degradation by factors I and H than ester-linked C3b.[16] Although iC3b cannot lead to formation of a C5 convertase, it can act as the complement ligand for the CR3 receptor on polymorphonuclear leukocytes and promote phagocytosis. Therefore, regulation of the relative amounts of amide and ester bound iC3b may influence the ultimate fate of the organism along with the degree of local inflammation that is elicited. The presence or absence of capsular sialic acid was recently shown to influence the amount of iC3b bound to Type III group B streptococci,[17] but sialylation of SS gonococci did not increase binding of iC3b. Our data indicated that gonococcal sialylation *in vitro* did not change the overall amount of iC3b bound to different phenotypes[2] nor did it apparently influence the binding of C3 via amide linkages. This may in part be related to the smaller amount of sialic acid present on the gonococcal surface compared to the group B streptococcal capsule.

Outer membrane reduction modifiable protein (Rmp) or protein III (PIII) is a highly conserved protein that is surface exposed and expressed by all strains of gonococci.[18] Because antibodies against certain Rmp epitopes have been reported to promote complement-mediated bactericidal activity,[19] Rmp might hold promise as a potential vaccine candidate. However, we previously showed that blocking antibodies in normal human serum directed against OmpA-shared Rmp sequences block complement-dependent killing (by immune serum) of *N. gonorrhoeae*. In this study, we examined the immune response directed against Rmp in DGI. We found that, overall, Rmp antibody increases after DGI, but that portion directed against Rmp that is shared with OmpA is minimally stimulated. Blocking antibody in human immune serum was mostly directed at the upstream disulfide loop of Rmp (the non-OmpA-shared portion). In DGI immune serum, the blocking effect of OmpA-directed Rmp antibody was overshadowed by disulfide loop-directed antibody.

The risk of transmission of *N. gonorrhoeae* to women exposed to infected men did not increase with increased exposure in accordance with a constant risk probability model (data not shown). For the transmission of *N. gonorrhoeae,* our investigations strongly suggested that an increased level of antibody to the gonococcal Rmp (PIII) was significantly associated with an increased rate of transmission. This suggests that the proposed blocking function of this antibody may enhance the risk of infection by *N. gonorrhoeae*. Lower antibody levels to Por and LOS were strongly implicated as risk factors for transmission, but the combination of all these antibody levels (inversely for Rmp), which may predict the level of bactericidal activity against gonococci,[6] strengthens the association of antibody level and protection against this infection.

SUMMARY

N. gonorrhoeae differentially subvert the effectiveness of complement (C) and alter the inflammatory responses elicited in human infection. Disseminated (DGI) isolates typically resist killing by normal serum (are serum-resistant), inactivate more C3b (to iC3b preferentially bound via amide linkages), generate less C5a, and result in less inflammation at local sites. Pelvic inflammatory disease isolates are serum-sensitive, inactivate less C3b (while maintaining active C3b via stable amide linkages), generate more C5a, and result in more inflammation at local sites. Sialylation of SS gonococci, presumed to occur *in vivo,* converts them to serum-resistant, but it does not change the patterns of C3b inactivation and therefore may not affect local inflammation.

IgG antibody directed against gonococcal reduction modifiable protein (Rmp) blocks C-mediated killing of *N. gonorrhoeae.* Anti-Rmp blocking antibodies may harbor specificity for OmpA sequences shared with other neisserial species or Enterobacteriaceae or may be directed against unique Rmp upstream cysteine loop specific sequences, or both. Preexisting antibodies directed against Rmp facilitate transmission of gonococcal infection to exposed women; exclusion of highly immunogenic Rmp antigens from vaccine candidates may be important.

ACKNOWLEDGMENTS

We thank Jo Ellen Schweinle for providing ^{125}I-C3 used in these studies, and Dipanita Gupta for assistance in preparing the manuscript.

REFERENCES

1. DENSEN, P., S. GULATI & P. RICE. 1987. J. Clin. Invest. **80:** 78–87.
2. McQUILLEN, D. P., D. B. JANI & P. A. RICE. 1991. *In* Neisseriae 1990. M. Achtman, P. Kohl, C. Marchal, G. Morelli, A. Seiler & B. Thiesen, eds.: 353–358. Walter de Gruyter & Co. Berlin, Germany.
3. GITLIN, J. D., F. S. ROSEN & P. J. LACHMANN. 1975. J. Exp. Med. **141:** 1221–1226.
4. RICE, P. A. & D. L. KASPER. 1977. J. Clin. Invest. **60:** 1149–1158.
5. HOOK, E. W., A. OLSEN & T. M. BUCHANAN. 1984. Infect. Immun. **43:** 706–709.
6. RICE, P. A., H. E. VAYO, M. R. TAM & M. S. BLAKE. 1986. J. Exp. Med. **164:** 1735–1748.
7. GULATI, S., P. A. RICE, M. S. BLAKE, S. K. SARAFIAN, S. A. MORSE, M. J. QUENTIN-MILLET & F. ARMINJON. 1991. *In* Neisseriae 1990. M. Achtman, P. Kohl, C. Marshal, G. Morelli, A. Seiler & B. Thiesen, eds.: 229–234. Walter de Gruyter & Co. Berlin, Germany.
8. GOTSCHLICH, E. C., M. SEIFF & M. S. BLAKE. 1987. J. Exp. Med. **165:** 471–482.
9. RICE, P. A. 1989. Clin. Micro. Rev. **2:** S112–117.
10. GAITHER, T. H., C. H. HAMMER & M. M. FRANK. 1979. J. Immunol. **123:** 1195–1204.
11. WETZLER, L. M., E. C. GOTSCHLICH, M. S. BLAKE & J. M. KOOMEY. 1989. J. Exp. Med. **169:** 2199–2209.
12. SWANSON, J., L. W. MAYER & M. R. TAM. 1982. Infect. Immun. **38:** 668–672.
13. LYTTON, E. J. & M. S. BLAKE. 1986. J. Exp. Med. **164:** 1749–1759.
14. BLAKE, M. S. & E. C. GOTSCHLICH. 1982. Infect. Immun. **82:** 277–283.
15. JOINER, K. A., L. F. FRIES, M. A. SCHMETZ & M. M. FRANK. 1985. J. Exp. Med. **162:** 877–889.
16. PUENTES, S. M., D. M. DWYER, P. A. BATES & K. A. JOINER. 1989. J. Immunol. **143:** 3743–3949.
17. MARQUES, M. B., D. L. KASPER, M. K. PANGBURN & M. R. WESSELS. 1992. Infect. Immun. **60:** 3986–3993.
18. JUDD, R. C. 1982. Infect. Immun. **37:** 622–663.
19. VIRJI, M., K. ZAK & J. E. HECKELS. 1987. J. Gen. Micro. **133:** 3393–3407.

The Cell Biology of *Listeria monocytogenes* Infection (Escape from a Vacuole)

DANIEL A. PORTNOY AND SIAN JONES

Department of Microbiology
University of Pennsylvania School of Medicine
Philadelphia, Pennsylvania 19104-6076

Intracellular pathogens are responsible for a devastating amount of morbidity and mortality worldwide. Surprisingly, our understanding of the molecular and cellular basis of intracellular parasitism is still in its infancy. Such an understanding will undoubtedly lead to effective measures for prevention and treatment. The lack of progress in this area is due, in part, to the difficulty in cultivating many of these pathogens and to the lack of useful genetic systems. This provides much of the rationale for the use of *Listeria monocytogenes* as a model intracellular pathogen amenable to both genetic and biochemical analysis. In addition, *L. monocytogenes* is a significant public health problem and a serious pathogen which threatens pregnant women, their offspring, and immunocompromised individuals.[1,2]

Intracellular pathogens can be classified into one of two broad groups.[3,4] One group is comprised of organisms that are enclosed by a host vacuolar membrane. Intravacuolar pathogens have been shown in some cases to prevent acidification of the vacuole and/or fusion of the vacuole with lysosomes. However, little is known about the cell biology of these processes, the regulation of vacuolar gene expression, and the specific mechanisms of nutrient acquisition. The second group of intracellular pathogens, which includes *L. monocytogenes,* consists of parasites that escape from the vacuolar confines and grow directly within the cytoplasm of the host cell. A common feature in both groups of intracellular pathogens is the necessity of dealing effectively with the potentially hostile environment of the host vacuole. Interestingly, a strategy adopted by at least four different intracytoplasmic pathogens is the production of hemolytic activity associated with escape from the vacuole. This includes a contact hemolysin for *Shigella flexneri,*[5] phospholipase A_2 in *Rickettsia prowazekii,*[6] and a pore-forming hemolysin for *Trypanosoma cruzi*[7] and for *L. monocytogenes.*[8] The *L. monocytogenes* hemolysin, listeriolysin O (LLO), is the major focus of this chapter.

Whereas *L. monocytogenes* is an important and dangerous human pathogen, it is also a great model system to study many aspects of host-parasite interactions. Indeed, *L. monocytogenes* has been used by immunologists for decades as a model pathogen in the study of cell-mediated immunity in mice.[9] Although it was once thought that immunity to *L. monocytogenes* could be entirely explained by the generation of activated macrophages, it is now clear that the immune response to *L. monocytogenes* is multifactorial, encompassing both an innate immune response[10] and an acquired response. In the absence of an acquired immune response, as in SCID mice, the animals are not killed, but they harbor the bacteria chronically even though a large proportion of macrophages are activated. It seems that the role of T cells is to recognize infected cells and to mediate their destruction by direct cytotoxicity or by the secretion of cytokines. It is also clear that antibody plays no measurable role in resistance to infection. Mice that survive a challenge with live *L. monocytogenes* are subsequently immune, whereas those challenged with dead bacteria are not immune. Interestingly, mice challenged with live nonhemolytic bacteria also fail to induce protective immunity.[11] To understand these observations requires an understanding of the cell biology of infection, which is to be described.

CELL BIOLOGY OF INFECTION

L. monocytogenes infects almost all adherent cells, but the efficiency of entry has a 4-log range. In primary macrophages and macrophage-like cell lines, 10–20 bacteria/cell can readily be achieved in a 30-minute infection. In contrast, infection of mouse L-cell fibroblasts is approximately 10,000 times less efficient. However, regardless of the cell type, the intracellular doubling time is approximately 1 hour. Intracellular growth assays rely on gentamicin which kills extracellular bacteria but has little or no measurable effect on intracellular bacteria.[12,13]

As just stated, *L. monocytogenes* enters almost all adherent cells. The mechanism of entry in nonphagocytic cells is thought to involve the activity of the membrane protein internalin,[14] but little is yet known concerning its precise mode of action. In macrophages, entry is partially mediated by the complement receptor CR3.[15]

The survival of internalized bacteria is dependent on the cell type. *In vivo,* after intravenous infection, it is believed that *L. monocytogenes* is first ingested by resident macrophages, such as the Kupffer cells in the liver, where the majority of the bacteria are killed. *In vitro,* many of the bacteria are killed by peritoneal macrophages,[16] but the relative contribution of oxidative and nonoxidative killing mechanisms has not been sorted out. Internalized bacteria are initially found in host-derived vacuoles or phagosomes.[13,17,18] Surprisingly, we still know little about the properties of the *L. monocytogenes*-containing vacuole. For example, we do not know if the vacuole is acidic or if it fuses with host lysosomes. However, it is currently believed that *L. monocytogenes* cannot grow within the host vacuole, as mutants that cannot escape the vacuole fail to grow.[13,17]

One of the primary aspects of *L. monocytogenes* pathogenesis is the ability to escape from a host vacuole. This is studied by examining thin sections of infected cells by electron microscopy. Using the appropriate fixation techniques, it is feasible to quantitate the number of bacteria in vacuoles *versus* those in the cytoplasm.[18] Evidence indicates that the *L. monocytogenes* hemolysin, LLO, is largely responsible for this event. First of all, mutants that fail to express LLO are found trapped in the vacuole,[13,17,18] fail to grow,[13,17,19] and are avirulent.[13,20,21] Introduction of the structural gene encoding LLO on a multicopy plasmid restores hemolytic activity and virulence.[22] Introduction of the structural gene encoding LLO into *Bacillus subtilis* confers on this normally nonpathogenic bacterium the ability to escape the vacuole of J774 cells.[23] This experiment had to be performed in a phagocytic cell line, because the hemolytic *B. subtilis* is not invasive of nonphagocytic cells. Taken together, these data support the premise that LLO is largely responsible for lysis of the host vacuole. However other observations suggest that LLO is not acting alone, and in some cell types, such as Henle 407 or Hela cells, LLO is not even necessary for escape from the vacuole or for subsequent growth.[13]

Once *L. monocytogenes* enters the cytoplasm, rapid growth ensues. Indeed, the bacteria continue to grow with an intracellular doubling time of approximately 1 hour for 8 hours or longer. The precise nutritional requirements for intracytoplasmic growth are not known, but so far, none of the auxotrophs tested has had a severe growth defect.[24] Our current thinking is that generally the cytoplasm of most mammalian cells is a rich medium. Thus, aromatic amino acid and purine auxotrophs of *L. monocytogenes* are capable of intracytoplasmic growth and are still virulent in contrast to analogous mutants in *Salmonellae* and *Yersiniae*.[24] We believe that these data are consistent with the concept that *L. monocytogenes* inhabits an intracytoplasmic niche *in vivo*.

Shortly after *L. monocytogenes* enters the cytoplasm, the bacteria become enshrouded by host actin filaments.[18,25] After a few divisions, the actin filaments become polarized to one end of the bacteria. The bacteria utilize a host system of actin-based motility to move through the cytoplasm of the host at rates that range from less than 0.1 to 1.5 μ/sec.[26,27] It appears that the rate of movement equals the rate of actin polymerization, and the data are consistent with the idea that actin polymerization provides the driving force for bacterial movement.[26–28] As an aside, it is interesting that *L. monocytogenes* has emerged as a model system to study host mechanisms of actin-based motility. Most importantly, Theriot *et al.*[29] recently described that *L. monocytogenes* can undergo actin-based motility in cell-free extracts derived from *Xenopus* oocytes. This is the first *in vitro* model for actin-based motility and is sure to have a large impact on that field.

The contribution of *L. monocytogenes* in the mediation of actin-based motility can be traced to the bacterial ActA protein.[29–34] Mutants with insertions or deletions in *actA* are absolutely defective for the nucleation of host actin filaments, and an in-frame deletion in *actA* was 3 logs less virulent for mice.[34] The *actA* gene predicts a protein of 610 amino acids which contains a signal sequence, a region of four proline-rich repeats, and a hydrophobic stretch of amino acids at its carboxy terminus which may serve the role of a membrane anchor.[30,32] The protein has a surface-associated polarized distribution[31,33] and can be removed from the bacterial surface with SDS under conditions that do not result in lysis of the bacteria. Although the *actA* gene predicts a protein with a molecular mass of 67 kD, it migrates on SDS-PAGE at an apparent molecular mass greater than 90 kD. The ActA protein is the major SDS-extractable bacterial protein labeled with ^{35}S-methionine during intracellular growth.[34] Furthermore, the ActA protein migrates as a triplet of bands only during intracellular growth. The higher molecular mass bands result from phosphorylation of ActA in the cytoplasm of the host cells.[34] The significance of the intracellular modification of ActA is not known, but we speculate that it may modulate its intracellular activity.

It is not yet known how ActA mediates nucleation of host actin filaments or actin-based motility, but suggestive evidence indicates that the actin monomer binding protein profilin may be involved. Because profilin is known to bind to polyproline and ActA contains four proline-rich repeats, it was suggested that ActA might contain a profilin binding site(s). Indeed, Theriot *et al.*[29] provided evidence that profilin localizes at the rear end of moving bacteria. In addition, depletion of profilin from *Xenopus* extracts resulted in the cessation of bacterial movement. Interestingly, the bacteria still nucleated actin filaments in the profilin-depleted extracts, but were never seen to have actin-based tails.[29] These data suggest that ActA may have more than one activity, one involved in actin filament nucleation and another in binding profilin which may facilitate movement. Lastly, efforts to demonstrate actin filament nucleation or profilin binding *in vitro* have largely been unsuccessful.[18,29,35]

The actin-based motility of *L. monocytogenes* has attracted considerable attention from the cell biology community, yet the role of intracellular motility is undoubtedly used by the bacteria as a prelude to cell-to-cell spread. Wild-type *L. monocytogenes* spread readily from cell to cell, but the precise mechanism is unknown. However, it appears that the mechanism allows the bacteria to spread from one cell to another without contact with the extracellular medium. Therefore, in the presence of extremely bactericidal concentrations of gentamicin, the wild-type bacteria can propagate the infection, whereas an *actA* mutant is killed sometime after approximately eight bacterial divisions.[34] Similarly, the *actA* mutant makes extremely small plaques in monolayers of mouse L cells. Observation of infected cells by light microscopy revealed that *L. monocytogenes* is often seen at the tip of filopodial-like extensions (FIG. 2, panel A). It was proposed that these structures are somehow recognized by neighboring cells and phagocytosed.[18] This model predicts that the bacteria would be found in double-membrane vacuoles, and this has been observed. *L. monocytogenes* expresses two distinct phospholipases C[36–41] which probably play a role in cell-to-cell spread. Indeed, evidence was provided that a mutant in *plcB*, which encodes a broad-range phospholipase C, was defective in escape from a double membrane vacuole.[42] Also, mutants that have in-frame deletions in both *plcA* and *plcB* make small plaques in tissue culture (Smith and Portnoy, unpublished observations). However, the mutants still show considerable spreading, perhaps mediated by LLO.

FURTHER STUDIES ON THE ROLE OF LISTERIOLYSIN O

The cell biology of *L. monocytogenes* infection is clearly complex and can be divided broadly into three stages: life in a vacuole, life in the cytoplasm, and cell-to-cell spread. This chapter focuses on escape from the phagocytic vacuole. This is of fundamental importance in our understanding of the pathogenesis of *L. monocytogenes* as well as other intracytoplasmic pathogens. In addition, even pathogens that reside in a vacuole must survive and acquire nutrients within the vacuole, so our studies using *L. monocytogenes* may have significance for intravacuolar pathogens as well.

As just mentioned, LLO is largely responsible for the escape of *L. monocytogenes* from a vacuole. LLO is a member of a large family of hemolysins found in gram-positive bacteria. This family is known as the sulfhydryl-activated, oxygen-labile cytolysins.[43] All of the hemolysins in this family have a single unique cysteine which renders them susceptible to reversible inactivation by oxidation. However, the cysteine can be changed to an alanine without affecting its activity.[44,45] Based on studies using streptolysin O (SLO), their mechanism of action is thought to involve binding of monomers to membrane cholesterol followed by oligomerization of 20–80 monomers

TABLE 1. Characteristics of the Four Strains Used in This Study

Strain	Hemolytic Units[a]	LD_{50}[b]
10403S (wild-type)	640	2×10^4
DP-L1044 (*hly::Tn917*)	0	5×10^8
DP-L1044 (pAM401::*hly*)	640	2×10^5
DP-L1044 (pAM401::*pfo*)	640	2×10^8

[a] Hemolytic units determined at pH 5.5 after growth in Luria broth.

[b] LD_{50} determined in BALB/c mice after intravenous infection.

into ring and arc-like structures.[46] However, it should be pointed out that the mechanism of action of LLO could be significantly different from that of SLO.

The pH optimum of LLO is 5.6.[8] This observation fits quite well with the notion that LLO acts in a host vacuole that is likely acidic. However, the related hemolysins, streptolysin O (SLO) and perfringolysin O (PFO), are also fully active at pH 5.6.[47] Also, LLO and PFO have the same specific activity at pH 5.6. Therefore, it was not surprising that *B. subtilis* expressing PFO was able to lyse the phagocytic vacuole and enter the cytoplasm.[47] The question that arises from these studies is, what, if anything, is unique about LLO? Could any related hemolysin functionally replace LLO if expressed appropriately? To answer these questions, we set out to replace LLO with PFO and evaluate the effects.

RESULTS

Cloning and Expression of PFO in L. monocytogenes. To replace LLO with PFO, we decided to clone the structural gene encoding PFO downstream from the promoter for the structural gene encoding LLO. (The structural gene encoding LLO is called *hly*.) This was accomplished using PCR technology and resulted in a construct containing the −35 and −10 regions from *hly* and the ribosome binding site and PFO structural gene (*pfo*) from *Clostridium perfringens*. This construct was cloned into the gram-positive/ gram-negative shuttle plasmid pAM401[48] and transformed into a strain of *L. monocytogenes* that had a transposon insertion within *hly*. As a control, the entire *hly* gene was also cloned into pAM401 and transformed into the LLO minus strain of *L. monocytogenes*. The four strains used for the remainder of this study and their relevant characteristics are shown in TABLE 1.

Characterization of the PFO-Expressing Strain of L. monocytogenes. As previously reported,[22] introduction of *hly* into an LLO minus strain restores full hemolytic activity and almost full virulence (TABLE 1). The observation that *hly* on a plasmid did not restore the strain to full virulence is probably due to the presence of the *hly* promoter on multicopy which may titrate the essential transcription factor PrfA.[49] As expected, introduction of *pfo* into *L. monocytogenes* also restored the strain to full hemolytic activity, although the activity was identical when tested at pH 5.5 or 7.0 as reported.[47] However, in contrast to *hly*, *pfo* did not restore the virulence of the

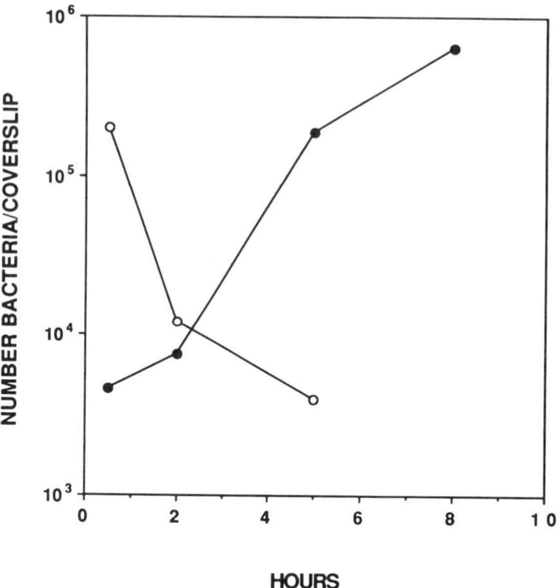

FIGURE 1. Growth of *L. monocytogenes* strains in the J774 macrophage-like cell line. *Closed circles:* wild-type strain 10403S growing within the J774 cells; *open circles:* the LLO negative strain with *pfo* cloned on a plasmid. The strain was rapidly killed presumably by the gentamicin; gentamicin was added to a final concentration of 50 μg/ml at T = 1.

strain. Indeed, *L. monocytogenes* expressing PFO in place of LLO was essentially avirulent. Why?

The properties of the strains were evaluated both in the J774 macrophage-like cell line and in primary cultures of mouse bone marrow-derived macrophages. Initially, J774 cells were examined after 1 hour of infection by electron microscopy. The results clearly showed that the PFO-expressing strain had escaped from the vacuole into the cytoplasm (data not shown). Surprisingly, evaluation of colony-forming units revealed that whereas the wild-type strain grew normally, the PFO-containing strain showed a dramatic loss in colony-forming units during the first 2 hours after infection (FIG. 1). This is in contrast to the LLO minus strain which does not grow in J774 cells, but does not die.[50] The most likely explanation for these results is that PFO somehow allows gentamicin to enter the infected J774 cells and is consequently killed. Examination of infected bone marrow-derived macrophages supports this model (FIG. 2). Whereas the wild-type strain can be seen in healthy cells in the process of spreading, most of the cells harboring the PFO-expressing strain have lysed. Taken together, these data indicate that PFO is capable of mediating lysis of the vacuole, but it results in the death of the host cell.

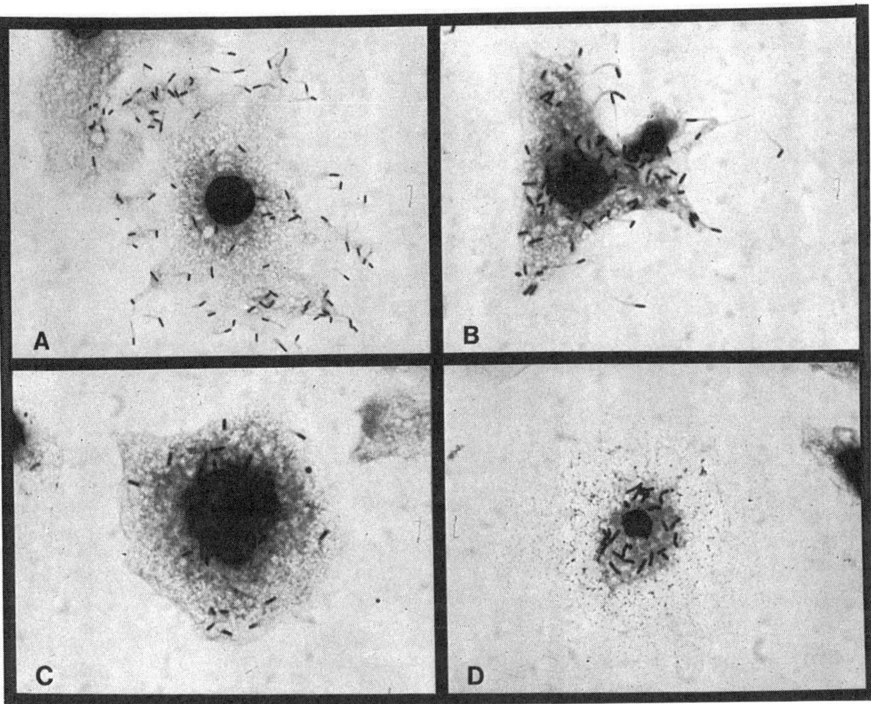

FIGURE 2. Light micrographs depicting infection of bone marrow-derived macrophages after 8 hours of infection. (**A**) 10403S; (**B**) LLO negative strain with *hly* on a plasmid; (**C** and **D**) LLO negative strain with *pfo* contained on a plasmid. Approximately 80% of the cells appeared as in **D**.

DISCUSSION

The results of this study indicate that PFO can replace LLO with regard to hemolytic activity and escape from a vacuole but not with regard to virulence or growth in cells. The explanation appears to be that PFO-expressing *L. monocytogenes* kill their host cell. Just as a parasite does not want to kill its host, an intracellular pathogen does not want to kill its host cell. Thus one of the unique features of LLO is that it is apparently nontoxic to host cells.

There are a number of possible reasons that PFO kills infected host cells. It is possible that gene expression is not regulated appropriately inside of host cells. It is not currently known if LLO is normally expressed once *L. monocytogenes* reaches the cytoplasm. It is possible that a repressor blocks its expression and that our construct is somehow insensitive to this repression. We tried to avoid this scenario by cloning *pfo* downstream from the *hly* promoter, but we cannot rule this out. Also, the current construct is present on a multicopy plasmid. We are currently in the process of introducing *pfo* onto the chromosome in single copy.

Another possible explanation of the toxicity of PFO is its pH optimum. Unlike LLO which is relatively inactive at pH 7.4, PFO is fully active at both pH 5.5 and 7.4. Therefore, it is possible that LLO is nontoxic because it is inactive in the neutral pH of the cytoplasm whereas PFO is fully active. Thus, *L. monocytogenes* may have adopted a strategy for compartmentalizing activities which is used by the host cell. For example, lysosomal hydrolases have pH optima in the acidic range, which may be a mechanism for preventing host cell damage.

Another possibility for the toxic effect of PFO may relate to its half-life in the cytoplasm. It is known that the half-life of proteins can vary from 2 minutes to greater than 10 hours. The most critical issue in determining the half-life of a protein is its NH_2-terminal amino acid, referred to as the N-end rule.[51] Based on the predicted amino acid sequence of LLO and PFO, neither would have a long half-life in the cytoplasm of host cells, yet it is certainly possible that their half-lives would differ. As an aside, it is interesting to note that the predicted NH_2-terminus of ActA would predict that it would be stable in the cytoplasm of mammalian cells. Indeed, pulse chase experiments have indicated that it is stable for hours (unpublished observations). Preliminary experiments looking for LLO in the cytoplasm have not been successful, possibly because it is degraded or simply not expressed.

It is premature to conclude which of the foregoing scenarios explains the toxicity of PFO. We favor a model in which all may be involved. LLO is clearly an essential determinant of pathogenesis and is likely to be regulated at multiple levels, both at the transcriptional and at the posttranscriptional level. In the near future, we will specifically examine all of the possibilities just discussed.

REFERENCES

1. FARBER, J. M. & P. I. PETERKIN. 1991. *Listeria monocytogenes,* a food-borne pathogen. Microbiol. Rev. **55:** 476-511.
2. GELLIN, B. G. & C. V. BROOME. 1989. Listeriosis. *J. Am. Med. Assoc.* **261:** 1313-1320.
3. FALKOW, S., R. R. ISBERG & D. A. PORTNOY. 1992. The interaction of bacteria with mammalian cells. Annu. Rev. Cell Biol. **8:** 333-363.
4. MOULDER, J. M. 1985. Comparative biology of intracellular parasitism. Microbiol. Rev. **49:** 298-337.
5. SANSONETTI, P. J., A. RYTER, P. CLERC, A. T. MAURELLI & J. MOUNIER. 1986. Multiplication of *Shigella flexneri* within HeLa cells: Lysis of the phagocytic vacuole and plasmid-mediated contact hemolysis. Infect. Immun. **51:** 461-469.
6. WINKLER, H. H. 1990. *Rickettsia* species (as organisms). Annu Rev. Microbiol. **44:** 131-153.
7. ANDREWS, N. W., C. K. ABRAMS, S. L. SLATIN & G. GRIFFITHS. 1990. A *T. cruzi*-secreted protein immunologically related to the complement component C9: Evidence for membrane pore-forming activity at low pH. Cell **61:** 1277-1287.
8. GEOFFROY, C., J. L. GAILLARD, J. E. ALOUF & P. BERCHE. 1987. Purification, characterization, and toxicity of the sulfhydryl-activated hemolysin listeriolysin O from *Listeria monocytogenes*. Infect. Immun. **55:** 1641-1646.
9. KAUFMANN, S. H. E. 1993. Immunity to intracellular bacteria. Annu. Rev. Immunol. **11:** 129-163.
10. PORTNOY, D. A. 1992. Innate immunity to a facultative intracellular bacterial pathogen. Current Opinion Immunol. **4:** 20-24.

11. BERCHE, P., J. GAILLARD & P. J. SANSONETTI. 1987. Intracellular growth of *Listeria monocytogenes* as a prerequisite for in vivo induction of T cell-mediated immunity. J. Immunol. **138:** 2266-2271.

12. HAVELL, E. A. 1986. Synthesis and secretion of interferon by murine fibroblasts in response to intracellular *Listeria monocytogenes*. Infect. Immun. **54:** 787-792.

13. PORTNOY, D. A., P. S. JACKS & D. J. HINRICHS. 1988. Role of hemolysin for the intracellular growth of *Listeria monocytogenes*. J. Exp. Med. **167:** 1459-1471.

14. GAILLARD, J. L., P. BERCHE, C. FREHEL, E. GOUIN & P. COSSART. 1991. Entry of *L. monocytogenes* into cells is mediated by internalin, a repeat protein reminiscent of surface antigens from gram-positive cocci. Cell **65:** 1127-1141.

15. DREVETS, D. A. & P. A. CAMPBELL. 1991. Roles of complement and complement receptor type 3 in phagocytosis of *Listeria monocytogenes* by inflammatory mouse peritoneal macrophages. Infect. Immun. **59:** 2645-2652.

16. PORTNOY, D. A., R. D. SCHREIBER, P. CONNELLY & L. G. TILNEY. 1989. Gamma interferon limits access of *Listeria monocytogenes* to the macrophage cytoplasm. J. Exp. Med. **170:** 2141-2146.

17. GAILLARD, J. L., P. BERCHE, J. MOUNIER, S. RICHARD & P. SANSONETTI. 1987. *In vitro* model of penetration and intracellular growth of *Listeria monocytogenes* in the human enterocyte-like cell line Caco-2. Infect. Immun. **55:** 2822-2829.

18. TILNEY, L. G. & D. A. PORTNOY. 1989. Actin filaments and the growth, movement, and spread of the intracellular bacterial parasite, *Listeria monocytogenes*. J. Cell Biol. **109:** 1597-1608.

19. KUHN, M., S. KATHARIOU & W. GOEBEL. 1988. Hemolysin supports survival but not entry of the intracellular bacterium *Listeria monocytogenes*. Infect. Immun. **56:** 79-82.

20. GAILLARD, J. L., P. BERCHE & P. SANSONETTI. 1986. Transposon mutagenesis as a tool to study the role of hemolysin in the virulence of *Listeria monocytogenes*. Infect. Immun. **52:** 50- 55.

21. KATHARIOU, S., P. METZ, H. HOF & W. GOEBEL. 1987. Tn916-induced mutations in the hemolysin determinant affecting virulence of *Listeria monocytogenes*. J. Bacteriol. **169:** 1291-1297.

22. COSSART, P., M. F. VINCENTE, J. MENGAUD, F. BAQUERO, J. C. PEREZ-DIAZ & P. BERCHE. 1989. Listeriolysin O is essential for virulence of *Listeria monocytogenes:* Direct evidence obtained by gene complementation. Infect. Immun. **57:** 3629-3636.

23. BIELECKI, J., P. YOUNGMAN, P. CONNELLY & D. A. PORTNOY. 1990. *Bacillus subtilis* expressing a haemolysin gene from *Listeria monocytogenes* can grow in mammlian cells. Nature **345:** 175-176.

24. MARQUIS, H., H. G. A. BOUWER, D. J. HINRICHS & D. A. PORTNOY. 1993. Intracytoplasmic growth and virulence of *Listeria monocytogenes* auxotrophic mutants. Infect. Immun. **61:** 3756-3760.

25. MOUNIER, J., A. RYTER, M. COQUIS-RONDON & P. J. SANSONETTI. 1990. Intracellular and cell-to-cell spread of *Listeria monocytogenes* involves interaction with F-actin in the enterocytelike cell line Caco-2. Infect. Immun. **58:** 1048-1058.

26. THERIOT, J. A., T. J. MITCHISON, L. G. TILNEY & D. A. PORTNOY. 1992. The rate of actin-based motility of intracellular *Listeria monocytogenes* equals the rate of actin polymerization. Nature **357:** 257-260.

27. DABIRI, G. A., J. M. SANGER, D. A. PORTNOY & F. S. SOUTHWICK. 1990. *Listeria monocytogenes* moves rapidly through the host cytoplasm by inducing directional actin assembly. Proc. Natl. Acad. Sci. **87:** 6068-6072.

28. SANGER, J. M., J. W. SANGER & F. S. SOUTHWICK. 1992. Host cell actin assembly is necessary and likely to provide the propulsive force for intracellular movement of *Listeria monocytogenes*. Infect. Immun. **60:** 3609-3619.

29. THERIOT, J. A., J. ROSENBLATT, D. A. PORTNOY, P. J. GOLDSCHMIDT-CLERMONT & T. J. MITCHISON. 1994. Involvement of profilin in the actin-based motility of Listeria monocytogenes in cells and in cell-free extracts. Cell **74:** 505-517.

30. KOCKS, C., E. GOUIN, M. TABOURET, P. BERCHE, H. OHAYON & P. COSSART. 1992. *L. monocytogenes*-induced actin assembly requires the *act*A gene product, a surface protein. Cell **68:** 521-531.

31. KOCKS, C., R. HELLIO, P. GOUNON, H. OHAYON & P. COSSART. 1993. Polarized distribution of *Listeria monocytogenes* surface protein ActA at the site of directional actin assembly. J. Cell Sci. **105:** 699-710.

32. DOMANN, E., J. WEHLAND, M. ROHDE, S. PISTOR, M. HARTL, W. GOEBEL, M. LEIMEISTER-WACHTER, M. WUENSCHER & T. CHAKRABORTY. 1992. A novel bacterial virulence gene in *Listeria monocytogenes* required for host cell microfilament interaction with homology to the proline-rich region of vinculin. EMBO J. **11:** 1981-1990.

33. NIEBUHR, K. *et al.* 1993. Localization of the ActA polypeptide of *Listeria monocytogenes* in infected tissue culture cell lines: ActA is not associated with actin "comets." Infect. Immun. **61:** 2793-2802.

34. BRUNDAGE, R. A., G. A. SMITH, A. CAMILLI, J. A. THERIOT & D. A. PORTNOY. 1993. Expression and phosphorylation of the *Listeria monocytogenes* ActA protein in mammalian cells. Proc. Natl. Acad. Sci. USA. **90:** 11890-11894.

35. TILNEY, L. G., D. J. DeROSIER, A. WEBER & M. S. TILNEY. 1992. How *Listeria* exploits host cell actin to form its own cytoskeleton. II. Nucleation, actin filament polarity, filament assembly, and evidence for a pointed end capper. J. Cell Biol. **118:** 83-93.

36. LEIMEISTER-WACHTER, M., E. DOMANN & T. CHAKRABARTY. 1991. Detection of a gene encoding a phosphatidylinositol specific phospholipase C that is co-ordinately expressed with listeriolysin in *Listeria monocytogenes*. Mol. Microbiol. **5:** 361-366.

37. MENGAUD, J., C. BRAUN-BRETON & P. COSSART. 1991. Identification of phosphatidylinositol-specific phospholipase C activity in *Listeria monocytogenes:* A novel type of virulence factor? Mol. Microbiol. **5:** 367-372.

38. CAMILLI, A., H. GOLDFINE & D. A. PORTNOY. 1991. *Listeria monocytogenes* mutants lacking phosphatidylinositol-specific phospholipase C are avirulent. J. Exp. Med. **173:** 751-754.

39. GEOFFROY, C., J. RAVENEAU, J. BERETTI, A. LECROISEY, J.-A. VAZQUES-BOLAND, J. E. ALOUF & P. BERCHE. 1991. Purification and characterization of an extracellular 29-kilodalton phospholipase C from *Listeria monocytogenes*. Infect. Immun. **59:** 2382-2388.

40. GOLDFINE, H. & C. KNOB. 1992. Purification and characterization of *Listeria monocytogenes* phosphatidylinositol-specific phospholipase. C. Infect. Immun. **60:** 4059-4067.

41. GOLDFINE, H., N. C. JOHNSTON & C. KNOB. 1993. The non-specific phospholipase C of *Listeria monocytogenes:* Activity on phospholipids in Triton X-100 mixed micelles and in biological membranes. J. Bacteriol. **175:** 4298-4306.

42. VAZQUEZ-BOLAND, J.-A., C. KOCKS, S. DRAMSI, H. OHAYON, C. GEOFFROY, J. MENGAUD & P. COSSART. 1992. Nucleotide sequence of the lecithinase operon of *Listeria monocytogenes* and possible role of lecithinase in cell-to-cell spread. Infect. Immun. **60:** 219-230.

43. SMYTH, C. J. & J. L. DUNCAN. 1978. Thiol-activated (oxygen-labile) cytolysins. *In* Bacterial toxins and cell membranes. J. Jeljaszewicz & T. Wasstrom, eds. **1:** 129-183. Academic Press Inc. New York.

44. PINKNEY, M., E. BEACHEY & M. KEHOE. 1989. The thiol-activated toxin streptolysin O does not require a thiol group for cytolytic activity. Infect. Immun. **57:** 2553-2558.

45. MICHEL, E., K. A. REICH, R. FAVIER, P. BERCHE & P. COSSART. 1990. Attenuated mutants of the intracellular bacterium *Listeria monocytogenes* obtained by single amino acid substitutions in listeriolysin O. Mol. Microbiol. **4:** 2167-2178.

46. BHAKDI, S. & J. TRANUM-JENSEN. 1986. Membrane damage by pore-forming cytolysins. Microb. Pathog. **1:** 5-14.

47. PORTNOY, D. A., R. K. TWETEN, M. KEHOE & J. BIELECKI. 1992. Capacity of listeriolysin O, streptolysin O, and perfringolysin O to mediate growth of *Bacillus subtilis* within mammalian cells. Infect. Immun. **60:** 2710-2717.

48. WIRTH, R., F. Y. AN & D. B. CLEWELL. 1986. Highly efficient protoplast transformation system for *Streptococcus faecalis* and a new *Escherichia coli-S. faecalis* shuttle vector. J. Bacteriol. **165:** 831-836.

49. CAMILLI, A., L. G. TILNEY & D. A. PORTNOY. 1993. Dual roles of *plc*A in *Listeria monocytogenes* pathogenesis. Mol. Microbiol. **8:** 143-157.

50. SUN, A. N., A. CAMILLI & D. A. PORTNOY. 1990. Isolation of *Listeria monocytogenes* small-plaque mutants defective for intracellular growth and cell-to-cell spread. Infect. Immun. **58:** 3770-3778.

51. VARSHAVSKY, A. 1992. The N-end Rule. Cell **69:** 725-735.

Identification of Genes Involved in the Resistance of Mycobacteria to Killing by Macrophages[a]

SATHISH MUNDAYOOR [b,c] AND
THOMAS M. SHINNICK [d]

[b]Biotechnology Division
Godrej Soaps, Inc.
Bombay, India

[d]Division of Bacterial and Mycotic Diseases
Centers for Disease Control and Prevention
Atlanta, Georgia 30333

The diseases resulting from infections with *Mycobacterium* species have plagued mankind since prehistoric times. Tuberculosis, which is caused by *Mycobacterium tuberculosis,* was the leading cause of death for adults in the United States at the turn of the century, and at the height of the tuberculosis epidemic in Europe, tuberculosis was known as the White Death or the Captain of Death.[1] Hansen disease (leprosy), which is caused by *Mycobacterium leprae,* has been feared even more.[2] These diseases are still important sources of morbidity and mortality in the world, with particularly devastating effects in the developing and tropical countries.[3-5] Hansen disease afflicts 5–6 million individuals worldwide and causes crippling deformities in untreated cases.[3] Almost 2 billion persons are, or have been, infected with *M. tuberculosis,* and about 3 million persons die each year from tuberculosis.[4] This makes tuberculosis the leading cause of death due to a single infectious agent, accounting for about 25% of all preventable deaths in the world.[4] Tuberculosis has also reemerged as an important public health problem in many developed countries.[5] In the United States, the number of tuberculosis cases reported to the Centers for Disease Control and Prevention has steadily increased from a low of ~22,000 cases in 1984 to 26,673 cases in 1992.[6] This increase has been accompanied by outbreaks of tuberculosis caused by *M. tuberculosis* strains resistant to many of the commonly used antituberculosis drugs.[7]

Many of the clinical manifestations of Hansen disease and tuberculosis are the result of interactions between the mycobacteria and the host's immune system, and an important aspect of these interactions is that *M. leprae* and *M. tuberculosis* actually survive and replicate within the host's phagocytic cells, primarily within macrophages (reviewed in refs. 8–13). The pathogen-macrophage interaction is critical in determin-

[a]This work was supported in part by a grant from the UNDP/World Bank/WHO Programme for Vaccine Development.

[c]Address for correspondence: T. M. Shinnick, Ph.D., Mailstop G35, Centers for Disease Control and Prevention, 1600 Clifton Road, NE, Atlanta, GA 30333.

ing the establishment of infection, the containment of infection at the initial focus of infection, progression or regression of the infection, and the host's immune response to the invading mycobacterium. Indeed, the survival of these pathogens in the human host depends on their ability to produce gene products that counteract the bactericidal activities of macrophages.

In general, monocytes and macrophages of the mononuclear phagocyte series phagocytize and kill microorganisms using a variety of oxygen-dependent and oxygen-independent killing mechanisms (reviewed in refs. 14–16). For example, contact and phagocytosis can stimulate a metabolic burst which generates superoxide ions and H_2O_2. The lysosomal enzyme myeloperoxidase uses H_2O_2 and chloride ions to produce hypochlorous ions which are potent antimicrobial agents. Oxygen-independent killing mechanisms may include (1) digestion by lysozymes, proteases, or lipases, (2) chelation of iron, or (3) exposure to granular cationic proteins or reactive nitrogen intermediates. The phagocytized pathogens encounter these microbicidal agents following acidification of the phagosome and fusion with lysosomes. Although these processes are clearly present in the professional phagocytic cells, the precise mechanism(s) used to kill the phagocytized pathogen remains to be firmly established.

Intracellular pathogens, on the other hand, can survive and actually multiply while within the phagocytic cells. These pathogens include bacteria from the genera *Mycobacterium, Brucella, Legionella, Salmonella, Shigella,* and *Yersinia* and protozoa from the genera *Leishmania, Toxoplasma,* and *Trypanosoma,* and they have evolved a variety of strategies to avoid the killing processes of phagocytic cells.[15–21] For example, *Toxoplasma gondii* avoids the phagocytic pathway entirely by a receptor-mediated invasion into the endosomal compartment of the phagocytic cell.[22] Other strategies include (1) killing of phagocytic cells, (2) prevention of an oxidative burst, acidification, or phagosome-lysosome fusion, (3) production of enzymes such as superoxide dismutase that interfere with antimicrobial processes, (4) presence of a lipid or polysaccharide coat that shields the parasite from degradative enzymes, and (5) impairment of macrophage or T-cell functions involved in establishing a cellular immune response. Although the specific processes evaded by some of the intracellular pathogens have been identified, the molecular mechanisms of the resistance to killing remain to be elucidated.

With respect to the intracellular survival of mycobacteria in macrophages, much effort has gone into describing the mycobacterium-macrophage interaction at the light and electron microscopic levels, the time course of survival and multiplication of various *Mycobacterium* species in various types of cells and macrophages, and the effect of activation and exposure to various lymphokines on the ability of macrophages to restrict the growth of mycobacteria.[12,13,17–19] For example, the uptake of *M. leprae* and *M. tuberculosis* by human monocytes is primarily mediated by complement component C3 and complement receptor.[23,24] During phagocytosis, *M. leprae,* but not *M. tuberculosis,* inhibits an oxidative burst.[25] Once inside the macrophage, *M. leprae,* and perhaps *M. tuberculosis,* can escape from the phagosome into the cytoplasm[26–28] and thereby avoid the bactericidal activities found in phagosomes and phagolysosomes. Inhibition of the acidification of the phagosome and of phagosome-lysosome fusion has also been suggested to be important in the intracellular survival of both species.[29–31] The mechanism of fusion inhibition is unclear, but it appears to be mediated by cyclic AMP, polyanions, or ammonia.[32] Both *Mycobacterium* species are relatively resistant to oxidative killing systems, but they are susceptible to reactive nitrogen intermediates.[33,34] Mycobacteria produce superoxide dismutase and catalase, which may inactivate reactive oxygen molecules. Mycobacterial surface products such as phenolic glycolipids, lipoarabinomannans, and sulfolipids may also protect the organisms from killing by scavenging reactive oxygen molecules or by modulating macrophage activation.[19,30,35] A capsule-like structure called the "electron transparent zone" has been observed surrounding pathogenic mycobacteria within phagocytic cells and may represent yet another defense mechanism.[36] A key step in sorting out these proposed survival mechanisms will be the identification of the mycobacterial genes and gene products required for, or involved in, resistance to killing by macrophages.

For other intracellular pathogens, two basic approaches have been used to identify genes involved in intracellular survival. One approach was to isolate mutants that have decreased ability to survive in macrophages. For example, Fields *et al.*[37] isolated > 80 transposon mutants of *Salmonella typhimurium* that were more susceptible to killing by macrophages than the wild-type strain. The mutations affected many different genes and processes including purine biosynthesis, amino acid auxotrophy, serum sensitivity, lipopolysaccharide biosynthesis, and colony morphology. One group of mutations affected *phoP* and caused increased sensitivity to defensins.[38] Many of the mutations affected survival or killing processes that have not yet been characterized. Similar mutagenesis strategies have also been used to study the roles of specific genes in intracellular survival. For example, site-directed mutations in the *Legionella pneumophila mip* gene resulted in decreased ability to infect U937 macrophages and decreased virulence in a guinea pig model.[39]

A second strategy involved a recombinant DNA approach to identify the genes of a pathogen which confer a particular virulence-associated feature to a nonpathogenic strain. For example, Isberg and Falkow[40] passed a cosmid library of *Yersinia pseudotuberculosis* genomic DNA in *Escherichia coli* through the Hep 2 cell line to identify recombinant *E. coli* that could invade the epithelial cells. Using similar systems, invasion genes have been isolated from *Y. enterocolitica, Salmonella typhi, Salmonella typhimurium,* and *Shigella flexneri* (reviewed in ref. 41). This approach has also been used to study specific genes thought to be involved in intracellular growth, such as the listeriolysin O gene from *Listeria monocytogenes*. For example, expression of listeriolysin in *Bacillus subtilis* was sufficient to allow the *Bacillus* recombinant to escape from the phagosome into the cytoplasm and multiply intracellularly, whereas wild-type *Bacillus* bacteria were rapidly killed by macrophages.[42] This result may be of particular interest for studies on mycobacteria, which also express a hemolytic activity[43] and perhaps escape into the cytoplasm.[26–28.]

In the studies reported here, we used a strategy analogous to that of Isberg and Falkow[40] to isolate and characterize mycobacterial genes that can endow a normally susceptible bacterium with an enhanced ability to resist killing by macrophages. To do this, recombinant DNA libraries of *M. leprae* genomic DNA in *E. coli* were passed through macrophages to enrich for recombinant *E. coli* bacteria with increased resistance to killing. To isolate the recombinant clones that actually displayed the desired phenotype of increased survival, the clones arising from the enrichment process were assayed individually to determine their kinetics of survival in macrophages.

MATERIALS AND METHODS

Bacteria, Macrophages, Plasmids, and Recombinant DNA Libraries. The bacterial strains used in these studies were *E. coli* strains JM105 and DH5α and *Mycobacterium smegmatis* strain LR500. The *E. coli* strains were maintained on LB medium (Difco Laboratories, Detroit, MI) and the *M. smegmatis* strains were maintained on trypticase soy agar (TSA, Difco). A bone marrow derived macrophage cell line from A/J mice (*bcg*[r]) was used which displays many of the relevant properties of macrophages such as phagocytosis, antigen presentation, activation, and free radical production.[44,45] The line was provided by Dr. R. Little (Washington University, St. Louis, MO) and maintained in 75% Dulbecco's Modified Eagle's Medium (Gibco BRL, Gaithersburg, MD) with high glucose/high bicarbonate, 10% fetal calf serum (HyClone Laboratories Inc., Logan, UT), 5% horse serum (Gibco BRL), and 10% L-cell conditioned medium.[44]

A recombinant DNA library of *M. leprae* genomic DNA in the pHC79 cosmid vector[46] was provided by Dr. J. Clark-Curtiss (Washington University, St. Louis, MO). A recombinant DNA library of *M. leprae Bam*HI fragments was made by digesting *M. leprae* genomic DNA to completion with *Bam*HI (New England Biolabs, Beverly, MA) and inserting the fragments into *Bam*HI-cleaved and phosphatased pUC19 (New England Biolabs). Subclones were made in pUC19 or pJC85 (provided by Dr. J. Crawford, CDC, Atlanta, GA) using standard molecular biology techniques.[47] The plasmid pJC85 is a mycobacterium-*E. coli* shuttle vector which contains the mycobacterial origin of replication from pAL5000, the *E. coli* origin of replication and the multiple cloning site from pUC18, and a gene encoding kanamycin resistance as a selectable marker in both *E. coli* and *M. smegmatis* (J. Crawford, personal communication).

Enrichment Protocol. An 0.5-ml portion of an overnight culture of a recombinant DNA library (~1 × 10⁹ bacteria) was added to ~10⁷ macrophages, and phagocytosis was allowed to proceed for 1 hour at 37°C. The unphagocytized bacteria were removed by gentle washing with prewarmed Hanks' Balanced Salt Solution (HBBS, Gibco BRL). The cells were then incubated in fresh medium supplemented with 100 μg/ml gentamycin for 5 hours at 37°C. The macrophages were lysed by treatment with 1% Triton X-100 in water and dilutions of the lysate were plated on LB agar containing the appropriate antibiotic (10 μg tetracycline/ml for the cosmid recombinants and 33 μg ampicillin/ml for the pUC19 recombinants). After overnight incubation at 37°C, the resulting colonies were harvested and pooled. The suspension was diluted with LB broth containing the appropriate antibiotic, grown to an OD$_{600}$ of 0.3–0.4, and used to infect a fresh macrophage culture. A total of three of these cycles of enrichment were performed, except in the third cycle, the infected macrophage culture was incubated overnight in media containing gentamycin before lysis.

Kinetics of Survival in Macrophages. The time courses of survival of the individual clones in macrophages were determined in a manner similar to the enrichment protocol, except the infected macrophages were lysed at various times after phagocytosis and viable intracellular bacteria were enumerated by plating portions of the lysate on solid medium (LB agar for *E. coli* or TSA for *M. smegmatis*) containing the appropriate antibiotics.

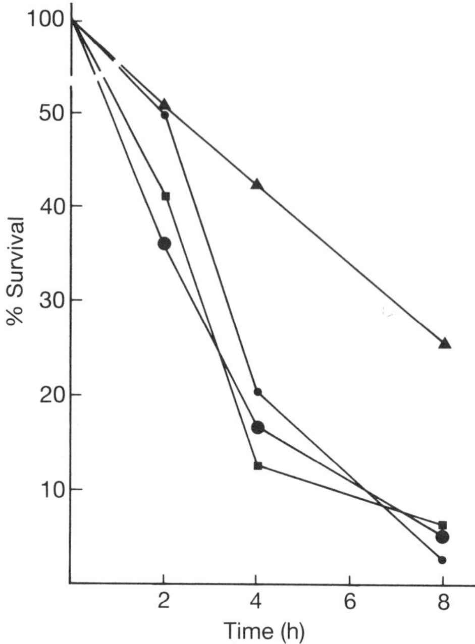

FIGURE 1. Survival of *E. coli* cosmid clones in macrophages. Approximately 4 × 10^6 *E. coli* JM105(pC101) (■), JM105(pC102) (●), JM105(pC103) (▲), or JM105(pHC79) (●) bacteria were mixed with ~10^6 macrophages, and phagocytosis was allowed to occur for 1 hour. Unphagocytized bacteria were removed by washing with HBBS. Fresh medium with 100 μg gentamycin/ml was added (time zero, t$_o$) and the cultures were incubated at 37°C. At t$_o$ and the indicated times, replicate cultures were lysed and the bacteria plated on LB agar containing 10 μg tetracycline/ml. Survival is indicated as 100 × [CFU at t$_x$ ÷ CFU at t$_o$].

RESULTS

Studies with the M. leprae *Cosmid Library.* Twenty-two clones were recovered from the *M. leprae* cosmid library in *E. coli* after the third cycle of enrichment. Cosmid DNA was isolated from each clone and a restriction enzyme analysis performed. Twenty-one clones contained mycobacterial DNA and one was the parent cosmid without any insert. Ten clones displayed unique, nonoverlapping restriction fragment patterns for the mycobacterial inserts, whereas 11 clones displayed 1 of 3 repeated restriction fragment patterns. The patterns represented by the cosmids pC101, pC102, and pC103 were present in 3, 3, and 5 recombinant clones, respectively.

Because passing the bacteria through macrophages simply enriches for enhanced survival, three clones were assayed individually to identify ones that actually displayed enhanced survival. The kinetics of survival in macrophages for *E. coli* cells carrying cosmids pC101, pC102, or pC103 or the cosmid vector pHC79 are shown in FIGURE 1. For these studies, time zero is defined as the end of the 1-hour incubation period for phagocytosis. The extent of phagocytosis was similar for each of the four strains tested as determined by microscopic examination of stained cultures (data not shown). *E. coli* carrying pHC79, pC101, or pC102 were rapidly killed by the macrophages. In contrast, *E. coli* carrying pC103 displayed significantly enhanced survival compared with the strain carrying the parent cosmid.

To ensure that the enhanced survival of the strain carrying pC103 was due to the presence of the cosmid as opposed to an unrelated mutation in the *E. coli* chromosome, pC103 was isolated by standard procedures and transformed into *E.*

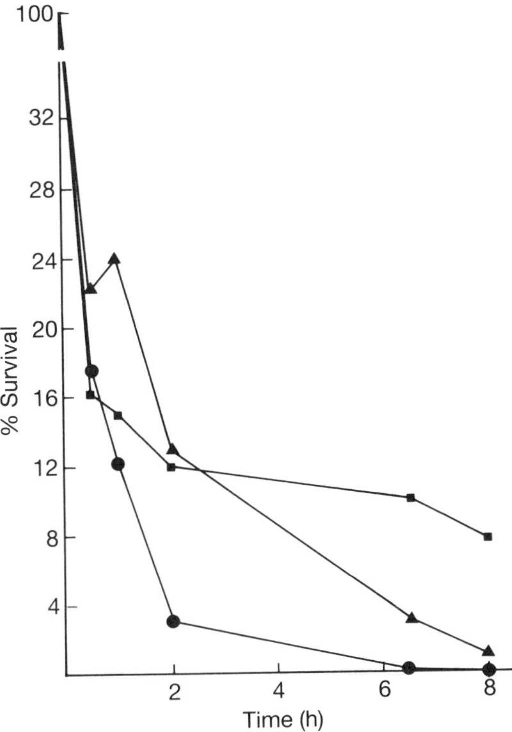

FIGURE 2. Survival of *E. coli* plasmid clones in macrophages. Strains JM105(pHD207) (■), JM105(pHD211) (▲), or JM105(pUC19) (●) were assayed as described in the legend to FIGURE 1 except the bacteria were plated on LB agar containing 33 μg ampicillin/ml.

coli strains JM105 and DH5α. The new transformants displayed the same pattern of increased intracellular survival as the original isolate (data not shown).

Because the initial studies involved plating the recovered bacteria on LB-agar containing tetracycline, we asked if the increased survival of strains carrying pC103 was due simply to increased stability of the plasmid by plating portions of the macrophage lysates onto LB media with and without tetracycline. For each time point, the number of colonies on the LB-tetracycline plates was equal to the number of colonies on the LB plates (data not shown).

Currently, we are in the process of subcloning the gene or genes from the ~32-kb mycobacterial DNA insert in cosmid pC103 in order to define and characterize the gene(s) in greater detail. The other cosmid clones resulting from the enrichment process have not yet been assayed individually.

Studies with the M. leprae *Plasmid Library.* Using a similar enrichment protocol, two additional clones were isolated from a recombinant DNA library made by cloning *M. leprae BamHI* genomic fragments into pUC19. These *E. coli* recombinants were designated pHD207 and pHD211, and each clone exhibited somewhat increased survival in the macrophage cell line compared to the *E. coli* cells carrying the parent plasmid (FIG. 2). In three independent experiments, *E. coli* cells carrying pHD211 displayed greater survival than did those carrying pHD207 at the early time points, whereas those carrying pHD207 had demonstrably higher survival at later time points.

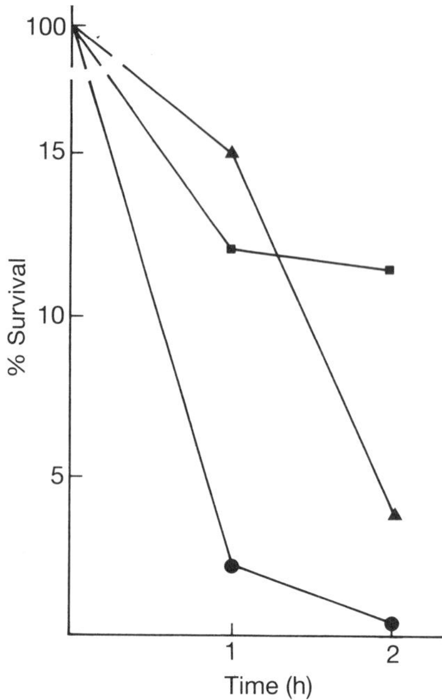

FIGURE 3. Survival of *M. smegmatis* transformants. *Mycobacterium smegmatis* strains LR500(pHD2001) (▲), LR500(pHD2003) (■), or LR500(pJC85) (●) were assayed for survival as described in the legend to FIGURE 1 except ~6 × 10⁵ bacteria were used to infect the macrophages and the bacteria were plated on TSA containing 10 μg kanamycin/ml.

The mycobacterial DNA inserts in these plasmids were 2.2 kb (pHD207) and 0.5 kb (pHD211). To look more closely at the possible effects of the genes carried by these plasmids on the survival of a mycobacterium in macrophages, as opposed to the survival of *E. coli* in macrophages, the mycobacterial DNA inserts of pHD207 and pHD211 were subcloned into the *E. coli*-mycobacterium shuttle vector pJC85. The resulting constructs pHD2001 (0.5-kb insert from pHD211) and pHD2003 (2.2-kb insert from pHD207) were then electroporated into *M. smegmatis* strain LR500. Individual transformants were single-colony purified and their time courses of survival in macrophages were determined as just described (FIG. 3). *M. smegmatis* LR500 cells carrying the parent plasmid pJC85 were killed rapidly by the macrophages, whereas the strains carrying the recombinant constructs demonstrated greater resistance to killing by the macrophages. The mycobacterial strain with pHD2003 displayed greater survival than did the one carrying pHD2001 at an early time point and less survival at later time points, results similar to those obtained with the *E. coli* recombinants.

DISCUSSION

Theoretically, two types of clones could be recovered from the enrichment protocol. The predominant class should be clones that carry determinants which endow the recipient strains with an increased resistance to killing. That is, recombinant bacteria carrying genes that impart increased survival as a result of the direct effect of a gene product on resistance to killing by the macrophage should be preferentially isolated. These gene products may include previously identified mycobacterial proteins such as superoxide dismutase or catalase or ones involved in the inhibition of phagosome-lysosome fusion or escape into the cytoplasm. Detailed characterization of the fate of the recombinant bacteria in macrophages at the light and electron microscopic levels should enable us to identify possible mechanisms for the increased survival of the recombinants, which in turn should help elucidate the evasion processes used by the mycobacteria.

The enrichment protocol may also identify a second class of recombinant clones, ones that carry mycobacterial determinants involved in attachment or invasion or that produce products which increase phagocytosis. For example, although the phagocytosis of mycobacteria is primarily mediated by complement and complement receptor, some uptake is mediated by the terminal mannosyl residues on the mycobacterial lipoarabinomannan and the phagocyte's mannose receptors (Larry Schlesinger, personal communication). Hence, expression of mycobacterial gene products that could add mannosyl residues to a surface-exposed component on the recipient cell might increase the phagocytosis of the recombinant and thereby increase the recovery of that clone during the enrichment process. Similarly, the expressions of an ''invasion'' gene might increase the entrance of a recombinant into the macrophages and thereby increase its recovery. The possible involvement of invasion genes in the entrance of mycobacteria into eukaryotic cells was originally suggested by the work of Shepard[48] in which he showed that mycobacteria could invade *in vitro* cultured cells such as Hep 2 cells and fibroblasts.

One limitation of the enrichment scheme is that it will probably bias the recovery of clones towards ones that confer much improved survival. As such, the approach will not generate a random collection of the genes required for intracellular survival and will not allow an estimate of the number of genes involved in these processes. A second limitation of this approach is that it can effectively identify only genes that express positive effector molecules. Certain genes involved in the ability of mycobacteria to survive and multiply intracellularly probably will not be isolated by this approach. Such genes may include ones (1) required for scavenging essential metabolites (e.g., mycobactin), (2) involved in synthesis of components required for growth (e.g., thymidine, aromatic amino acids), (3) that modulate (up-regulate or down-regulate) other genes or operons, or (4) that are part of a multi-protein complex or pathway (e.g., enzymes required for cell wall biosynthesis). Nonetheless, the approach described in this report should identify an important class of genes and gene products and may provide important insights into the survival of mycobacteria within macrophages and potential new targets for combatting these important pathogens.

An additional limitation of the work reported here is that *E. coli* was used as the host cell for the initial isolation of the mycobacterial genetic elements that confer increased survival onto the bacterial host, and not all mycobacterial genes are efficiently expressed in *E. coli*.[49] Despite this limitation, we were able to identify at least three different genetic elements from *M. leprae* that appear to be involved in resistance to killing by macrophages. To circumvent this limitation, we are constructing mycobacterial genomic DNA libraries in *E. coli*-mycobacterium shuttle vectors and will repeat the enrichment process and screening using the new recombinant DNA libraries in *M. smegmatis.* This should enable us to identify additional genes involved in the resistance to killing by macrophages.

SUMMARY

The survival of *M. leprae* and *M. tuberculosis* in the human host is dependent upon their ability to produce gene products that counteract the bactericidal activities of macrophages. To identify such mycobacterial genes and gene products, recombinant DNA libraries of mycobacterial DNA in *E. coli* were passed through macrophages to enrich for clones carrying genes that endow the normally susceptible *E. coli* bacteria with an enhanced ability to survive within macrophages. Following three cycles of enrichment, 15 independent clones were isolated. Three recombinants were characterized in detail, and each confers significantly enhanced survival on *E. coli* cells carrying them. Two of the cloned genetic elements also confer enhanced survival onto *M. smegmatis* cells. Further characterization of these genes and gene products should provide insights into the survival of mycobacteria within macrophages and may identify new approaches of targets for combatting these important pathogens.

ACKNOWLEDGMENTS

We thank Drs. J. Clark-Curtiss, J. Crawford, C. H. King, and R. Little for providing essential materials for these studies and helpful discussions.

REFERENCES

1. DUBOS, R. & J. DUBOS. 1952. The White Plague: Tuberculosis, Man, and Society. Little, Brown, and Co. Boston, MA.
2. BROWNE, S. G. 1975. Some aspects of the history of leprosy: The leprosy of yesteryear. Proc. Roy. Soc. Med. **68:** 485–493.
3. NOORDEEN, S. K., L. L. BRAVO & T. K. SUDARESAN. 1992. Estimated number of leprosy cases in the world. Bull. W.H.O. **70:** 7–10.
4. SUDRE, P., G. TEN DAM & A. KOCHI. 1992. Tuberculosis: A global overview of the situation today. Bull. W.H.O. **70:** 149–159.
5. BLOOM B. R. & C. J. MURRAY. 1992. Tuberculosis: Commentary on a reemergent killer. Science **257:** 1055–1064.
6. CENTERS FOR DISEASE CONTROL AND PREVENTION. 1993. Tuberculosis morbidity–United States, 1992. Morbid. Mortal. Weekly Rep. **42:** 363.
7. DOOLEY, S. W., W. R. JARVIS, W. J. MARTONE & D. E. SNIDER, JR. 1992. Multidrug-resistant tuberculosis. Ann. Intern. Med. **117:** 257–259.
8. RIDLEY, D. S. 1988. Pathogenesis of Leprosy and Related Diseases. Wright. London.
9. DANNENBERG, A. M. 1987. Immune mechanisms in the pathogenesis of pulmonary tuberculosis. Rev. Infect. Dis. **11**(Suppl.2): S369–S378.
10. KAUFMANN, S. H. E. 1988. Immunity against intracellular bacteria: Biological effector functions and antigen specificity of T lymphocytes. Curr. Topics Microbiol. Immunol. **138:** 141–176.
11. ROOK, G. A. W. 1988. Role of activated macrophages in the immunopathology of tuberculosis. Br. Med. Bull. **44:** 611–623.

12. LOWRIE, D. B. 1983. Mononuclear phagocyte-mycobacterium interaction. *In* The Biology of the Mycobacteria. C. Ratledge & J. Stanford, eds. Vol. **2:** 235–278. Academic Press. London.

13. BIRDI, T. J. & N. H. ANTIA. 1989. The macrophage in leprosy: A review on the current status. Int. J. Lepr. **57:** 511–525.

14. GREEN S. J., M. S. MELTZER, J. B. HIBBS, JR. & C. A. NACY. 1990. Activated macrophages destroy intracellular *Leishmania major* amasitigotes by an L-arginine-dependent killing mechanism. J. Immunol. **144:** 278–283.

15. MIMS, C. A. 1990. The Pathogenesis of Infectious Disease. 3rd Ed. Academic Press. London.

16. HAAS, A. & W. GOEBEL. 1992. Microbial strategies to prevent oxygen-dependent killing by phagocytes. Free Rad. Res. Comm. **16:** 137–158.

17. RASTOGI, N., Ed. 1990. Killing intracellular mycobacteria: Dogmas and realities. Fifth Forum in Microbiology. Res. Microbiol. **141:** 191–270.

18. DRAPER, P. 1981. Mycobacterial inhibition of intracellular killing. *In* Microbial Perturbation of Host-Defences. F. O'Grady & H. Smith, eds.: 143–164. Academic Press. London.

19. GOREN, M. B. 1977. Phagocyte lysosomes: Interactions with infectious agents, phagosomes, and experimental perturbations in function. Annu. Rev. Microbiol. **31:** 507–533.

20. HORWITZ, M. A. 1988. Intracellular parasitism. Curr. Opin. Immunol. **1:** 41–46.

21. KAUFMANN, S. H. E. & M. J. REDDEHASE. 1989. Infection of phagocytic cells. Curr. Opinions Immunol. **2:** 43–49.

22. JOINER, K. A., S. FUHRMAN, H. M. MIETTINEN, L. H. KASPER & I. MELLMAN. 1990. *Toxoplasma gondii:* Fusion competence of parasitophorous vacuoles in Fc receptor-transfected fibroblasts. Science **249:** 641–646.

23. SCHLESINGER, L. S. & M. A. HORWITZ. 1990. Phagocytosis of leprosy bacilli is mediated by complement receptors CR1 and CR3 on human monocytes and complement component C3 in serum. J. Clin. Invest. **85:** 1304–1311.

24. SCHLESINGER, L. S., C. G. BELLINGER-KAWAHARA, N. R. PAYNE & M. A. HORWITZ. 1990. Phagocytosis of *Mycobacterium tuberculosis* is mediated by human monocyte complement receptors and complement component C3. J. Immunol. **144:** 2771–2780.

25. LAUNOIS, P., B. MAILLERE, A. DIEYE, J. L. SARTHOU & M. A. BACH. 1989. Human phagocytic oxidative burst activation by BCG, *M. leprae,* and atypical mycobacteria: Defective activation by *M. leprae* is not reversed by interferon gamma. Cell. Immunol. **124:** 168–174.

26. MOR, N. 1983. Intracellular location of *Mycobacterium leprae* in macrophages of normal and immunodeficient mice and the effect of rifampin. Infect. Immun. **42:** 802–811.

27. MYRVICK, Q. N., E. S. LEAKE & M. J. WRIGHT. 1984. Disruption of phagosomal membranes of normal aveolar macrophages by the H37Rv strain of *Mycobacterium tuberculosis.* Am. Rev. Resp. Dis. **129:** 322–328.

28. MCDONOUGH, K. A., Y. KRESS & B. R. BLOOM. 1993. Pathogenesis of tuberculosis: Interaction of *Mycobacterium tuberculosis* with macrophages. Infect. Immun. **61:** 2763–2773.

29. D'ARCY HART, P. 1982. Lysosome fusion responses of macrophages to infection: Behavior and significance. *In* Phagocytosis: Past and Future. M. L. Karnovsky & L. Bolis, eds.: 437–447. Academic Press. New York.

30. FREHEL, C. & N. RASTOGI. 1987. *Mycobacterium leprae* surface components intervene in the early phagosome-lysosome fusion inhibition event. Infect. Immun. **55:** 2916–2921.

31. CROWLE, A. J., R. DAHL, E. ROSS & M. H. MAY. 1991. Evidence that vesicles containing living, virulent *Mycobacterium tuberculosis* or *Mycobacterium avium* in cultured human macrophages are not acidic. Infect. Immun. **59:** 1823–1831.

32. D'Arcy Hart, P. & M. R. Young. 1991. Ammonium chloride, an inhibitor of phagosome-lysosome fusion in macrophages, concurrently induces phagosome-endosome fusion, and opens a novel pathway: Studies of a pathogenic mycobacterium and a nonpathogenic yeast. J. Exp. Med. **174:** 881–889.

33. Denis, M. 1991. Interferon-gamma treated murine macrophages inhibit growth of tubercle bacilli via the generation of reactive nitrogen intermediates. Cell. Immunol. **132:** 150–157.

34. Adams, L. B., S. G. Franzblau, Z. Varvin, J. B. Hibbs, Jr. & J. L. Krahenbuhl. 1991. L-arginine-dependent macrophage effector functions inhibit metabolic activity of *Mycobacterium leprae.* J. Immunol. **147:** 1642–1646.

35. Chan, J., T. Fujiwara, P. Brennan, M. McNeil, S. J. Turco, J.-C. Sibille, M. Snapper, P. Aisen & B. R. Bloom. 1989. Microbial glycolipids: Possible virulence factors that scavenge oxygen radicals. Proc. Natl. Acad. Sci. USA **86:** 2453–2457.

36. Draper, P. & R. J. W. Rees. 1970. Electron-transparent zone of mycobacteria may be a defence mechanism. Nature **228:** 860–861.

37. Fields, P., R. Swanson, C. Haidaris & F. Heffron. 1986. Mutants of *Salmonella typhimurium* that cannot survive within the macrophage are avirulent. Proc. Natl. Acad. Sci. USA **83:** 5189–5193.

38. Fields, P. I., E. A. Grossman & F. Heffron. 1989. A *Salmonella* locus that controls resistance to microbicidal proteins from phagocytic cells. Science **243:** 1059–1062.

39. Cianciatto, N., B. Eisenstein, C. Mody, G. Toews & N. Engleberg. 1990. A mutation in the *mip* gene results in an attenuation of *Legionella pneumophila* virulence. J. Infect. Dis. **162:** 121–126.

40. Isberg, R. R. & S. Falkow. 1985. A single locus encoded by *Yersinnia pseudotuberculosis* permits invasion of cultured animal cells be *Escherichia coli* K-12. Nature **317:** 262–264.

41. Finlay, B. B. & S. Falkow. 1989. Common themes in microbial pathogenicity. Microbiol. Rev. **53:** 210–230.

42. Bielecki, J., P. J. Youngman, P. Connelly & D. A. Portnoy. 1990. *Bacillus subtilis* expressing a hemolysin gene from *Listeria monocytogenes* can grow in mammalian cells. Nature **345:** 175–176.

43. King, C. H., M. Sathish, J. T. Crawford & T. M. Shinnick. 1993. Expression of contact-dependent cytolytic activity by *Mycobacterium tuberculosis* and isolation of the genomic locus that encodes the activity. Infect. Immun. **61:** 2708–2712.

44. Johnson, C. R., D. Kitz & R. Little 1983. A method for the derivation and continuous propagation of cloned murine bone marrow macrophages. J. Immunol. Methods **65:** 319–332.

45. Stewart, C. C., E. B. Walker, C. Johnson & R. Little. 1985. Clonal analysis of bone marrow and macrophage cultures. *In* Mononuclear Phagocytes. R. van Furth, ed.: 255–265. Martinus Nijhoff. Boston, MA.

46. Clark-Curtiss, J., W. Jacobs, M. Docherty, L. Ritchie & R. Curtiss. 1985. Molecular analysis of DNA and construction of genomic libraries of *Mycobacterium leprae.* J. Bacteriol. **161:** 1093–1102.

47. Sambrook, J., E. F. Fritsch & T. Maniatis. 1989. Molecular Cloning: A Laboratory Manual. 2nd Ed. Cold Spring Harbor Laboratory Press. Cold Spring Harbor, NY.

48. Shepard, C. C. 1958. A comparison of the growth of selected mycobacteria in HeLa, monkey kidney, and human amnion cells in tissue culture. J. Exp. Med. **107:** 237–246.

49. Jacobs, W. R., M. Docherty, R. Curtiss & J. Clark-Curtiss. 1986. Expression of *Mycobacterium leprae* genes from a *Streptococcus mutans* promoter in *Escherichia coli* K-12. Proc. Natl. Acad. Sci. USA **83:** 1926–1939.

Mechanisms and Strategies of Viral Antigenic Variation

THOMAS M. FOLKS

Retrovirus Diseases Branch
Division of Viral and Rickettsial Diseases
National Center for Infectious Diseases
Centers for Disease Control and Prevention
Atlanta, Georgia 30333

As the World Health Organization has reported, infectious diseases remain the leading cause of human death worldwide. Despite remarkable progress in medicine during the past years, new and reemerging infectious diseases continue to cause profound human suffering and adversely affect the economies of both industrialized and developing countries.[1,2] As commerce and travel move the world closer together at a rapid pace, distance can no longer be considered a safe insulator from infectious diseases. As Joshua Lederberg aptly stated the dilemma, "The microbe that felled one child in a distant continent yesterday can reach yours today and seed a global pandemic tomorrow."

In the 1992 Institute of Medicine report on new and reemerging infectious disease threats, the definition of emerging infectious microbe was described under four broad categories: (1) a new agent that has not been described; (2) an agent that has been present but previously has gone undetected; (3) an agent derived from an established disease and now determined as the cause; and (4) an agent that reappears following a decline in the incidence of disease.

Several factors may influence the emergence or reemergence of an infectious organism. First, microbial adaption over time may permit an organism to become established in an environment in which it could not previously exist. Second, population shifts such as migration may introduce susceptible hosts or carriers into a new region. Third, environmental disturbances or changes can result in a rearrangement of conditions that before were unfavorable for the organism's survival. Fourth, mutation of an agent whereby a change has imparted a variation can lead to the emergence of that agent. The discussion here will follow up primarily on several aspects of viral variation, including strategies that viruses rely on for variation and why understanding viral variation, especially in lentiviruses, is crucial to understanding their pathogenesis.

MECHANISMS OF VARIATION

The very short generation times coupled with large susceptible host populations and extremely high mutation frequencies provide some viruses with great potential for change. Curiously, this is especially true of RNA viruses because their mechanism for replication lacks efficient "proofreading." DNA-based agents have a much greater fidelity of replication, ensuring copy uniformity. RNA viruses, including influenza

TABLE 1. Viral Mechanisms to Generate Diversity

Mechanism	Viral Genome
Point mutation	RNA or DNA
Reassortment	RNA
Recombination	DNA
Defective-interfering particles	RNA or DNA

virus, vesicular stomatitis virus, foot-and-mouth disease virus, Newcastle disease virus, and rhinoviruses, and retroviruses are notorious for high mutation rates, resulting in genetic change.[3,4] Researchers examining ways to protect the host from primary infection are particularly interested in how genetic changes arise. Such changes are paramount to vaccine design so that proper estimates of stable protective regions can be objectively measured. Understanding viral genomic divergence also is useful in predicting genetic relatedness and unraveling evolutionary relationships of viruses.

The most common form of genetic change in any organism is point mutation, which usually occurs as a result of misincorporation of nucleotides during replication. Viruses are certainly no exception to this process, and they often extensively acquire or delete larger regions of their genome.

Four mechanisms are usually put forth to describe how viruses generate divergence (TABLE 1). As mentioned previously, mutations, usually in the form of single-point changes, are one of the most common mechanisms for producing variation, especially in RNA viruses. A number of factors contribute to this process, including inherent error frequencies, proofreading inadequacies, and high replication cycles. A second mechanism is dependent on the viruses' genomic arrangement. Segmented viruses possess discrete genomic segments independent of one another, much like chromosomes. These segments may reassort during replication, producing progeny virions with divergent phenotypes. Reassortment is a powerful creator of divergence, especially among viruses that can exchange genetic material between humans and animals (e.g., influenza A virus). A third mechanism, recombination, explains rearrangements within the viral genome. Recombination events can lead to deletions or duplications of viral genes as well as the acquisition of foreign genetic material. Recombination is not thought to play a major role in RNA virus divergence, at least in those RNA viruses without a DNA intermediate. However, all DNA viruses undergo some form of homologous recombination. The contribution of homologous recombination to natural virus variation is still unclear. A fourth mechanism of divergence deals with the creation of "defective interfering" (DI) viruses. These viruses are often derived from intramolecular recombination events, leading to significant deletions of viral replicative function. Such "particles" can interfere with homologous viruses or closely related viruses, resulting in wild-type progeny for recombination events.[3,5]

SURVIVAL STRATEGIES–WHY VIRUSES VARY

A successful infection is one in which an organism has the capability to exist in its host long enough to reproduce. Viruses have developed several strategies to prolong their existence within their host and successfully replicate. Viral divergence may occur within the primary host so that continuous reinfection is achieved or it may occur outside the host to assure host-to-host progeny expansion. The latter effect is observed, for instance, in respiratory infection when time between initial infection, replication, and shedding is short.[6]

Although viruses survive without the need to vary or with minimal mutation, including rubella, measles (recently found to have high field variation), mumps, and smallpox, variation is the key to survival for many agents. Probably the most common functional host event in which divergence plays a major antagonistic role is that of immune surveillance. This role, however, does not explain the only contribution that variation provides in a virus total strategic plan. For instance, the primary replication site or tissue tropism might vary because of genomic changes in viral promoters. Likewise, if tissue tropisms change, then glycosylation units may change, thus producing an altered phenotype.

By far, though, the significance of genomic variability lies in antigenic changes that present new three-dimensional structures to the ongoing immune response. No group of viruses has achieved the mastery of antigenic divergence better than the lentiviruses.

LENTIVIRUSES

Lentiviruses, a subfamily of retroviruses, are especially proficient in functional divergence, such as random fixation of neutral mutants and nonrandom fixation of mutants that may become advantageous for their survival. Antigenic changes rapidly occurring in the receptor-binding domain of these viruses contribute not only to their global geographic evolution[7] but also to their microscopic variation within communities.[8] Before describing antigenic variation of lentiviruses, I should first briefly define *retroviral* strategies of divergence. Probably the single most responsible mechanism for variation in retroviruses lies in its error-prone replication enzyme, reverse transcriptase. Incorporation errors of nucleotides in the *env* gene have been estimated to occur at between 2×10^{-2} and 3×10^{-3} per site per year.[9] This magnitude of divergence easily allows for rapid antigenic changes, especially in the envelope.

The major neutralizing domain of human immunodeficiency virus type 1 (HIV-1) has been shown to reside in the V_3 loop of the viral envelope (FIG. 1). This loop is an external glycoprotein that possesses the primary junction for receptor-binding and fusion.[10] Most variation in HIV as well as in two other studied lentiviruses, visna virus and equine infectious anemia virus,[11] is focused around the envelop protein. Selective pressures by the immune system are thought to be mainly responsible for the emergence of envelope variation *in vivo*. This selective drift among the lentiviruses is also responsible for the escape from neutralizing antibody protection observed in other viruses.[11] It should be noted that although the V_3 region of HIV-1 is an important neutralizing domain, other variable portions of the envelope are susceptible to mutation. Changes in these regions can also contribute significantly to the overall three-dimensional conformation of V_3.

Recently, much attention has been given to the consequences of antigenic variation and its contribution to biological variants in the disease-causing process of AIDS.

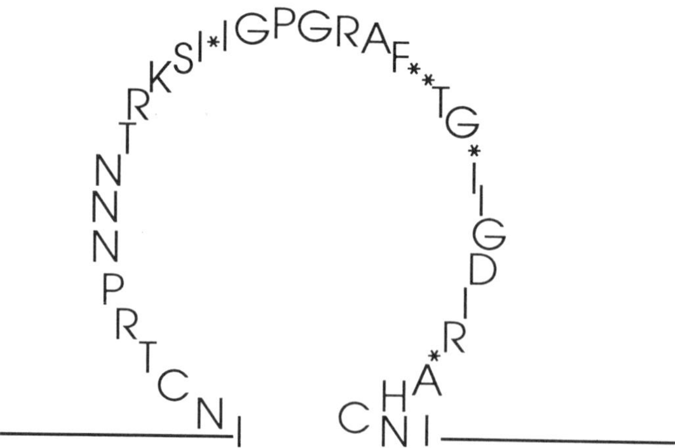

FIGURE 1. HIV-1 V_3 loop of external envelope. Asterisk (*) refers to hypervariable sites.

Two biological phenotypes have been described that basically define their cytopathic capabilities. These have been referred to as nonsyncytium-inducing (NSI) and syncytium-inducing (SI) strains.[12] Such strains seem to emerge within an individual at somewhat predicated times. Antigens present on the highly cytopathic SI strains tend to be potent stimulators of the humoral immune response and thus are rapidly cleared during the early acute phase of AIDS. This effect results in the emergence of the slower growing, less pathogenic NSI strains. Only during the later stages of HIV infection do the SI variants begin to reappear. This reactivation is thought to be due to a waning of the immune response that kept the cytopathic, rapidly growing SI strains dormant. As antigenic variants "out-run" the neutralizing immune response and deplete the peripheral lymphoid organs of helper lymphocytes, the SI strains reappear in high viral load.

This is not the only case in which antigenic variation and selection by the immune system results in phenotype emergence. While NSI *versus* SI selection is under way during the asymptomatic phase of HIV-1 infection, T-cell tropism *versus* monocytotropism is becoming established. These changes in tropism taking place *in vivo* may be responsible for important reservoirs that will later contribute to the long clinical latency period in AIDS.

CONCLUSION

I have reviewed some of the mechanisms by which viruses have evolved to antigenically modify themselves for survival. Changes at the genomic level are the most common mechanism of viral divergence. This process generally involves structural antigenic changes that require the protective immune response to evaluate a new foreign epitope. Such a response by specific immune cells is time dependent and thus must compete with the divergence mechanism of the virus. Obviously, classic vaccine development is dependent on our understanding of such divergence mechanisms, especially before we can ever hope to protect individuals against something as insidious as lentiviruses.

REFERENCES

1. NIAID. July 1991. Report of the Task Force on Microbiology and Infectious Disease. DHHS, PHS, NIH.
2. US Dept of HHS. 1990. Healthy People 2000. National Health Promotion and Disease Prevention Objectives. DHHS Publication No (PHS) 91-50213. US Government Printing Office. Washington, DC.
3. STRAUSS, E. G., J. H. STRAUSS & A. J. LEVINE. 1990. Virus evolution. *In* Virology, 2nd Ed. B. N. Fields, D. M. Knipe, R. M. Chanock, M. S. Hirsch, J. K. Melnick, T. P. Monath & B. Roizman, eds. Vol. **1:** 167-190. Raven Press. New York.
4. SMITH, D. B. & S. C. INGLIS. 1987. The mutation rate and variability of eukaryotic viruses: An analytical review. J. Gen. Virol. **68:** 2729-2740.
5. DOMINGO, E., J. J. HOLLAND & P. AHLQUIST, Eds. 1988. RNA Genetics: Variability of RNA Genomes. Vol 3. CRC Press, Inc. Boca Raton, FL.
6. MIMS, C. A. 1990. The Pathogenesis of Infectious Disease, 3rd Ed. Academic Press, Inc. New York.
7. BLATTNER, W. A. 1991. HIV epidemiology: Past, present, and future. FASEB J. **5:** 2340-2348.
8. OU, C. Y., C. A. CIESIELSKI, G. MEYERS, C. I. BANDEA, C.-C. LUO, B. T. M. KORBER, J. I. MULLINS, G. SCHOCHETMAN, R. L. BERKELMAN, A. N. ECONOMOU, J. J. WITTE, L. J. FURMAN, G. A. SATTEN, K. A. MacINNES, J. W. CORRAN, & H. W. JAFFEY. 1992. Molecular epidemiology of HIV transmission in a dental practice. Science **256:** 1165-1171.
9. HAHN, B. H., G. M. SHAW, M. E. TAYLOR, R. R. REDFIELD, P. D. MARKHAM, S. Z. SALAHUDDIN, F. WONG-STAAL, R. C. GALLO, E. S. PARKS & W. P. PARKS. 1986. Genetic variation in HTLV III/LAV over time in patients with AIDS and at risk for AIDS. Science **232:** 1548-1553.
10. LEVY, J. A. 1993. Pathogenesis of HIV infection. Microbiol. Rev. **57:** 183-289.
11. CLEMENTS, J. E., S. L. GDOVIN, R. C. MONTELARO & O. NARAYAN. 1988. Antigenic variation in lentiviral diseases. Ann. Rev. Immunol. **60:** 139-159.
12. TERSMETTE, M., J. M. A. LANGE, R. E. Y. DE GOEDE, R. DE WOLF, J. K. M. EEFTINK-SHATTENKERK, P. Th. A. SCHELLEKENS, R. A. COUTINHO, J. G. HUISMAN, J. GOUDSMIT & F. MIEDEMA. 1989. Differences in risk for AIDS and AIDS mortality associated with biological properties of HIV variants. Lancet **1:** 983-985.

Regulation of Cytokine Patterns in Leprosy[a]

PETER A. SIELING AND ROBERT L. MODLIN [b]

Division of Dermatology and
Department of Microbiology and Immunology
UCLA School of Medicine
Los Angeles, California 90024-1750

Leprosy, caused by the intracellular pathogen *Mycobacterium leprae,* provides an extraordinary window on immune regulation in infection. Leprosy is an ideal model because it presents as a spectrum of clinical manifestations that correlate with immune responses to the pathogen[1]: At one end of the spectrum, patients with tuberculoid leprosy typify the resistant response that restricts the growth of the pathogen. The number of lesions is few, but tissue and nerve damage is frequent. At the opposite end of this spectrum, patients with lepromatous leprosy represent extreme susceptibility to *M. leprae* infection. In lepromatous leprosy, the skin lesions are numerous and growth of the pathogen is unabated, resulting in many viable *M. leprae* throughout the skin lesions. These clinical presentations correlate with the level of cell-mediated immunity (CMI) against *M. leprae.* The standard measure of CMI to the pathogen is the Mitsuda reaction. Patients are challenged by intradermal injection of *M. leprae,* and induration is measured 3 weeks later. The test is positive in tuberculoid patients and negative in lepromatous patients.

Although the majority of immunologic studies in leprosy have been performed on peripheral blood lymphocytes, the focal point of the immune response to *M. leprae* is the tissue granuloma, a collection of lymphocytes and macrophages. To address questions concerning the immune mechanisms central to the pathogenesis of leprosy, we have used cellular and molecular approaches to define mechanisms of immunity and immunosuppression to the pathogen.

IMMUNOHISTOLOGY OF LESIONS

T-Cell Populations in Lesions

Monoclonal antibodies directed against T-cell subpopulations have enabled investigation of T cells *in situ,* in frozen sections of biopsy specimens, by immunohistologic techniques.[2-16] These studies indicate striking differences in the CD4:CD8 (T-hel-

[a]This work was supported by grants from the National Institutes of Health (AI 22553, AR 40312, and CA 09120) and the Heiser Trust.

[b]Address for correspondence: Robert L. Modlin, M.D., UCLA Division of Dermatology, 52-121 CHS, 10833 Le Conte Avenue, Los Angeles, CA 90024-1750.

per : T-suppressor) ratio at the poles of the leprosy spectrum. The data from all studies indicate that in tuberculoid leprosy lesions, the CD4 population predominates with a CD4:CD8 ratio of 1.9:1, whereas in lepromatous lesions the CD8 population predominates with a CD4:CD8 ratio of 0.6:1. The CD4:CD8 ratios in the lesions are independent of those in the blood of the patients, suggesting some selective migration of cells into, proliferation within, or retention in lesions.[17] Furthermore, it underscores the importance of studying those cells at the site of disease activity instead of in the peripheral blood.

Whereas the CD4:CD8 ratio is 2:1 both in the blood and in the lesions of tuberculoid patients, the tissue population does not represent a random filtrate from blood. The T-memory: T-naive ratio is 1:1 in blood but 14 : 1 in the lesions.[18] In contrast, in the lepromatous lesions, one half the CD4[+] cells belong to the T-naive subset. The majority of CD8[+] cells infiltrating lepromatous lesions are CD28[-], indicating that they are the T-suppressor cells, whereas CD8[+] cells of the T-cytotoxic phenotype (CD28[+]) predominate in the tuberculoid lesions.

Immunologic Microenvironments

The segregation of T-cell subsets into distinct microenvironments within the tuberculoid granuloma is intriguing. The immunohistologic studies reveal that CD4[+] cells are microanatomically associated with macrophages in the core of the granuloma, with CD8[+] cells restricted to the mantle surrounding the granuloma.[2,4,6,10,14] The CD4[+] cells present in the center of the granuloma are of the T-memory phenotype.[18] Inasmuch as they are located near macrophages, it is conceivable that they may play a role in mediating macrophage localization, activation, and maturation that leads to restriction or elimination of the pathogen. The T-naive cells are localized to the mantle surrounding the granuloma, near CD8[+] cells. In contrast, in lepromatous granulomas, the CD8[+] cells are admixed with macrophages and CD4[+] cells. Since these CD8[+] cells are of the T-suppressor phenotype, they may act to suppress the CMI response.

CD1

Langerhans cells, intraepidermal macrophages with a dendritic morphology, have antigen-presenting capabilities and share the CD1 epitope with immature thymocytes. The numbers of Langerhans cells in the epidermis of tuberculoid lesions are greater than those in lepromatous lesions.[4,19] CD1[+] Langerhans cells are present at the periphery of the tuberculoid granuloma.[4,9,14,20–22] These cells are infrequent in the granulomas of lepromatous patients.

CYTOKINE PATTERNS IN LESIONS

Detection of Cytokines in Situ

The immunoperoxidase technique has been used to detect IL-2, a lymphokine necessary for T-cell proliferation, in leprosy lesions.[9,14] The studies indicate that an order of magnitude greater number of IL-2 containing cells is present in tuberculoid lesions than in lepromatous lesions. Additional immunohistochemical studies revealed that IFN-γ,[23,24] IL-1β,[24] and TNF-α[24] positive cells are more numerous in tuberculoid than in lepromatous lesions.

The *in situ* hybridization technique allows for the microanatomic localization of mRNA coding for proteins in lesions. Since IFN-γ facilitates the intracellular killing of mycobacteria *in vitro* and *in vivo*,[25,26] leprosy skin biopsy specimens were examined for the presence of mRNA encoding this lymphokine.[27] Cells showing hybridization with an IFN-γ cDNA probe are more numerous in tuberculoid than lepromatous lesions, and the percentages of positive cells are similar to that seen using the anti-IL-2 monoclonal antibody. Furthermore, the presence of T cells of potential cytotoxic function was investigated using a riboprobe for an enzymatic marker associated with cytotoxic cells, serine esterase. Cells containing serine esterase mRNA are more numerous in tuberculoid lesions than in lepromatous lesions, indicating that T-cytotoxic cells may contribute to host defenses against mycobacterial infection by lysing infected targets.[28]

Detection of Cytokine mRNA by Polymerase Chain Reaction (PCR) Amplification

To more fully probe patterns of lymphokines in lesions at the extremes of the spectrum of leprosy, PCR amplification of cDNA derived by reverse transcription of lesion-extracted mRNA was performed using cytokine-specific primers.[29] Messenger RNAs encoding IL-2, IFN-γ, and lymphotoxin were detected at higher levels in tuberculoid lesions, but were virtually absent in lepromatous lesions. In contrast, IL-4, IL-5, and IL-10 mRNAs were present at higher levels in lepromatous than in tuberculoid lesions.

The distinctly different cytokine patterns in leprosy are strikingly parallel to the described Th1 and Th2 patterns that have been delineated in the mouse.[30] T cells that produce IL-2 and IFN-γ, termed Th1 cells, preferentially activate macrophages to kill intracellular pathogens. In contrast, T cells that produce IL-4, IL-5, and IL-10, termed Th2 cells, augment humoral responses and suppress CMI responses. These cytokine patterns, Th1 and Th2, correspond to resistant *versus* susceptible responses to infection in several murine models.[31–33] Therefore, the Type 1 cytokine mRNAs present in tuberculoid lesions might be involved in CMI to infection; those found to be increased in lepromatous lesions, Type 2 cytokines, might contribute to the immune unresponsiveness and elevated antibody levels.

FUNCTIONAL ACTIVITY OF T CELLS DERIVED FROM LESIONS

Although phenotyping offers intriguing hints regarding the activities of cells in leprosy lesions, direct examination of the immune function of cells in lesions may yield more substantial clues about their role in the pathogenesis of leprosy.

T-Helper Cells

T cells derived from tuberculoid lesions were expanded in the presence of IL-2 alone, to select for cells activated *in situ* by antigenic stimulation.[18] Such CD4$^+$ lines from tuberculoid leprosy lesions respond to the whole *M. leprae,* whereas CD4$^+$ lines from lepromatous lesions are unresponsive. These data indicate that CD4$^+$ lines from tuberculoid but not lepromatous lesions have been activated locally to express IL-2 receptors.

Tissue-extracted T cells have been analyzed by limiting dilution analysis to determine the precursor frequency of such antigen-reactive T cells.[18] Approximately 2% of T cells from tuberculoid leprosy lesions are capable of proliferation in response to *M. leprae,* whereas only 0.02% of peripheral blood cells are reactive to the same antigen.[18] Thus, there is a 100-fold enrichment in antigen-reactive T cells in tuberculoid lesions relative to blood.

To identify immunodominant antigens, *M. leprae*-specific T-cell lines were tested for their reactivity against *M. leprae* antigens separated on gradient SDS-PAGE gels, using the T-cell Western blot technique. Greatest reactivity was observed to proteins of molecular weight 7-10 kD and 16-18 kD.[34] Further immunologic analysis provided evidence that the *M. leprae* 10-kD antigen is a strong stimulator of T-cell responses.[35] Limiting dilution analysis performed in two *M. leprae*-reactive individuals indicated that approximately 1 of 3 *M. leprae*-reactive T-cell precursors responded to the *M. leprae* 10-kD antigen. Sequencing of the gene encoding the *M. leprae* 10-kD protein revealed significant homology with GroES stress protein of *Escherichia coli.*[36] The ability of the immune system to recognize stress proteins provides the ability to react with the wide variety of pathogens that express these antigens.

T-Suppressor Cells

Most patients with lepromatous leprosy exhibit normal CMI to a variety of mycobacterial antigens, including *M. tuberculosis,* but they are unresponsive to antigens of *M. leprae.* One possible hypothesis to explain this phenomenon is that one or a small number of unique epitopes associated with *M. leprae* are capable of inducing suppression of T-helper cell responses.[37–40] To examine this theory at the level of the skin lesion, CD8$^+$ cells were extracted from lesions.[17,41] CD8 lines derived from lepromatous but not tuberculoid lesions suppress mitogen and antigen responses of peripheral blood cells as well as CD4$^+$ clones only in the presence of *M. leprae.*[17] Therefore, the CD8$^+$ T-suppressor cells in lepromatous lesions may contribute to the unresponsiveness *in vivo* by their action on the microanatomically apposed CD4$^+$ population.

The suppressor activity of these CD8$^+$ cells appears to be restricted by MHC class II antigens, specifically HLA-DQ determinants.[41,42] The Ts clones express the T-cell receptor αβ heterodimer T-cell receptors on their cell surface.[43] Immunohistologic studies further demonstrated that the majority of CD8$^+$ cells in lepromatous lesions expressed the β chain of the T-cell receptor *in situ.*[43] The ability of these CD8$^+$ cells to mediate suppression is dependent on this T-cell receptor because suppression is blocked by monoclonal antibodies to the variable segment of the β chain.[42]

Cytokine Patterns of T-Cell Subsets

Analysis of T-cell clones derived from lesions and blood of patients with leprosy has revealed that the differing patterns of lymphokines found in skin lesions are produced by the predominant CD4 and CD8 subsets in these lesions. CD4[+] clones from tuberculoid patients are potent producers of IFN-γ and CD8[+] T-suppressor clones derived from lepromatous lesions characteristically produce IL-4 *in vitro*,[44] which may down-regulate the macrophage response to IFN-γ.[44] Suppressor activity could be abrogated by the addition of anti-IL-4 antibodies to the cultures. Finally, IL-4 may serve as an autocrine growth factor for these CD8[+] T-suppressor cells.[45] It is a well-known immunologic generalization that a dichotomy exists between antibodies to a pathogen and cell-mediated immunity. Lepromatous leprosy patients, lacking CMI, have significantly higher levels of anti-*M. leprae* antibodies than do tuberculoid patients. These data can best be reconciled by appreciating that IL-4 has the capacity not only to enhance antibody formation, but also to suppress multiple components of CMI responses.

REGULATION OF CYTOKINE PATTERNS

One of the many factors that may bias the cytokine response is the cytokine milieu. We have investigated the role of several cytokines in contributing to the major cytokine profiles.

Immunosuppressive Role of IL-10

To define the regulatory role of IL-10 in the immune response to infection, we studied *in vitro* responses to *M. leprae*.[45] *M. leprae* triggered IL-10 release from PBMC of patients and healthy donors; the predominant source of the IL-10 was found to be macrophages. Stimulation of PBMC in the presence of neutralizing anti-IL-10 monoclonal antibodies indicated that endogenous IL-10 production inhibited PBMC proliferation and release of TNF-α, GM-CSF, and IFN-γ. While it is likely that additional cytokines contribute to immunosuppression, these data suggest that in addition to IL-4, IL-10 contributes to immunosuppression in human infectious disease. These data provided functional evidence for anti-IL-10 in up-regulating CMI and Th1 responses in human infection.

Immunostimulatory Role of IL-7

IL-7 is a T-cell growth and differentiation factor that is reported to be produced in the thymus and spleen as well as by keratinocytes. We investigated IL-7 mRNA expression by PCR and found stronger expression in tuberculoid than in lepromatous lesions.[46] IL-7 receptor mRNA, the membrane-bound form, was also more strongly expressed in tuberculoid lesions. We detected IL-7 mRNA in *M. leprae*-stimulated PBMC and in cultured keratinocytes, especially after culture with IFN-γ. Finally, rIL-7 supported the growth of T cells which had been stimulated by *M. leprae in vitro.* These results indicate that the IL-7 is released in leprosy lesions in response to the local production of IFN-γ and may potentiate T-cell responses *in situ.*

Regulatory Role of IL-12

IL-12 is the most potent T-cell growth factor described. To investigate the role of IL-12 in *M. leprae*-specific T-cell responses, we performed *in vitro* studies using rIL-12 and anti-IL-12 antibodies.[47] Anti-IL-12 almost completely abrogated *M. leprae*-specific T-cell responses in responder patients. Although rIL-12 had no effect on resting T cells or *M. leprae*-specific T-cell responses of responder patients, rIL-12 was able to significantly augment T-cell responses to *M. leprae in vitro* in nonresponder patients to credible stimulation indices of approximately 10-fold.

IL-12 has been shown to direct T cells in a primary response towards a Th1 cytokine pattern.[48,49] However, it is unclear whether IL-12 can bias a T-cell response by preferential expansion of previously committed Th1 cells. To address this, *M. leprae*-specific T-cell clones of the CD4+ Type 1 or CD8+ Type 2 cytokine pattern were cultured in the presence of rIL-12 or rIL-2 as a control. rIL-12 induced T-cell proliferation of CD4+ Type 1 but not CD8+ Type 2 cells. Both sets of clones proliferated to rIL-2. Therefore, IL-12 promoted the expansion of T cells with an established Type 1 but not a Type 2 cytokine pattern.

T-CELL RECEPTOR POPULATIONS IN LESIONS

The majority of T cells have a T-cell receptor (TCR) heterodimer composed of α and β chains, with a smaller population expressing TCR composed of γ and δ chains. The TCR complex is composed of variable (V), diversity (D), joining (J), and constant region gene segments that define the antigen specificity of the T cell. The role of TCR subpopulations in contributing to the pathogenesis of infection has been explored in leprosy.

TCR Vβ Gene Usage

Identification of predominant V gene families used in αβ T cells infiltrating leprosy lesions was accomplished using quantitative PCR. We examined the TCRβ repertoire in reversal reaction lesions as a model for DTH responses to pathogens *in situ.*[50] The striking finding was that T cells expressing Vβ6 were overrepresented in the lesions of reversal reaction patients as compared to blood and pre-DTH lesions from the same patients. Analysis and predicted amino acid sequence of the Vβ6 PCR product derived from lesions indicated clonal selection of these TCRs by antigen, followed by local oligoclonal expansion. The limited diversity further indicates that a limited set of antigens is recognized in the reversal reaction response.

To further assess the distribution of Vβ6 TCRs in leprosy, TCR Vβ repertoire was analyzed in nine tuberculoid and nine lepromatous lesions and PBMC from the same individuals.[51] We found a predominance of Vβ6 TCRs in tuberculoid lesions compared to PBMC, but not in lepromatous lesions. TCRs encoded by the Vβ6.1-

6.4 subfamilies were overrepresented in 7 of 9 tuberculoid lesions but only 1 of 9 lepromatous lesions ($p < 0.005$). Furthermore, TCRs encoded by Vβ6.5, 6.8, and 6.9 subfamilies were overrepresented in 4 of 9 tuberculoid but 0 of 9 lepromatous lesions ($p < 0.025$). Finally, TCRs encoded by Vβ6.6 and 6.7 subfamilies were overrepresented in 5 of 9 tuberculoid as well as 3 of 9 lepromatous lesions ($p > 0.05$). These results further indicated an association with the Vβ6-encoded TCR in lesions of leprosy characterized by CMI against the pathogen.

TCR γδ Cells

It has been suggested that T cells bearing γδ antigen receptors function as a first line of defense against infectious pathogens. The frequency of cells bearing TCR γδ or TCR αβ in leprosy lesions was compared using immunoperoxidase staining of skin biopsy specimens with specific monoclonal antibodies.[52] TCR γδ T cells comprised 25-35% of infiltrating CD3[+] T cells in both Mitsuda reactions and reversal reactions, compared to approximately 5% of the CD3[+] cells in lesions of other forms of the disease. Since the Mitsuda reaction is a DTH response to *M. leprae,* and the reversal reaction is a naturally occurring DTH response to *M. leprae,* the data suggest that TCR γδ cells may be involved in the DTH response with active granuloma formation rather than in the more chronic and/or immunologically unresponsive leprosy lesions.

The γδ T-cell lines derived from skin lesions and peripheral blood of patients with leprosy proliferated in response to *M. leprae.*[52] Such γδ T cells produced high levels of IFN-γ, characteristic of the Type 1 pattern, and TNF-α.[53] Striking macrophage aggregation and cell division were seen in cultures of bone marrow-derived macrophages containing GM-CSF with supernatants of activated TCR γδ cells, but not those containing supernatants of nonstimulated TCR γδ cells or either component alone.[52] This activity was blocked using a neutralizing antibody to TNF-α and could be restored by the addition of rTNF-α.[53] γδ T cells may contribute to the granulomatous response via the release of Type 1 cytokines and through the production of TNF-α.

TCR αβ Double-Negative Cells

T cells bearing an αβ TCR but devoid of the accessory molecules CD4 and CD8 (double negative, DN) were identified recently in peripheral blood and skin of normal individuals. Double-negative T cells are not restricted by classical MHC molecules; rather they recognize antigen in the context of a nonpolymorphic MHC class I-like molecule, CD1. The role of αβ[+] CD4[-] and CD8[-] T cells in the immune response to human infection was investigated in leprosy. Double-negative T cells were derived from lesions and blood of tuberculoid leprosy patients and shown to be *M. leprae*-reactive and CD1-restricted. Four of five DN T-cell lines produced IFN-γ (median value 436 pg/ml) and no IL-4 (median <20 pg/ml) characteristic of the Type 1 pattern. Finally, IL-10 inhibited CD1 expression and antigen presentation (>80%) to DN T cells. These data suggest that DN T cells promote effective cell-mediated immunity at the site of infection.

CONCLUSION

The skin lesions of leprosy provide a window for directly studying immune responses to a pathogen. Analysis of the local immune responses in these lesions revealed distinct T-cell and cytokine patterns that correlate with resistance *versus* susceptibility to infection. Modulation of T-cell and cytokine responses *in vitro* have provided new rationales for devising therapeutic strategies.

REFERENCES

1. RIDLEY, D. S. & W. H. JOPLING. 1966. Classification of leprosy according to immunity. A five-group system. Int. J. Lepr. **34:** 255–273.

2. MODLIN, R. L., F. M. HOFMAN, C. R. TAYLOR & T. H. REA. 1982. In situ characterization of T lymphocyte subsets in leprosy granulomas [letter]. Int. J. Lepr. **50:** 361–362.

3. VAN VOORHIS, W. C., G. KAPLAN, E. N. SARNO, M. A. HORWITZ, R. M. STEINMAN, W. R. LEVIS, N. NOGUEIRA, L. S. HAIR, C. R. GATTASS, B. A. ARRICK & Z. A. COHN. 1982. The cutaneous infiltrates of leprosy: Cellular characteristics and the predominant T-cell phenotypes. N. Engl. J. Med. **307:** 1593–1597.

4. MODLIN, R. L., F. M. HOFMAN, C. R. TAYLOR & T. H. REA. 1983. T lymphocyte subsets in the skin lesions of patients with leprosy. J. Am. Acad. Dermatol. **8:** 182–189.

5. MODLIN, R. L., F. M. HOFMAN, P. R. MEYER, O. P. SHARMA, C. R. TAYLOR & T. H. REA. 1983. In situ demonstration of T lymphocyte subsets in granulomatous inflammation: Leprosy, rhinoscleroma and sarcoidosis. Clin. Exp. Immunol. **51:** 430–438.

6. NARAYANAN, R. B., L. K. BHUTANI, A. K. SHARMA & I. NATH. 1983. T cell subsets in leprosy lesions: In situ characterization using monoclonal antibodies. Clin. Exp. Immunol. **51:** 421–429.

7. MODLIN, R. L., J. F. GEBHARD, C. R. TAYLOR & T. H. REA. 1983. In situ characterization of T lymphocyte subsets in the reactional states of leprosy. Clin. Exp. Immunol. **53:** 17–24.

8. KATO, H., K. SANADA, M. KOSEKI & T. OZAWA. 1983. Identification of lymphocyte subpopulations in cutaneous lesions of leprosy. Nippon. Rai. Gakkai. Zasshi **52:** 126–132.

9. MODLIN, R. L., F. M. HOFMAN, D. A. HORWITZ, L. A. HUSMANN, S. GILLIS, C. R. TAYLOR & T. H. REA. 1984. In situ identification of cells in human leprosy granulomas with monoclonal antibodies to interleukin 2 and its receptor. J Immunol. **132:** 3085–3090.

10. WALLACH, D., B. FLAGEUL, M. A. BACH & F. COTTENOT. 1984. The cellular content of dermal leprous granulomas: An immuno-histological approach. Int. J. Lepr. **52:** 318–326.

11. SARNO, E. N., G. KAPLAN, F. ALVARANGA, N. NOGUEIRA, J. A. PORTO & Z. A. COHN. 1984. Effect of treatment on the cellular composition of cutaneous lesions in leprosy patients. Int. J. Lepr. **52:** 496–500.

12. NARAYANAN, R. B., S. LAAL, A. K. SHARMA, L. K. BHUTANI & I. NATH. 1984. Differences in predominant T cell phenotypes and distribution pattern in reactional lesions of tuberculoid and lepromatous leprosy. Clin. Exp. Immunol. **55:** 623–628.

13. MODLIN, R. L., A. C. BAKKE, S. A. VACCARO, D. A. HORWITZ, C. R. TAYLOR & T. H. REA. 1985. Tissue and blood T-lymphocyte subpopulations in erythema nodosum leprosum. Arch. Dermatol. **121:** 216–219.

14. LONGLEY, J., A. HAREGEWOIN, T. YEMANEBERHAN, T. W. VAN DIEPEN, J. NSIBAMI, D. KNOWLES, K. A. SMITH & T. GODAL. 1985. *In vivo* responses to *Mycobacterium leprae:* Antigen presentation, interleukin-2 production, and immune cell phenotypes in naturally occurring leprosy lesions. Int. J. Lepr. **53:** 385–394.

15. MODLIN, R. L., V. MEHRA, R. JORDAN, B. R. BLOOM & T. H. REA. 1986. *In situ* and *in vitro* characterization of the cellular immune response in erythema nodosum leprosum. J. Immunol. **136:** 883–886.

16. NILSEN, R., R. N. MSHANA, Y. NEGESSE, G. MENIGISTU & B. KANA. 1986. Immunohisto-chemical studies of leprous neuritis. Lepr. Rev. **57**(suppl. 2): 177–187.

17. MODLIN, R. L., V. MEHRA, L. WONG, Y. FUJIMIYA, W. CHANG, D. A. HORWITZ, B. R. BLOOM, T. H. REA & P. K. PATTENGALE. 1986. Suppressor T lymphocytes from lepromatous leprosy skin lesions. J. Immunol. **137:** 2831–2834.

18. MODLIN, R. L., J. MELANCON-KAPLAN, S. M. M. YOUNG, C. PIRMEZ, H. KINO, J. CONVIT, T. H. REA & B. R. BLOOM. 1988. Learning from lesions: Patterns of tissue inflammation in leprosy. Proc. Natl. Acad. Sci. USA **85:** 1213–1217.

19. REA, T. H., J.-Y. SHEN & R. L. MODLIN. 1986. Epidermal keratonocyte Ia expression, Langerhans cell hyperplasia and lymphocytic infiltration in skin lesions of leprosy. Clin. Exp. Immunol. **65:** 253–259.

20. NARAYANAN, R. B., L. K. BHUTANI, A. K. SHARMA & I. NATH. 1984. Normal numbers of T6 positive epidermal langerhans cells across the leprosy spectrum. Lepr. Rev. **55:** 301–308.

21. COLLINGS, L. A., M. F. WATERS & L. W. POULTER. 1985. The involvement of dendritic cells in the cutaneous lesions associated with tuberculoid and lepromatous leprosy. Clin. Exp. Immunol. **62:** 458–467.

22. KAPLAN, G., A. NUSRAT, M. D. WITMER, I. NATH & Z. A. COHN. 1987. Distribution and turnover of Langerhans cells during delayed immune responses in human skin. J. Exp. Med. **165:** 763–776.

23. VOLC-PLATZER, B., H. STEMBERGER, T. LUGER, T. RADASZKIEWICZ & G. WIEDERMANN. 1988. Defective intralesional interferon-gamma activity in lepromatous leprosy. Clin. Exp. Immunol. **71:** 235–240.

24. ARNOLDI, J., J. GERDES & H.-D. FLAD. 1990. Immunohistologic assessment of cytokine production of infiltrating cells in various forms of leprosy. Am. J. Pathol. **137:** 749–753.

25. ROOK, G. A. W., J. STEELE, L. FRAHER, S. BARKER, R. KARMALI & J. O'RIORDAN. 1986. Vitamin D_3, gamma interferon, and control of proliferation of *Mycobacterium tuberculosis* by human monocytes. Immunology **57:** 159–163.

26. NATHAN, C. F., G. KAPLAN, W. R. LEVIS, A. NUSRAT, M. D. WITMER, S. A. SHERWIN, C. K. JOB, C. R. HOROWITZ, R. M. STEINMAN & Z. A. COHN. 1986. Local and systemic effects of intradermal recombinant interferon-gamma in patients with lepromatous leprosy. N. Engl. J. Med. **315:** 6–15.

27. COOPER, C. L., C. MUELLER, T.-A. SINCHAISRI, C. PIRMEZ, J. CHAN, G. KAPLAN, S. M. M. YOUNG, I. L. WEISSMAN, B. R. BLOOM, T. H. REA & R. L. MODLIN. 1989. Analysis of naturally occurring delayed-type hypersensitivity reactions in leprosy by *in situ* hybridization. J. Exp. Med. **169:** 169: 1565–1581.

28. MUSTAFA, A. S. & T. GODAL. 1987. BCG induced CD4+ cytotoxic T cells from BCG vaccinated healthy subjects: Relation between cytotoxicity and suppression *in vitro.* Clin. Exp. Immunol. **69:** 255–262.

29. YAMAMURA, M., X.-H. WANG, J. D. OHMEN, K. UYEMURA, T. H. REA, B. R. BLOOM & R. L. MODLIN. 1992. Cytokine patterns of immunologically mediated tissue damage. J. Immunol. **149:** 1470–1475.

30. MOSMANN, T. R., H. CHERWINSKI, M. W. BOND, M. A. GIEDLIN & R. L. COFFMAN. 1986. Two types of murine helper T cell clones. I. Definition according to profiles of lymphokine activities and secreted proteins. J. Immunol. **136:** 2348–2357.

31. HEINZEL, F. P., M. D. SADICK, B. J. HOLADAY, R. L. COFFMAN & R. M. LOCKSLEY. 1989. Reciprocal expression of interferon gamma or interleukin 4 during the resolution or

progression of murine leishmaniasis. Evidence for expansion of distinct helper T cell subsets. J. Exp. Med. **169:** 59–72.

32. PEARCE, E. J., P. CASPAR, J.-M. GRZYCH, F. A. LEWIS & A. SHER. 1991. Downregulation of Th1 cytokine production accompanies induction of Th2 responses by a parasitic helmith, *Schistosoma mansoni*. J. Exp. Med. **173:** 159–166.

33. POND, L., D. L. WASSOM & C. E. HAYES. 1989. Evidence for differential induction of helper T cell subsets during *Trichinella spiralis* infection. J. Immunol. **143:** 4232–4237.

34. MEHRA, V., B. R. BLOOM, V. K. TORIGIAN, D. MANDICH, M. REICHEL, S. M. M. YOUNG, P. SALGAME, J. CONVIT, S. W. HUNTER, M. MCNEIL, P. J. BRENNAN, T. H. REA & R. L. MODLIN. 1989. Characterization of *Mycobacterium leprae* cell wall-associated proteins using T-lymphocyte clones. J. Immunol. **142:** 2873–2878.

35. MEHRA, V., B. R. BLOOM, A. C. BAJARDI, C. L. GRISSO, P. A. SIELING, D. ALLAND, J. CONVIT, X. D. FAN, S. W. HUNTER, P. J. BRENNAN, T. H. REA & R. L. MODLIN. 1992. A major T cell antigen of *Mycobacterium leprae* is a 10 kD heat-shock cognate protein. J. Exp. Med. **175:** 275–284.

36. HEMMINGSEN, S. M., C. WOOLFORD, S. M. VAN DER VIES, K. TILLY, D. T. DENNIS, C. P. GEORGOPOULOS, R. W. HENDRIX & R. J. ELLIS. 1988. Homologous plant and bacterial proteins chaperone oligomeric protein assembly. Nature **333:** 330–334.

37. MEHRA, V., L. H. MASON, J. P. FIELDS & B. R. BLOOM. 1979. Lepromin-induced suppressor cells in patients with leprosy. J. Immunol. **123:** 1813–1817.

38. MEHRA, V., L. H. MASON, W. ROTHMAN, E. REINHERZ, S. F. SCHLOSSMAN & B. R. BLOOM. 1980. Delineation of a human T cell subset responsible for lepromin-induced suppression in leprosy patients. J. Immunol. **125:** 1183–1188.

39. MEHRA, V., J. CONVIT, A. RUBINSTEIN & B. R. BLOOM. 1982. Activated suppressor T cells in leprosy. J. Immunol. **129:** 1946–1951.

40. NELSON, E. E., L. WONG, K. UYEMURA, T. H. REA & R. L. MODLIN. 1987. Lepromin-induced suppressor cells in lepromatous leprosy. Cell. Immunol. **104:** 99–104.

41. MODLIN, R. L., H. KATO, V. MEHRA, E. E. NELSON, F. XUE-DONG, T. H. REA, P. K. PATTENGALE & B. R. BLOOM. 1986. Genetically restricted suppressor T-cell clones derived from lepromatous leprosy lesions. Nature **322:** 459–461.

42. SALGAME, P., J. CONVIT & B. R. BLOOM. 1991. Immunological suppression by human CD8+ T cells is receptor dependent and HLA-DQ restricted. Proc. Natl. Acad. Sci. USA **88:** 2598–2602.

43. MODLIN, R. L., M. B. BRENNER, M. S. KRANGEL, A. D. DUBY & B. R. BLOOM. 1987. T-cell receptors of human suppressor cells. Nature **329:** 541–545.

44. SALGAME, P., J. S. ABRAMS, C. CLAYBERGER, H. GOLDSTEIN, J. CONVIT, R. L. MODLIN & B. R. BLOOM. 1991. Differing lymphokine profiles of functional subsets of human CD4 and CD8 T cell clones. Science **254:** 279–282.

45. SIELING, P. A., J. S. ABRAMS, M. YAMAMURA, P. SALGAME, B. R. BLOOM, T. H. REA & R. L. MODLIN. 1993. Immunosuppressive roles for interleukin-10 and interleukin-4 in human infection: *In vitro* modulation of T cell responses in leprosy. J. Immunol. **150:** 5501–5510.

46. SAKIMURA, L., M. YAMAMURA, P. A. SIELING, K. UYEMURA, D. TAHERY, J. L. OLIVEROS, B. J. NICKOLOFF, T. H. REA & R. L. MODLIN. 1993. Expression of interleukin-7 in the cell-mediated immune response to a human pathogen. Submitted for publication.

47. SIELING, P. A., X.-H. WANG, M. K. GATELY, J. L. OLIVEROS, P. F. BARNES, S. F. WOLF, M. YAMAMURA, Y. YOGI, K. UYEMURA, T. H. REA & R. L. MODLIN. 1993. IL-12 regulates T cell and cytokine responses in human infectious disease. Submitted for publication.

48. HSIEH, C., S. E. MACATONIA, C. S. TRIPP, S. F. WOLF, A. O'GARRA & K. M. MURPHY. 1993. Development of Th1 CD4+ T cells through IL-12 produced by Listeria-induced macrophages. Science **260:** 547–549.
49. MANETTI, R., P. PARRONCHI, M. G. GIUDIZI, M. PICCINNI, E. MAGGI, G. TRINCHIERI & S. ROMAGNANI. 1993. Natural killer cell stimulatory factor (interleukin 12 [IL-12]) induces T helper type 1 (Th1)-specific immune responses and inhibits the development of IL-4-producing Th cells. J. Exp. Med. **177:** 1199–1204.
50. WANG, X.-H., J. D. OHMEN, K. UYEMURA, T. H. REA, M. KRONENBERG & R. L. MODLIN. 1993. Selection of T-lymphocytes bearing limited T-cell receptor β chains in the response to a human pathogen. Proc. Natl. Acad. Sci. USA **90:** 188–192.
51. WANG, X., L. GOLKAR, K. UYEMURA, J. D. OHMEN, L. G. VILLAHERMOSA, T. T. FAJARDO, J. R. V. CELLONA, G. P. WALSH & R. L. MODLIN. 1993. T cells bearing Vbeta6 T-cell receptors in the cell-mediated immune response to mycobacterium leprae. Submitted for publication.
52. MODLIN, R. L., C. PIRMEZ, F. M. HOFMAN, V. TORIGIAN, K. UYEMURA, T. H. REA, B. R. BLOOM & M. B. BRENNER. 1989. Lymphocytes bearing antigen-specific gamma/delta T-cell receptors in human infectious disease lesions. Nature **339:** 544–548.
53. BARNES, P. F., J. S. ABRAMS, S. Z. LU, P. A. SIELING, T. H. REA & R. L. MODLIN. 1993. Patterns of cytokine production by mycobacterium-reactive human T-cell clones. Infect. Immun. **61:** 197–203.

Role of α/β T and γ/δ T Cells in Innate and Acquired Immunity

H. KIRK ZIEGLER, MARIANNE J. SKEEN, AND
KEVIN M. PEARCE

Department of Microbiology and Immunology
Emory University School of Medicine
Atlanta, Georgia 30322

T-lymphocyte subpopulations can be classified according to the differential expression of T-cell receptors, surface markers, adhesion molecules, cytokines, and their receptors. One distinction is in the expression of T-cell surface molecules such as CD4 and CD8. The binding of CD4 to class II MHC molecules or CD8 to class I MHC molecules is thought to create a requisite stabilizing "bridge" between the antigen-presenting cell and the responding T cell as well as a conduit of transducing signals. Class I MHC molecules displayed on a variety of cells are involved in antigen presentation to CD8[+] T cells, whereas class II MHC molecules, expressed on a more restricted spectrum of cell types such as macrophages and B cells, serve as recognition molecules for CD4[+] T cells. As such, the appropriate interactions of CD8[+] cytotoxic T cells with infected cells and CD4[+] helper cells with B cells and macrophages are facilitated.

T cells of the CD4[+] subset can also be subdivided into at least two major types by their patterns of cytokine production. TH1 cells secrete gamma-interferon (INF-γ) and interleukin-2 (IL-2), whereas TH2 cells produce IL-4, IL-5, IL-6, and IL-10.[1,2] These differences in lymphokine secretion correlate with functional specialization. TH1 cells are involved in delayed-type hypersensitivity reactions and macrophage activation,[3] whereas TH2 cells may be more important for helping B cells respond with expression of certain antibody isotypes.[4] Differential regulation of these subsets plays an important role in infectious disease,[5] transplantation reactions,[6] and hypersensitivity.[7]

Another newly recognized subdivision of T cells is based on the differential expression of T-cell receptors (TCR). The TCR is expressed in association with the CD3 protein complex that plays an important role in TCR surface expression and signal transduction. The antigen-specific TCR is a disulfide bond-linked heterodimer composed of an alpha (α) chain paired with a beta (β) or a gamma (γ) chain associated with a delta (δ) chain. Very early in T-cell development, cells become committed to express either α or β chain gene products **or** γ and δ proteins. As such, distinct T-cell lineages are generated that express either the α/β or the γ/δ TCR. These cell subsets are termed α/β T cells and γ/δ T cells. During the last several years it has become apparent the α/β T cells differ from γ/δ T cells in several fundamental ways. These are summarized in TABLE 1.

The recognition of antigen by α/β T cells depends on the processing and presentation of antigens by either class I or class II MHC proteins. Antigen-presenting cells

53

TABLE 1. T-Cell Receptor Expression and Characteristics of α/β and γ/δ T Cells

Characteristic	α/β T Cells	γ/δ T Cells
Tissue localization	Blood, spleen, lymph node	Skin, gut epithelium, peritoneum
Phylogeny	Less "primitive" birds	More "primitive" mammals
Ontogeny	Later expression, thymus-dependent	Early expression, thymus-independent
TCR diversity	Large number of variable segments	Smaller number of segments
Surface markers	CD4$^+$ or CD8$^+$ Thy1$^+$	CD4$^-$/CD8$^+$ or$^-$ Thy1$^+$ or$^-$
Antigens	Peptide products of processing	HSP, peptides, CHO?
Presenting molecules	Class I/II MHC	MHC? Nonclassical MHC?
Function	Cytokines. Help. Killing.	Cytokines? Help? Killing

make antigenic determinants or epitopes available for interaction with T lymphocytes through a series of intracellular events termed antigen-processing.[8,9] For class II MHC presentation pathways, these antigen-processing events involve endocytosis of antigen into acidic intracellular compartments in which antigens are solubilized, unfolded, and/or fragmented by proteolysis and then bound by MHC gene products synthesized by the antigen-presenting macrophages and transported to the cell surface.[10–13] Processing is also required for presentation via class I MHC molecules, but this pathway is favored when antigen is endogenous to the antigen-presenting cells and may involve cytosolic trafficking compartments where antigen fragments are bound to class I MHC proteins in the endoplasmic reticulum prior to transport to the cell surface.[14] The ability of MHC molecules to bind antigenic peptides in a selective manner accounts for immune response (Ir) gene control.[15,16] Crystallographic analysis indicates that the MHC molecule appears to have a peptide-binding pocket on the top surface that is formed by polymorphic domains.[17] Two helical regions border the presumed peptide-binding groove over a floor of a beta-sheet. The antigenic peptide may fit into the groove like a "hotdog in a bun." The peptide-MHC complex displayed on the cell surface is recognized by a specific interaction with the α/β TCR. The cross-linking of the TCR (and the CD3 complex), together with other accessory molecules,[18–20] leads to activation of T lymphocytes with respect to proliferation, expression of cytolytic function, and cytokine production.[21] In addition to MHC–peptide–TCR interactions, adhesion molecules, membrane IL-1, and other costimulatory signals (such as CD28 and B7 interactions) can also play important roles in T-cell activation.[19,22,23] The growth of α/β T cells is driven in an autocrine fashion primarily by the cytokine IL-2 produced predominately by CD4$^+$ (and CD8$^+$) T cells.

In contrast, antigen recognition by γ/δ T cells is poorly understood. Little is known about the presenting molecules used, the antigens recognized, and the pathways of antigen processing relevant for activation of γ/δ T cells. Although γ/δ T-cell cloned lines from the spleen recognize antigen in association with class II MHC,[24] other γ/δ T cells appear to recognize nonpolymorphic class I MHC molecules such as TL[24,25] or surface molecules such as CD1.[26] Some investigators find MHC restriction,[27,28] whereas others do not.[29–31] Inasmuch as few studies have successfully defined the recognition requirements of γ/δ T cells, it is difficult to establish any general rules. The only consensus is that γ/δ T cells are fundamentally different from α/β

T cells. Generalizations about the antigens recognized by γ/δ T cells are difficult to make with certainty. Recognition of carbohydrate antigens was suggested.[32,33] Several intriguing observations suggest that γ/δ T cells recognize epitopes of stress proteins or heat shock proteins shared by microbes and mammals.[27,34] The role of these cross-reactions among these conserved molecules in autoimmune disease was suggested.[35–37] These results also produced interesting speculations about a primitive surveillance system in which γ/δ T cells discriminate stressed from nonstressed cells. This could occur in "front line" defense reactions that occur in tissues rich in γ/δ T cells such as the skin and intestinal epithelium. Suggestive evidence that microbial products are the stress-inducing agents relevant in this system has been presented, but more detailed evaluation is needed. The predominance of γ/δ T cells at sites of infection with *Mycobacteria* and *Listeria,* for example, is in keeping with these ideas (refs. 28 and 30 and this manuscript). Nothing is currently known about the processing pathways relevant to the function of γ/δ T cells.

One particularly intriguing aspect of γ/δ T cells is their distinctive tissue localization. Although γ/δ T cells represent a relatively minor T-cell population in lymphoid organs, γ/δ T cells predominate in mouse epidermis,[38] intestinal epithelium,[39] lung,[40] and female reproductive organs.[41] The association with epithelial tissue at sites of first contact with foreign antigens implicates γ/δ T cells in "frontline" defense reactions or homeostatic mechanisms unique to the self-nonself interface. This feature of γ/δ T cells together with their association with infectious lesions must be critical to their unique purpose and central to our understanding of the mechanisms of γ/δ T-cell function.

The expression of γ/δ TCRs in terms of ontogeny and diversity is related to tissue localization.[42] In the fetal thymus, γ/δ T cells first begin to appear on day 14 of gestation, and until about day 18 they represent the major population of T cells in the thymus. Expression of particular V-region gene segments occurs in distinct waves of development with Vγ3 expressed initially. Such developing T cells apparently seed into particular epithelial tissue, resulting in a preferential usage of V-region segments in individual sites. For example, in the skin of adult mice, the γ/δ T cells are essentially nonpolymorphic in that most if not all skin γ/δ T cells express Vγ3. Similarly, Vγ5 and Vδ4 predominate in the intestine. Interestingly, intestinal γ/δ T cells are present in athymic mice, suggesting a thymus-independent development.[43] The small numbers of γ/δ T cells in the lymph nodes use Vγ2 and many other gene segments and therefore appear more diverse than do the epithelial γ/δ T cells. The relation between tissue site and V-gene usage may suggest that γ/δ T cells recognize structures unique to the tissue site. Such structures may be either certain presenting molecules (e.g., nonclassical class I MHC), tissue-specific self-antigens (e.g., keratinocyte stress proteins), and/or microbial antigens (e.g., GroES/GroEL). Studies with transgenic mice indicate, however, that V-region usage of γ/δ T cells cannot account entirely for the homing patterns of these cells.[44] The preferential expression of γ/δ T cells can theoretically be due to the selective homing and/or proliferation of cells controlled by factors unique to γ/δ T cells and a particular site or experimental condition such as microbial infection. Such controlling factors include homing receptors, antigens or superantigens, presenting molecules, accessory molecules, and cytokines. These questions will be answered only when a more thorough

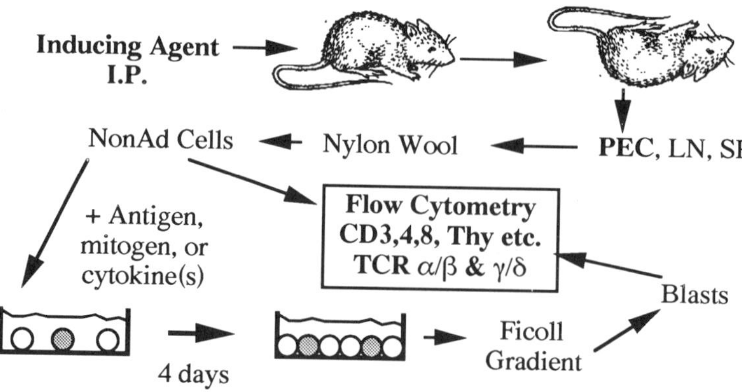

FIGURE 1. Regulation of T-cell receptor (TCR) expression. The protocol used for analysis of α/β T cells and γ/δ T cells after injection of bacteria (usually *Listeria*) or other inducing agents is illustrated. For details see refs. 45 and 46. (LN = lymph node cells; PEC = peritoneal exudate cells; SP = spleen cells.)

understanding of the phenotype, function, and activation requirements of γ/δ T cells is achieved.

RESULTS AND DISCUSSION

Tissue Localization, Phenotype, and Induction of γ/δ T Cells by Microbial Products. We monitored TCR expression in secondary lymphoid organs and the peritoneal cavity as illustrated in FIGURE 1 and detailed in references 45 and 46. Mice (C3H) were injected with various inducing agents, and nonadherent peritoneal exudate cells, lymph node cells, and spleen cells were analyzed by flow cytometry. Lymphocyte populations were analyzed with monoclonal antibodies specific for CD3, the α/β TCR, and the γ/δ TCR (and other surface markers). Cell populations were analyzed on the day of harvest or after culture for 4 days in the presence of antigens, mitogens, or cytokines.

Peritoneal γ/δ T cells represent ~12% of the CD3+ cells in the peritoneal cavity, in contrast to the <2% expression in the spleen or lymph node. The frequency of CD3+ cells and in particular γ/δ TCR+ T cells was increased following injection of *Listeria,* resulting in a 2- to 4-fold increase in frequency and a 5- to 25-fold increase in the number of peritoneal γ/δ T cells. Stimulation of the induced peritoneal T cells with *Listeria* antigens or concanavalin A (ConA) *in vitro* caused further increases in the number and frequency of γ/δ T cells, resulting in 44 and 66% γ/δ T cells in the blast population, respectively. This γ/δ T-cell induction after *Listeria in vivo* and mitogen *in vitro* was noted in the peritoneum but not in either the spleen or lymph nodes. Thus, the peritoneal cavity is relatively rich in γ/δ T cells, and induction by bacteria is localized to the site of the initial infection.

The kinetics of induction of peritoneal γ/δ T cells was followed after intraperitoneal injection of *Listeria* or lipopolysaccharide (LPS).[45,46] Injection of *Listeria* produced an increase in the number of γ/δ T cells at day 7 with a maximal response at day 10. The frequency of γ/δ T cells was significantly increased at day 7 with continued increases until day 14. This high frequency of γ/δ T cells was maintained for at least 6 weeks (e.g., 30% at day 42). The response to LPS was faster with a peak increase in number and frequency 3 days after injection. Another toxin, listeriolysin-O (LLO), also produced rapid increases in γ/δ T cells. This heightened frequency of γ/δ T cells was very long-lived, suggesting an almost permanent change in the α/β to γ/δ T-cell ratio in this tissue site.

Both α/β and γ/δ peritoneal T cells were analyzed for expression of Thy-1, CD4, CD8, PGP1, and CD45R. Peritoneal α/β T cells showed a typical phenotype of > 95% Thy-1[+], 37% CD4[+], and 19% CD8[+] (data not shown). In contrast, peritoneal γ/δ T cells from normal mice were 29% Thy-1[+], and they were essentially negative (<0.5%[+]) for CD4 and CD8. Consistent with an activation phenotype, all γ/δ T cells express PGP1, and 68% are CD45R lo. Injection of *Listeria* increased Thy-1 expression to 66%[+], but other markers were unchanged. The CD4 and CD8 negative phenotype of peritoneal γ/δ T cells is similar to that of γ/δ T cells found in the skin and lymphoid tissue, but differs from the CD8[+] phenotype of γ/δ T cells in the intestinal epithelium.[47] In keeping with other studies with gut γ/δ T cells, Thy-1 expression may represent an activation marker whose expression is driven by microbial stimulation.[43] Unlike the preferential expression of Vγ2 in lymph nodes, Vγ3 in skin, and Vδ4 in intestine, γ/δ T cells in the peritoneal cavity show no detectable expression of these V-gene segments. This is evidenced by the finding that the appropriate monoclonal antibodies stain less than 1% of peritoneal γ/δ T cells induced by either *Listeria* or LPS. As such, the peritoneal T cells may represent either a novel, as yet undefined, V-segment preference or a diverse polyclonal population of T cells.

To survey the range of inducing agents operative in the peritoneal cavity, we followed the increases in γ/δ T cells following injection of bacterial pathogens, microbial toxins, inflammatory agents, mitogens, and antigens. TABLE 2 summarizes our findings, illustrating the number of peritoneal γ/δ T cells per mouse as well as the frequency of γ/δ T cells after stimulation *in vitro* for 4 days with the mitogen ConA. Intraperitoneal injection of several bacterial strains caused marked increases in γ/δ T cells including gram-positive organisms such as *Listeria monocytogenes* and the mycobacterium strain bacillus Calmette-Guérin (BCG) as well as Gram-negative bacteria such as *Escherichia coli* and *Salmonella typhimurium*. Subcutaneous injection of *Listeria* or mycobacteria in complete Freund's adjuvant did not increase significantly the expression of γ/δ T cells in the peritoneal cavity, indicating the localized nature of the induction. The requirement for virulent exotoxin-producing *Listeria* organisms was indicated by the finding that neither heat-killed *L. monocytogenes* (HKLM) nor avirulent hemolysin-negative *Listeria* (Hly-LM)[48] induced γ/δ T cells. Isolated listeriolysin-O (LLO), the major hemolysin secreted by virulent *Listeria*, caused γ/δ T-cell induction when injected intraperitoneally. The importance of exotoxin production was also noted with gram-negative bacteria inasmuch as Hly+ *E. coli* was superior to Hly-*E. coli* in producing a more profound increase in the number of γ/δ T cells and in maintaining increased γ/δ T-cell frequency *in vitro*. The role of bacterial endotoxins was apparent by the induction of γ/δ T cells following intraperitoneal injection of LPS. Like other activation parameters of LPS, induction

TABLE 2. Induction of Gamma/Delta T-Cell Receptor-Expressing Peritoneal T Cells by Virulent Bacteria and Their Toxins[a,b]

Injection	Fresh T Cells (γ/δ^+ cells [n] per mouse)	Con A Blasts (frequency of γ/δ^+ cells)
10 Days prior to harvest		
PBS ip	-	-
Hly⁺ LM ip (3,000)	++++	++++
Hly⁻ LM ip (3,000)	-	-
Heat-killed LM ip (100,000,000)	-	-
Hly⁺ LM sc (3,000)	-	-
Peptone ip (1.5 ml of 10%)	+	-
LLO 215-234 sc in CFA (50 µg)	-	-
OVA sc in CFA (50 µg)	-	-
SRBCs ip (100,000,000)	-	-
ConA (100 µg) ip	++	-
BCG ip (1,000,000)	+++	+
Hly⁺ EC ip (1,000,000)	+++	++
Hly⁻ EC ip (1,000,000)	++	+
ST ip (1,000,000)	++	+
ST ip (100,000,000)	++	+++
LPS (1 µg) in C3Heb/FeJ Mice ip	++++	+++
3 Days prior to harvest		
PBS ip	-	-
Hly⁺ LM ip (3,000)	-	-
LPS (1 µg) in C3Heb/FeJ Mice ip	++	++
LPS (1 µg) in C3H/HeJ Mice ip	-	nt
rLLO (400 units) ip	++++	+
Peptone (1.5 ml of 10%) ip	-	-
ConA (100 µg) ip	+	-
PHA (35 µg) ip	+	-
rIFNg (5,000 units bid) ip	-	-
NaIO4 (1 mg) ip	++	-
Poly I : C (100 µg) ip	-	-

ABBREVIATIONS: BCG = bacillus Calmette-Guérin; CFA = complete Freund's adjuvant; ConA = concanavalin A; EC = *Escherichia coli;* Hly = hemolysin; LLO = listeriolysin O; LM = *Listeria monocytogenes;* LPS = lipopolysaccharide; OVA = ovalbumin; PBS = phosphate-buffered saline solution; PHA = phytohemagglutinin; SRBC = sheep red blood cells; ST = *S. typhimurium.*

[a]Plus symbols represent the relative magnitude of induction of γ/δ T cells.

[b]Adapted from Skeen and Ziegler. 1993. J. Exp. Med. **178:** 971.

of γ/δ T cells by LPS was under *lps* gene control because no increases were observed in LPS-hyporesponsive mice (C3H/HeJ). Thus, profound induction of peritoneal γ/δ T cells was mediated by virulent bacteria and their exotoxins and endotoxins.

The significance of microbial stimulation is underscored by the fact that strong induction was not observed with common peritoneal inflammatory stimulants such as peptone or routinely used antigens such as ovalbumin in complete Freund's adjuvant subcutaneously or a particulate antigen such as sheep red blood cells intraperitoneally. While intraperitoneal injection of polyclonal T-cell activators such phytohemagglutinin, ConA, or sodium periodate (NaIO$_4$) resulted in some increases in the number of γ/δ T cells at the injection site, an increased frequency of γ/δ T cells was not maintained following stimulation *in vitro*. Furthermore, induction of γ/δ T cells did not necessarily accompany other known induction events in the peritoneal cavity such as up-regulation of class II MHC-expressing macrophages or natural killer cells. For example, neither intraperitoneal injection of gamma interferon (which caused induction of macrophage MHC expression) nor injection of poly I : C (which dramatically increased natural killer cells) resulted in significant changes in peritoneal γ/δ T cells. Collectively, our results and others represent strong evidence that bacterial infection is intimately and uniquely associated with profound regulation of γ/δ T cells.[45,49,50]

***Activation of γ/δ T Cells* in Vitro.** We evaluated the requirements for the selective expansion of γ/δ T cells *in vitro*. Starting with a population of α/β and γ/δ peritoneal T cells induced by *Listeria in vivo*, the absolute numbers of both α/β and γ/δ subsets were monitored following culture with various combinations of immobilized anti-TCR antibodies, bacterial antigens, mitogens, cytokines, and accessory cells (FIGS. 1 and 2). *Listeria* antigens such as HKLM or LLO "presented by" macrophages increased expansion of γ/δ T cells, which may be in part due to the cytokine elaboration by both macrophage accessory cells and activated α/β T cells. The conclusion that activation of α/β T cells can result in expansion of γ/δ T cells is supported by the finding that expansion of γ/δ T cells occurs in the presence of immobilized anti-TCR antibody specific for the α/β T-cell subset present in coculture or across a cell-impermeable barrier. Staphylococcal enterotoxin B, a Vβ8-specific superantigen, also causes expansion of γ/δ T cells in coculture with α/β T cells. In contrast, neither anti-α/β TCR antibody nor staphylococcal enterotoxin B will cause the proliferation of **purified** γ/δ T cells.[45,46]

To understand the activation requirements and growth control of peritoneal α/β and γ/δ T cells, we established the conditions for cell purification with magnetic beads or tissue culture plates coated with antibody to the TCR.[45,46] The proliferative ability of purified α/β and γ/δ T cells was examined by thymidine incorporation. Isolated γ/δ T cells showed a significant response to ConA and HKLM. It is clear from this and other experiments that a T-cell response to HKLM was associated with both γ/δ and α/β T cells. Similar conclusions resulted from experiments in which IFN-γ production rather than proliferation was used as a readout for T-cell activation. Both α/β and γ/δ T cells produced IFN-γ on stimulation with HKLM or anti-TCR antibody in the presence of macrophages[46,51] (TABLE 3). However, isolated γ/δ T cells did not elaborate IL-2 even when stimulated with anti-γ/δ TCR antibody (TABLE 3). This apparent lack of an IL-2 autocrine pathway may account for the growth dependency of γ/δ T cells on activated α/β T cells.

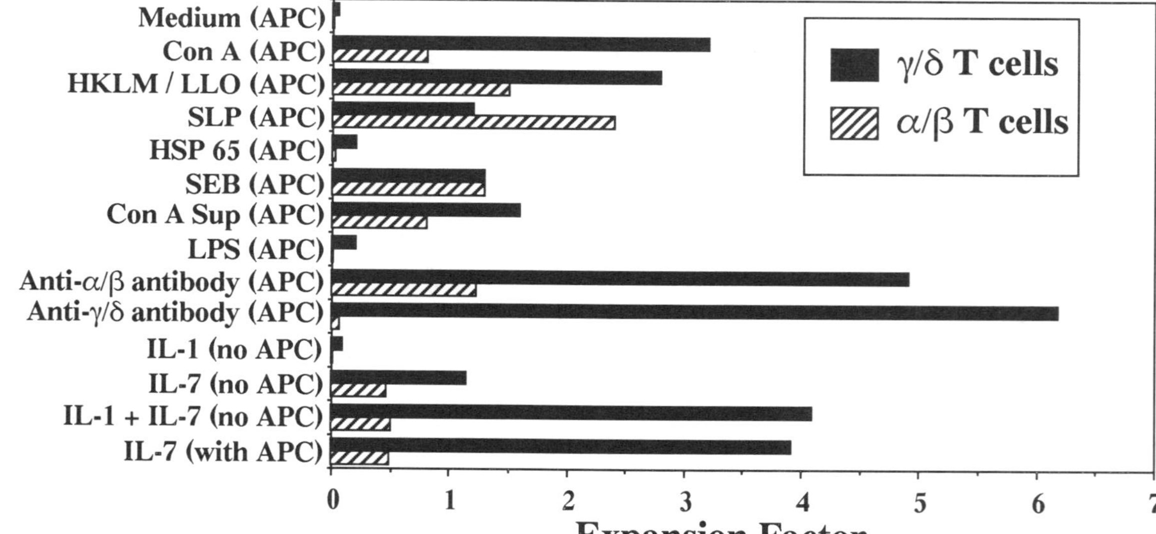

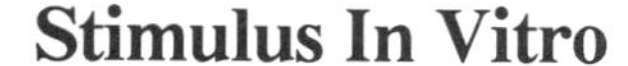

FIGURE 2. Requirements for expansion of γ/δ T cells *in vitro*. Expansion can result from activation of α/β T cells and the presence of cytokines (IL-1 and IL-7). Peritoneal exudate cells from *Listeria*-injected mice (after 10 days) were cultured *in vitro* with the indicted stimulus. The number of α/β T cells and γ/δ T cells (as determined by cell counting and flow cytometry) recovered after a 4-day culture was used to calculate expansion factors as described.[46] For example, a factor of 2 represents twice the number of T cells recovered as compared to the number placed initially in culture.

TABLE 3. Cytokine Production by α/β and γ/δ T cells[a]

Stimulus *in Vitro*	Purified γ/δ T Cells		Purified α/β T Cells	
	IFN-γ (U/ml)	IL-2 (cpm × 10³)	IFN-γ (U/ml)	IL-2 (cpm × 10³)
Medium	0	0.04	0	0.71
HKLM	28.5	0.07	38.6	23.44
LPS	3.5	0.03	0	0.15
Immob. anti-γ/δ TCR mAb	16.5	0.08	0	0.28
Immob. anti-γ/β TCR mAb	5.3	0.12	101.2	26.49
Medium (allogeneic APC)	0	0.04	0	1.15
HKLM (allogeneic APC)	17.1	0.02	8.3	3.52

ABBREVIATIONS: APC = antigen-presenting cells; HKLM = heat-killed *L. monocytogenes;* LPS = lipopolysaccharide; mAb = monoclonal antibody; TCR = T-cell receptor.

[a]Peritoneal T cells from *Listeria*-injected mice were purified as previously described.[45,46] Purified T cells (300,000/ml) were cultured 24 hours with syngeneic (unless noted otherwise) peritoneal macrophages as APCs and the indicated stimulus. Supernatants were tested for the indicated cytokine. IFN-γ was determined by dual antibody capture ELISA relative to a standard curve. IL-2 was determined using the HT-2 cell line bioassay. Relative amounts of IL-2 are expressed as tritiated thymidine incorporation. Note that γ/δ T cells elaborate IFN-γ but not IL-2, whereas α/β T cells make both cytokines. Also note that γ/δ T cells can respond with both syngeneic and allogeneic accessory cells.

The α/β T cells were responsive to anti-α/β TCR antibody and the antigen HKLM in the presence of either macrophages or irradiated spleen cells, whereas the γ/δ T cells reacted to HKLM only in the presence of macrophages.[46] The response of isolated α/β T cells was predictable in terms of specificity and MHC restriction and in keeping with previous studies. In contrast, isolated γ/δ T cells responded to LPS (TABLE 3), did not show clear antigen specificity,[46] and responded very well with allogeneic macrophages[46] (TABLE 3). These results suggest a fundamental difference in the response requirements of α/β and γ/δ T cells.

Another striking difference was the ability of γ/δ T cells, but not α/β T cells to respond to IL-7 in the presence of macrophage accessory cells.[46] Several of the known macrophage-derived cytokines were tested for synergy with IL-7. Tumor necrosis factor and IL-6 appeared to have no effect while IL-1 was active. The synergy between IL-1 and IL-7 was striking in that minimal proliferative responses were observed with either cytokine alone. Under these conditions, the synergistic effects of IL-1 and IL-7 were observed with the γ/δ T cells with only a minimal effect on isolated α/β T cells.[46] We also found that IL-7 together with macrophage antigen-presenting cells or a mixture of IL-1 and IL-7 can cause expansion of γ/δ T cells in unseparated populations of cells, as illustrated in FIGURE 2. Because of the selective effects of IL-7 on γ/δ T cells, the possibility exists that local production of IL-1 and IL-7 may account for epithelial tissue distribution and induction of γ/δ T cells at sites of infection. The testing of these hypotheses will require more information on the cellular sources and regulation of IL-7 production.

TABLE 4. Proliferation and Gamma-Interferon Production by γ/δ T Cells in Response to Cytokines and Bacteria[a]

Stimulus *in Vitro*	Response of Purified γ/δ T cells	
	IFN-γ	Proliferation
Medium	-	-
IL-1	+	-
IL-2	-	+
IL-7	-	+
IL-12	-	-
TNFα	-	-
IL-1 plus IL-2	++	+++
IL-1 plus IL-7	++	++++
IL-1 plus IL-12	++++	++
IL-1 plus IL-7 plus IL-12	++++	+++
IL-2 plus IL-12	+	+++
IL-7 plus IL-12	+	++
TNFα plus IL-12	-	-
Macrophages plus IL-12	nt	+++
Macrophages plus medium	-	-
Macrophages plus HKLM	++	+++
Macrophages plus HKLM plus anti–IL-12 antibody	-	-
Macrophages plus HKLM plus control antibody	++	+++

[a]Purified γ/δ T cells were cultured 24 hours with the indicated stimulus. Twenty-four–hour supernatants were tested for IFN-γ by dual antibody capture ELISA relative to a standard curve. Proliferation was determined after a 4-day culture and monitored by tritiated thymidine incorporation. Plus signs indicate relative amounts of interferon production or proliferation: ++++ represents interferon production of about 60–80 U/ml and proliferation of about 10,000–20,000 cpm. (Adapted in part from ref. 46.)

We examined the response of isolated γ/δ T cells to a variety of cytokines using both proliferation and IFN-γ production as readouts for activation (TABLE 4). Ultimately we found that γ/δ T cells proliferated in response to IL-2, IL-7, and IL-12 in the presence of macrophages or IL-1[46] (TABLE 4). Production of IFN-γ was elicited with several mixtures of cytokines but most notably with a mixture of IL-1 and IL-12. These results indicate that γ/δ T cells are poised to receive cytokine signals (IL-1 and IL-12) from activated macrophages. Given this finding we examined the response of γ/δ T cells to macrophages and HKLM and found that both proliferation and IFN-γ production could be inhibited by neutralizing antibodies to IL-12. As such, the apparent response of γ/δ T cells from *Listeria*-infected mice to HKLM was likely due to cytokine signaling rather than only a TCR-mediated antigen recognition event. This conclusion was also supported by the fact that drugs such as cyclosporine and FK506 (which inhibit TCR-mediated events rather that cytokine responses) would only partially inhibit the response to HKLM and macrophages (data not shown). Thus, although the role of cytokines in γ/δ T-cell activation is further

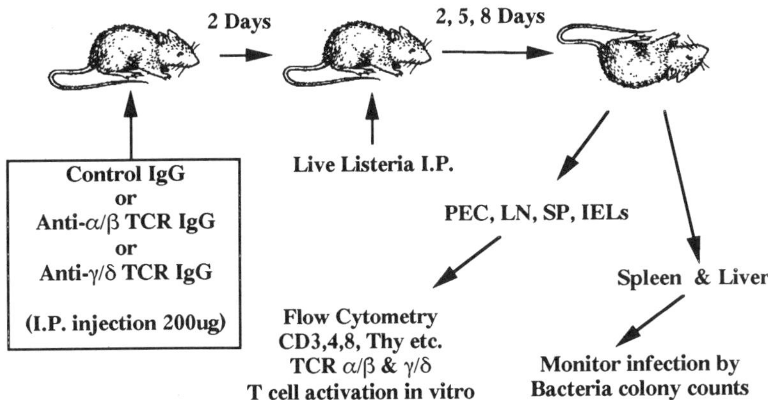

FIGURE 3. Depletion of α/β and γ/δ T cells *in vivo*. The protocol used to deplete mice of T-cell subsets is illustrated. For specific details see legend to TABLE 5 and reference 45; for abbreviations, see legend to FIGURE 1.

defined by these studies, the TCR specificity remains unclear. It is interesting to note that production of IL-1 and IL-12 by bacteria and the resulting production of IFN-γ by γ/δ T cells may contribute to an immune deviation toward a TH1 pathway[52] (FIG. 5). In this regard we noted that depletion of γ/δ T cells *in vivo,* as will be described, results in an increase in the IL-4 produced by spleen cells stimulated with either ConA or immobilized anti-α/β TCR antibody.

***Depletion of Either* α/β *or* γ/δ *T Cells* in Vivo *Impairs Resistance to Infection with* Listeria.** T-cell subsets were depleted by intraperitoneal injection of anti-TCR monoclonal antibody prior to the injection of *Listeria* 2 days later. Both the phenotype of T-cell subsets and the extent of bacterial infection were monitored on days 2, 5, and 8 following injection of *Listeria* (FIG. 3). Injection of anti-TCR monoclonal antibody results in subset-specific depletion which remained effective throughout the course of the experiment.[45] In fact, depletion persisted at least 30 days with no additional antibody injections.

This treatment had a profound effect on the resistance to *Listeria* infection. In the group depleted of γ/δ T cells, there is a clear indication that a severe reduction in the numbers of γ/δ T cells allows for persistence and an increased magnitude of a *Listeria* infection (TABLE 5). Resistance to *Listeria* infection was also apparent when the survival of groups of mice was followed, as illustrated in FIGURE 4. Mice depleted of γ/δ T cells died very soon after challenge as compared to mice depleted of α/β T cells or control mice. These results may indicate that γ/δ T cells are involved in the initial events that control bacterial infection. The role of both α/β T cells and γ/δ T cells was also noted when LD_{50} determinations were made. Depletion of either subset reduced the lethal dose about 10-fold. Depletions of γ/δ T cells also had a profound effect on the resistance to *Listeria* infection on intragastric challenge (TABLE 5). This route of infection may mimic the clinical infection that results from contaminated foods and may indicate a role for intestinal epithelial γ/δ T cells in early defensive reactions.

TABLE 5. Depletion of α/β and γ/δ T Cells *in Vivo* Alters Resistance to Infection with Listeria[a]

Treatment[1]	Mouse Number	Bacteria per Spleen ($\times$ 10,000)		
		Primary IG Challenge[2]	Primary IP Challenge[3]	Secondary IP Challenge[4]
Control IgG	1	5	0.10	0.03
	2	5	0.60	0.75
	3	21	0.01	1.1
	4	23	8.00	13.6
	5	1	2.20	0.48
	6	0	2.50	nt
	7	1	3.70	nt
Anti-α/β TCR IgG	1	2,300	6	6,000
	2	12,000	90	2,420
	3	Dead	15,000	9,700
	4	900	130	5,460
	5	92	340	2,550
	6	69	98	nt
	7	7,000	10,000	nt
Anti-γ/δ TCR IgG	1	180	400	0.05
	2	24	2.9	0.25
	3	Dead	140	8.3
	4	Dead	38	0.5
	5	200	19	3.4
	6	20	4.9	nt
	7	20	58	nt

[a]Three different experiments are shown. (1) Mice were treated with purified IgG (200 μg/ mouse ip) of either control normal hamster IgG (Control IgG), H57 mAb (anti-α/β TCR IgG), or GL3 mAb (anti-γ/δ TCR IgG). (2) Two days later mice were infected with 10^8 viable Listeria intragastrically (IG) using a stomach tube. On day 5 (mouse 1, 2, and 3) or day 6 (mouse 4, 5, 6, and 7), Listeria colony counts were determined from plated lysates of spleen. Deaths occurred on day 4 or 5 after infection. (3) Mice were challenged intraperitoneally (ip) with 6 $\times$ 10^3 Listeria and spleen lysates plated after 5 days. (4) Mice were primed with a sublethal dose of Listeria (9 $\times$ 10^3 per mouse 4 weeks before antibody treatment and then challenged with 10^6 Listeria ip and lysates were tested 4 days after infection. (Adapted in part from ref. 45.)

In contrast to effects on primary resistance to infection with *Listeria*, γ/δ T cells appeared to have little or no effect in secondary challenges with *Listeria*. Mice were immunized by sublethal infection with *Listeria* about 30 days prior to depletion of T-cell subsets and then challenged with bacteria. In this case, only depletion of α/β T cells had a dramatic effect on infection. Therefore, the memory response was primarily mediated by α/β T cells[46,55] (TABLE 5). Our results and others indicate that γ/δ T cells are strongly up-regulated by infection and that depletion of γ/δ T cells

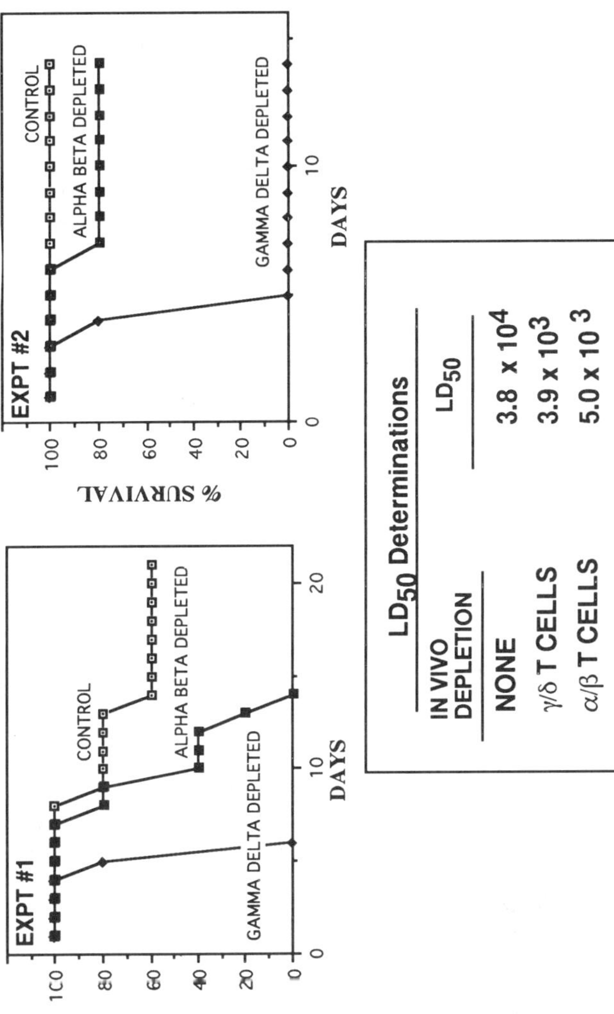

FIGURE 4. Survival times and LD$_{50}$ determinations indicate that γ/δ T cells play an important role in resistance to infection by L. monocytogenes. Groups of five mice were analyzed for survival after an LD$_{40}$ dose of *Listeria* (Expt. 1) or a sublethal injection of bacteria (Expt. 2). Depletions with antibody were as shown in FIGURE 3 and TABLE 5. LD$_{50}$ determinations were as previously described.[48] Note the rapid death in mice depleted of γ/δ T cells.

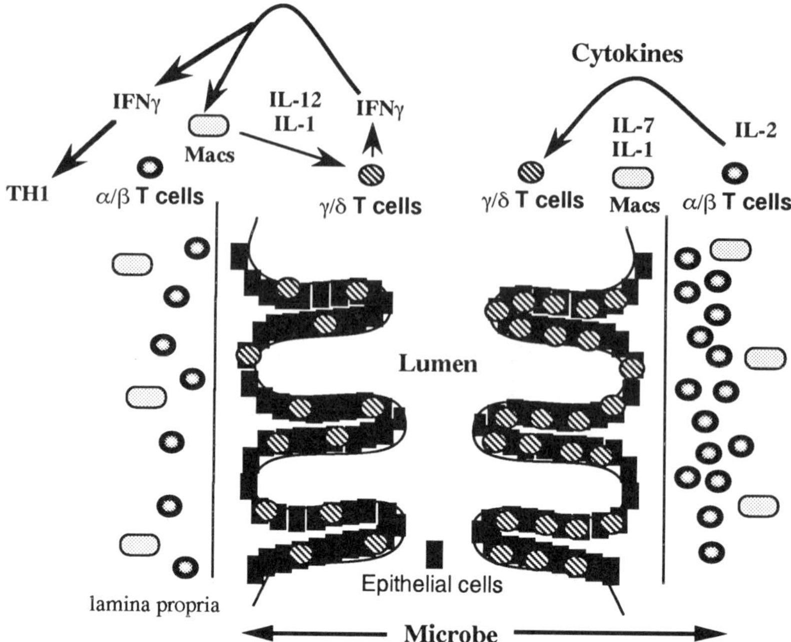

FIGURE 5. Cytokine cascade and intercellular interactions. A schematic representation of the tissue organization and potential cytokine production in the small intestine is shown. See text for discussion.

in vivo with specific antibody or by gene-knockout procedures impairs resistance to primary exposure to *Listeria*.[45,53–55] These results suggest a critical role for γ/δ T cells in the innate frontline defensive reactions to microbial infection.

Mechanism of Action of γ/δ T Cells? When the data on tissue expression and induction of γ/δ T cells are considered collectively together with the cytokine responses and intercellular interactions operative with macrophage and T cells, the schematic illustrated in FIGURE 5 can be generated. It is apparent that γ/δ T cells exist in epithelial tissue at sites of first contact with invading microbial pathogens, an example being the cellular organization of the small intestine as illustrated. The γ/δ T cell was shown to be a cellular source of IFN-γ[51] (TABLES 3 and 4), and this cytokine is clearly a potent macrophage-activating agent for antimicrobial defenses. Apparently γ/δ T cells respond to macrophage-derived cytokines IL-1 and IL-12 with vigorous production of IFN-γ. Both IL-1 and IL-12 are induced by exposure of macrophages to bacteria.[52] As such, an activation pathway can be envisioned in which invading bacteria cause macrophage production of IL-1 and IL-12 which in turn activates γ/δ T cells to produce IFN-γ which then induces the full activation of macrophages to permit the efficient destruction of bacteria. The initial burst of IFN-γ production generated in this way may also bias the response to the TH1 cell differentiation which would mediate further macrophage activation and lymphocyte recruitment via IFN-γ and IL-2. In this scheme, γ/δ T cells are not only dependent on activation of other cell types but also able to regulate the function of both macrophages and other T cells.

The proliferative capacity of γ/δ T cells may also be regulated by cytokines produced by both macrophages, α/β T cells, and possibly epithelial cells. Our experiments indicate that γ/δ T cells do not generate IL-2 for an autocrine pathway. Instead, γ/δ T cells proliferate preferentially to IL-1 and IL-7 (and both α/β and γ/δ T cells proliferate in response to IL-1 and IL-2). One could speculate that because of this dependency, γ/δ T cells in epithelial tissue do not proliferate vigorously in response to antigen. This may provide a necessary dampened reactivity in the epithelial tissue where foreign antigen concentrations may be relatively high and an ongoing inflammatory response may be more damaging than protective. If, however, the microbe breaches the epithelium to cause activation of the α/β T cells, macrophages, and IL-7-producing cells that remain undefined, then the cytokines produced would amplify the activities and proliferative capacity of γ/δ T cells. This mechanism takes into account the dependency of γ/δ T cells on other cell types and may further suggest that γ/δ T cells play a negative regulatory role in epithelial tissue. In this regard we have noted that acute depletion of γ/δ T cells with antibody *in vivo* (as just described) enhances the response of α/β T cells to specific immunization and abrogates the tolerance that normally results from the oral administration of large doses of soluble antigen (Pearce and Ziegler, manuscript in preparation). Thus, γ/δ T cells appear to play both defensive and regulatory roles in response to ingested material, and clearly the defensive functions must be reconciled with the requirement for tolerance to ingested proteins and to the maintenance of epithelial tissue integrity. The precise mechanism(s) by which γ/δ T cells exert these diverse immunologic effects remains to be determined.

REFERENCES

1. MOSMANN, T. R. & R. L. COFFMAN. 1989. TH1 and TH2 cells: Different patterns of lymphokine secretion lead to different functional properties. Ann. Rev. Immunol. **7:** 145–173.

2. CHERWINSKI, H. C., J. H. SCHUMACHER, K. D. BROWN & T. R. MOSMANN. 1987. Two types of mouse helper T cell clone. 3. Further differences in lymphokine synthesis between TH1 and TH2 clones revealed by RNA hybridization, functionally monospecific bioassays and monoclonal antibodies. J. Exp. Med. **166:** 1229–1244.

3. CHER, D. J. & T. R. MOSMANN. 1987. Two types of murine helper T cell clone. 2. Delayed-type hypersensitivity is mediated by TH1 clones. J. Immunol. **138:** 3688–3694.

4. COFFMAN, R. L., B. W. SEYMOUR, D. A. LEBMAN, *et al.* 1988. The role of helper T cell products in mouse B cell differentiation and isotype regulation. Immunol. Rev. **102:** 5–28.

5. SCOTT, P., R. L. NATOVITZ, R. L. COFFMAN, E. PEARCE & A. SHER. 1988. Immunoregulation of cutaneous leishmaniasis. T cell lines that transfer protective immunity or exacerbation belong to different T helper subsets and respond to distinct parasite antigens. J. Exp. Med. **168:** 1675.

6. PAPP, I., K. J. WIEDER, T. SABLINSKI, P. J. O'CONNELL, E. L. MILFORD, T. B. STROM & J. W. KUPIEC-WEGLINSKI. 1992. Evidence for functional heterogeneity of rat CD4+ T cells *in vivo*. Differential expression of IL-2 and IL-4 mRNA in recipients of cardiac allografts. J. Immunol. **148:** 1308–1314.

7. CHER, D. J. & T. R. MOSSMAN. 1987. Two types of murine helper T cell clone. II. Delayed-type hypersensitivity is mediated by TH1 clones. J. Immunol. **138:** 3688-3692.

8. UNANUE, E. R., D. I. BELLER, C. Y. LU & P. M. ALLEN. 1984. Antigen presentation: Comments on its regulation and mechanism. J. Immunol. **132:** 1-5.

9. CHESTNUT, R. S., S. COLON & H. M. GREY. 1982. Requirements for the processing of antigen by antigen-presenting B cells. I. Functional comparison of B cell tumors and macrophages. J. Immunol. **129:** 2382-2388.

10. YEWDELL, J. W. & J. R. BENNINK. 1990. The binary logic of antigen processing presentation to T cells. Cell **62:** 203-205.

11. ZIEGLER, H. K. & E. R. UNANUE. 1982. Decrease in macrophage antigen catabolism by ammonia and chloroquine is associated with inhibition of antigen presentation to T cells. Proc. Natl. Acad. Sci. USA **79:** 175-178.

12. ZIEGLER, H. K., C. A. ORLIN & C. W. CLUFF. 1987. Differential requirements for the processing and presentation of soluble and particulate bacterial antigens by macrophages. Eur. J. Immunol. **17:** 1287-1291.

13. UNANUE, E. R. 1984. Antigen-presenting function of the macrophage. Ann. Rev. Immunol. **2:** 395-428.

14. BRODSKY, F. M. & L. E. GUAGLIARDI. 1991. The cell biology of antigen processing. Ann. Rev. Immunol. **9:** 707-744.

15. BABBITT, D., P. ALLEN, G. MATSUEDA, E. HABER & E. UNANUE. 1985. Binding of immunogenic peptides to Ia histocompatibility molecules. Nature **317:** 359-361.

16. BUUS, S., A. SETTE, S. COLON, D. JENIS & H. GREY. 1986. Isolation and characterization of antigen-Ia complexes involved in T cell recognition. Cell **47:** 1071-1077.

17. BROWN, J. H., T. JARDETZKY, J. C. GORGA, L. J. STERN, R. G. URBAN, J. L. STROMINGER & D. C. WILEY. 1993. Three-dimensional structure of the human class II histocompatibility antigen HLA-DR1. Nature **364:** 33-39.

18. SPITS, H., J. BORST, C. TERHORST & J. E. DEVRIES. 1982. The role of T cell differentiation markers in antigen-specific and lectin-dependent cellular cytotoxicity mediated by T8+ and T4+ human cytotoxic T cell clones directed at class I and class II MHC antigens. J. Immunol. **129:** 1563-1569.

19. WEAVER, C. T. & E. R. UNANUE. 1986. T cell induction of membrane IL-1 on macrophages. J. Immunol. **137:** 3868.

20. ASHWELL, J. D., M. K. JENKINS & R. H. SCHWARTZ. 1988. Effect of gamma radiation on resting B lymphocytes. II. Functional characterization of the antigen-presentation defect. J. Immunol. **141:** 2536-2544.

21. BIERER, B. E., B. P. SLECKMAN, S. E. RATNOFSKY & S. J. BURAKOFF. 1989. The biological roles of CD2, CD4, and CD8 in T-cell activation. Ann. Rev. Immunol. **7:** 579-599.

22. JANEWAY, C. W. JR. 1992. The T cell receptor as a multicomponent signalling machine: CD4/CD8 coreceptors and CD45 in T cell activation. Ann. Rev. Immunol. **10:** 645-674.

23. LINSLEY, P. S., W. BRADY, L. GROSMAIRE, A. ARUFFO, N. K. DAMLE & J. A. LEDBETTER. 1991. Binding of the B cell activation antigen B7 to CD28 costimulates T cell proliferation and interleukin 2 mRNA accumulation. J. Exp. Med. **173:** 721-730.

24. BLUESTONE, J. A., R. Q. CRON, M. COTTERMAN, B. A. HOULDEN & L. A. MATIS. 1988. Structure and specificity of T cell receptor g/d on major histocompatibility complex antigen-specific CD3+, CD4-, CD8-T lymphocytes. J. Exp. Med. **168:** 1899-1916.

25. ITO, K., L. VAN KAER, M. BONNEVILLE, S. HSU, D. B. MURPHY & S. TONEGAWA. 1990. Recognition of the product of a novel MHC TL region gene (27b) by a mouse gamma delta T cell receptor. Cell **62:** 549-561.

26. PORCELLI, S., M. B. BRENNER, J. L. GREENSTEIN, S. P. BALK, C. TERHORST & P. A. BLEICHER. 1989. Recognition of cluster of differentiation 1 antigen by CD4-CD8-cytolytic T lymphocytes. Nature **341:** 447-449.

27. HAREGEWOIN, A., G. SOMAN, R. C. HAM & R. W. FINBERG. 1989. Human γ/δ+ T cells respond to mycobacterial heat-shock protein. Nature **340:** 309-312.

28. MODLIN, R. L., C. PIRMEZ, F. M. HORMAN, V. TORIGAN, K. UYEMURA, T. H. REA, B. R. BLOOM & M. B. BRENNER. 1989. Lymphocytes bearing antigen-specific γ/δ T cell receptors accumulate in human infectious disease lesions. Nature **339:** 544-548.

29. KABELITZ, D., A. BENDER, S. SCHONDELMAIER, B. SCHOEL & S. H. E. KAUFMANN. 1990. A large fraction of human peripheral blood γ/δ+ T cells is activated by *Mycobacterium tuberculosis* but not by its 65-kDa heat shock protein. J. Exp. Med. **171:** 667-669.

30. HOLOSHITZ, J., F. KONING, J. E. COLIGAN, J. DE BRUYN & S. STROBER. 1989. Isolation of CD4-CD8-*Mycobacteria* reactive T lymphocyte clones from rheumatoid arthritis synovial fluid. Nature **339:** 226-229.

31. JANIS, E. M., S. H. E. KAUFMANN, R. H. SCHWARTZ & D. M. PARDOLL. 1989. Activation of $\gamma\delta$ T cells in the primary immune response to *Mycobacterium tuberculosis*. Science **244:** 713-716.

32. STROMINGER, J. L. 1989. The $\gamma\delta$ T cell receptor and Class 1b MHC-related proteins: Enigmatic molecules of immune recognition. Cell **57:** 895-898.

33. PFEFFER, K., B. SCHOEL, H. GULLE, S. H. E. KAUFMANN & H. WAGNER. 1990. Primary responses of human T cells to mycobacteria: A frequent set of γ/δ T cells are stimulated by protease-resistant ligands. Eur. J. Immunol. **20:** 1175-1179.

34. O'BRIEN, R. L. & W. BORN. 1991. Heat shock proteins as antigens for $\gamma\delta$ T cells. Semin. Immunol. 81-87.

35. VAN EDEN, W., J. E. R. THOLE, R. VAN DER ZEE, A. NOORDZIJ, J. D. A. VAN EMBDEN, E. J. HENSEN & I. R. COHEN. 1988. Cloning of the mycobacterial epitope recognized by T lymphocytes in adjuvant arthritis. Nature **331:** 171-173.

36. LAMB, J. R., V. BAL, P. MENDEZ-SAMPERIO, A. MEHLERT, A. SO, J. ROTHBARD, S. JINDAL, R. A. YOUNG & D. B. YOUNG. 1989. Stress proteins may provide a link between the immune response to infection and autoimmunity. Int. Immunol. **1:** 191-196.

37. HAREGEWOIN, A., B. SINGH, R. S. GUPTA, & R. W. FINBERG. 1991. A mycobacterial heat-shock protein-responsive gamma delta T cell clone also responds to the homologous human heat-shock protein: A possible link between infection and autoimmunity. J. Infect. Dis. **163:** 156-160.

38. ASARNOW, D. M., W. A. KUSIEL, M. BONYHADI, R. E. TIGELAAR, P. W. TUCKER & J. P. ALLISON. 1988. Limited diversity of gamma delta antigen receptor genes of Thy-1+ dendritic epidermal cells. Cell **55:** 837-847.

39. GOODMAN, T. & L. LEFRANCOIS. 1988. Expression of the γ/δ T cell receptor on intestinal CD8+ intraepithelial lymphocytes. Nature **333:** 855-858.

40. AUGUSTIN, A., R. T. KUBO & G.-K. SIM. 1989. Resident pulmonary lymphocytes expressing the γ/δ T-cell receptor. Nature **340:** 239-241.

41. ITOHARA, S., A. G. FARR, J. J. LAFAILLE, M. BONNEVILLE, Y. TAKAGAKI, W. HAAS & S. TONEGAWA. 1990. Homing of a γ/δ thymocyte subset with homogeneous T-cell receptors to mucosal epithelia. Nature **343:** 754-757.

42. ALLISON, J. P. & W. L. HAVRAN. 1991. The immunobiology of T cells with invariant $\gamma\delta$ antigen receptors. Ann. Rev. Immunol. **9:** 679-705.

43. DEGEUS, B., M. VAN DEN ENDEN, C. COOLEN, L. NAGELKERKEN, P. VAN DER HEIJDEN & J. ROZING. 1990. Phenotype of intraepithelial lymphocytes in euthymic and athymic mice: Implications for differentiation of cells bearing a CD3-associated γ,δ T cell receptor. Eur. J. Immunol. **20:** 291-298.

44. BONNEVILLE, M., S. ITOHARA, E. G. KRECKO, P. MOMBAERTS, I. ISHIDA, M. KATSUKI, A. BERNS, A. G. FARR, C. A. JANEWAY, JR. & S. TONEGAWA. 1990. Transgenic mice

demonstrate that epithelial homing of gamma/delta T cells is determined by cell lineages independent of T cell receptor specificity. J. Exp. Med. **171:** 1015-1026.

45. SKEEN, M. J. & H. K. ZIEGLER. 1993. Induction of murine peritoneal γ/δ T cells and their role in resistance to bacterial infection. J. Exp. Med. **178:** 971-975.

46. SKEEN, M. J. & H. K. ZIEGLER. 1993. Intercellular interactions and cytokine responsiveness of peritoneal α/β and γ/δ T cells from Listeria-infected mice: Synergistic effects of IL-1 and IL-7 on γ/β T cells. J. Exp. Med. **178:** 985-996.

47. LEFRANCOIS, L. & T. GOODMAN. 1989. *In vivo* modulation of cytolytic activity and Thy-1 expression in TCR-γ/δ+ intraepithelial lyphocytes. Science **243:** 1716-1718.

48. SAFLEY, A. S., C. W. CLUFF, N. E. MARSHALL & H. K. ZIEGLER. 1991. Role of listeriolysin-o (LLO) in the T lymphocyte response to infection with *Listeria monocytogenes.* J. Immunol. **146:** 3604-3616.

49. OHGA, S., Y. YOSHIKAI, Y. TAKEDA, K. HIROMATSU & K. NOMOTO. 1990. Sequential appearance of γ/δ and α/β-bearing T cells in the peritoneal cavity during an i.p. infection with *Listeria monocytogenes.* Eur. J. Immunol. **29:** 533-538.

50. EMOTO, M., T. NAITO, R. NAKAMURA & Y. YOSHIKAI. 1993. Different appearance of γ/δ T cells during Salmonellosis between Ity^r and Ity^s mice. J. Immunol. **150:** 3411-3420.

51. YAMAMOTO, S., F. RUSS, H. C. TEIXEIRA, P. CONRADT & S. H. E. KAUFMANN. 1993. *Listeria monocytogenes*-induced gamma interferon secretion by intestinal intraepithelial γ/δ T cell lymphocytes. Infect. Immun. **61:** 2154-2161.

52. HSIEH, C.-S., S. E. MACATONIA, C. S. TRIPP, S. F. WOLF, A. O'GARRA & K. M. MURPHY. 1993. Development of TH1 CD4+ T cells through IL-12 produced by Listeria-induced macrophages. Science **260:** 547-549.

53. HIROMATSU, K., Y. YOSHIKAI, G. MATSUZAKI, S. OHGA, K. MURAMORI, K. MATSUMOTO, J. A. BLUESTONE & K. NOMOTO. 1992. A protective role of γ/δ T cells in primary infection with *Listeria monocytogenes* in mice. J. Exp. Med. **175:** 49-56.

54. ITOHARA, S., P. MOMBAERTS, J. LAFAILLE, J. IACOMINI, A. NELSON, A. R. CLARKE, M. L. HOOPER, A. FARR & S. TONEGAWA. 1993. T cell receptor δ gene mutant mice: Independent generation of α/β T cells and programmed rearrangements of γ/δ TCR genes. Cell **72:** 337-348.

55. MOMBAERTS, P., J. ARNOLDI, F. RUSS, S. TONEGAWA & S. H. E. KAUFMANN. 1993. Different roles of α/β and γ/δ T cells in immunity against an intracellular bacterial pathogen. Nature **365:** 53-56.

New Perspectives on Use of Thymic Factors in Immune Deficiency[a]

SUSANNA CUNNINGHAM-RUNDLES,[b,e,g]
MADELINE HARBISON,[c,e] SONIA GUIRGUIS,[d,e]
DAVID VALACER,[d,e] AND PAUL B. CHRETIEN[f]

*The Immunology Research Laboratory
Divisions of Hematology/Oncology,[b] Endocrinology,[c] and
Allergy/Immunology,[d] and
[e]Department of Pediatrics
The New York Hospital
Cornell University Medical College
New York, New York 10021*

*[f]The University of Maryland
Baltimore, Maryland*

The significance of the thymus gland as an endocrine organ producing various factors important for the development of the immune system was initially established in 1965 when DiGeorge[1] characterized a case of congenital absence of the thymus with fatal outcome, and in addition cited a previous historic letter from 1829 by Harrington[2] reporting a similar case. This description defined a syndrome and provided a connecting link between thymic hypoplasia and susceptibility to recurrent infection. Subsequently, there followed reports of successful reconstitution of immune deficiency by means of fetal thymus transplantation[3,4] and thymic factors.[5,6]

At the time of DiGeorge's discovery, the well-known previous work of Miller[7] and Good *et al.*[8] had shown that experimental, prenatal thymectomy caused severe immune defects. The result was described as a wasting syndrome characterized by recurrent and ultimately fatal infections. Reversal and resolution of these defects by implantation of thymic tissue in a millipore diffusion chamber from which cells could not enter or leave and even by thymic epithelial and stromal cells essentially free of lymphoid elements derived from thymic tissue were achieved.[9] This established the concept that factors made by thymic tissue act on lymphocytes derived from the bone marrow and cause their maturation into functionally mature cells.

The almost mysterious, vital potential of the thymus gland has had many historical references. Attempts to isolate thymic factors were documented as early as the end of the nineteenth century (reviewed in ref. 10). In 1935 Gregoire[10] reported that cortical regions of the thymus exposed to damaging levels of radiation were subsequently

[a]These studies were supported in part by National Institutes of Health NCI 29502, the Helena Rubenstein Foundation, and the Children's Blood Foundation.

[g] Address for correspondence: Dr. Susanna Cunningham-Rundles, The New York Hospital, Cornell University Medical Center, 1300 York Avenue, New York, New York 10021.

repopulated by circulating lymphocytes. Murine studies by Stutman et al.[11] were important in the demonstration that "committed" prethymic precursor T cells were formed from a pluripotent stem cell similar to those observed for other cellular lineages. Furthermore, Stutman[12] found that postthymic cells that had previously been influenced by intrathymic processing populated the bone marrow and lymphoid organs of mice. These cells retained the potential to repopulate and reconstitute an athymic mouse. Although these postthymic cells appeared not to need direct physical contact with thymic tissue, thymic humoral factors were essential and were required to promote maturation to mature T cells. These postthymic T cells appear to comprise a critical T-cell reserve that retains the potential to mature in the presence of thymic humoral factors.

The identity of an analogous population of cells in humans remains speculative. Interestingly, a recent report from Incefy et al.[13] showing restoration of thymic epithelial production of the thymic hormone thymulin following bone marrow transplantation for severe combined immune deficiency (SCID) suggests that the stimulus for thymic secretion requires a bone marrow-derived cell. Further indirect evidence of such an analogous postthymic T-cell population may be inferred from the relatively little effect of normal thymic atrophy on T-cell function in the mature animal[14] or in humans. As will be discussed, related evidence exists for a marrow donor postthymic T-cell response to residual host thymic factor in bone marrow reconstitution of congenital thymic absence.

The human thymus is a unique gland which appears to reach maximum size at 1 year of age and then progressively involutes.[15] The thymus is unusually sensitive to external environmental stimuli including stress or infections which may directly influence size. Involution of the thymus is a poorly understood process that may involve more than one mechanism, and in certain instances, such as lactation, involution is reversible. The issue of which normal developmental changes or events may affect thymic involution is controversial.[16] A recent report showing the existence of prolactin receptors on thymocytes[17] and other studies indicating thymic response to growth hormone and insulin-like growth factor-1[18] support the general concept that neuroendocrine modulation is highly significant for thymic activity. As the thymus becomes smaller, circulating levels of thymic hormones and thymic factors show a significant age-related decline.[19] Although an age-related decline is thought to be permanent, this may not always be true. Current understanding of the consequences of thymic atrophy during aging suggests that ultimately, loss of thymic influence, specifically thymic factors, is responsible for key aspects of immune senescence. However, Gravenstein et al.[20] showed that treatment of elderly men with thymosin α_1 (Tα_1) significantly augmented antibody responsiveness to influenza vaccine. These results suggest that the postthymic T-cell population remains capable of response to thymic factors.

During the late 1960s and 1970s several thymic factors were isolated and partially purified.[10,21] These biologically active fractions were studied in bioassays primarily designed to measure a single aspect of lymphocyte maturation in vitro and to test efficacy to reconstitute experimentally thymectomized animals in certain in vivo settings. Subsequently, various thymic fractions were used to treat patients with more or less clearly defined immune deficiencies for varying lengths of time. In addition, attempts were made to restore immune competence to the cancer patient using thymic factors as immunotherapeutic agents.

These efforts to treat primary and secondary immune deficiency were begun well before the advent of monoclonal antibodies or recombinant technology that has made possible analysis of specific lymphocyte subpopulations, growth factors, or cytokines and before biochemical and immunological characterization of thymic factors. Effects were often transient, and in primary immune deficiency, the introduction of bone marrow transplantation, intravenous gamma globulin, and cytokine treatment often appeared to offer a more direct approach to treatment. The complexities of these alternative treatments have also come to be appreciated. Now, as the importance of regulatory circuits as a third dimension to immune function can be studied more directly, it is possible to define selective use of thymic factors as well.

The following sections briefly outline current implications of accrued experience at the level of implications for mechanism and of therapeutic use of thymic factors in primary and secondary immune deficiency. Finally, we present current clinical experience in primary immune deficiency which suggests that thymic factors have significant use in restoring impaired immune host defense against potential microbial pathogenesis.

THYMIC FACTORS: CLUES TO MECHANISM OF ACTION

Thymically derived factors that have been identified and at least partially purified include **thymosin fraction 5 (TF-5); thymosin α_1, thymopoetin II (TP), facteur thymique serique (FTS),** now called **thymulin, thymic humoral factor (THF), and THFγ2.** There are also others that have not been as clearly defined. Although many of the known thymic factors have similar activities in certain biological assays and may contain trace amounts of other known thymic factors, it is likely that the defined thymic factors act essentially at different points in T-cell maturation and may be operationally separable.

Increasing evidence suggests that thymic epithelial or myoid cells produce a range of cytokines.[22] These include certain interleukins such as IL-1 (both alpha and beta), IL-6, IL-7, tumor necrosis factor alpha, granulocyte-colony stimulating factor (G-CSF), and macrophage-colony stimulating factor (M-CSF).[23-25] The conditions that elicit cytokine production by thymic cells need clarification. Some studies are based on thymically derived cell lines that may have undergone changes during the establishment period or reflect the response of a homogeneous population of cells *in vitro* rather than the more complex outcome of cellular interactions that may occur *in vivo*. Cytokines may be secreted endogenously by specific cells of the thymus, during particular stages of development, or by thymic cells activated in response to an exogenously derived signal. Thymocytes can be activated through different pathways reflecting mechanisms that involve distinct cell surface antigens as elegantly described by the extensive studies of Haynes and collaborators.[22] Use of these pathways may depend on cytokine signals and thymic factors. Reports of receptors on thymic cells, such as the prolactin receptor,[17] the observation of thymic response to growth hormone, and insulin-like growth factor-1[18] suggest several levels of regulatory control within the thymus.

Dardenne and Bach[26] showed that zinc is required for the biological activity of the thymic hormone thymulin. Furthermore, in intriguing new work, this group has shown that mild, oral zinc supplementation of the diet of aging mice could be used to stimulate thymic lymphocytes through regrowth of the thymus and an increase in thymic hormone production.[27] Other studies, such as those by Coto *et al.*,[28] demonstrated that IL-1 (both alpha and beta) which stimulates uptake of zinc by human thymic epithelial cells regulates the secretion of the zinc-thymulin complex, suggesting that zinc may be the connecting link between IL-1 and the thymic response.

The significance of altered cytokine patterns in the developing thymus is suggested from several sources. Studies in Down's syndrome show a connection between altered morphology of thymic cells characteristic of the syndrome and up-regulation of tumor necrosis factor and gamma interferon production.[29] Whether this is indeed specific to Down's syndrome or reflects cause and effect remains to be clarified. Cytokines produced outside the thymus may also critically influence thymic function as suggested by studies showing differential expression of receptors for epidermal growth factor and nerve growth factor on the normal human thymus and thymomas.[30] Efforts to identify specific breakpoints in primary immune deficiency likely will also clarify thymic factor and cytokine network interactions.

Efforts to use thymic factors to augment immune response also support a possible relationship to cytokine activity. Thus, $T\alpha_1$ has been found to potentiate IL-2 induced cytotoxicity in mice[31] and the antitumor activity of IL-2 in Lewis lung carcinoma.[32] These findings *in vivo* are in agreement with related data *in vitro* suggesting that this synthetic thymic hormone acts to activate natural killer cells by enhancing IL-2 production and by up-regulating IL-2 receptor expression.[33] Crude thymic extracts such as thymostimulin are also effective, as shown by Lin *et al.*[34] who were able to enhance both IL-2 and gamma interferon (INF-γ) production of cord blood lymphocytes from infants with congenital thymic deficiency.

Recently, thymic factors such as thymic extract, thymopeptide, and thymic factor x were used successfully in clinical trials of chronic hepatitis B. Thymic factors do not appear to have any direct antiviral activity. The studies of Mutchnick *et al.*[35] with TF-5 and $T\alpha_1$ suggest that the beneficial clinical effects may be related to increased peripheral blood lymphocyte counts, increased CD3[+]T and CD4[+]T lymphocyte subsets, and increased *in vitro* production of INF-γ.

In summary, current studies indicate that thymic factors may act through cytokine network interaction perhaps by altering cytokine balance. The types of cytokine reactivity patterns, recently defined as a T-helper type 1 or type 2 response,[36] may be useful in future studies of thymic factors, because in general thymic factors may potentiate a T-helper type 1 response as characterized by increased production of IL-2 and INF-γ.

THYMIC FACTOR REPLACEMENT IN PRIMARY IMMUNE DEFICIENCY

Wara *et al.*[5,37] were the first to show that poor lymphocyte proliferative response to allogeneic stimulation in the mixed lymphocyte culture reaction *in vitro* in patients with primary immune deficiency could be restored with the addition of TF-5 *in vivo*.

Over several years, patients with a range of immune deficiency disorders including SCID, DiGeorge syndrome, ataxia telangiectasia, chronic mucocutaneous candidiasis, disseminated histiocytosis X, Hyper-IgE syndrome, Wiskott Aldrich, and combined immune deficiency were treated. Some patients showed marked improvement as determined by lymphocyte functional response *in vitro* and resolution of clinically significant infections including herpes, streptococcus pneumonia, and candidiasis. In some cases improvement was transient; in others, when treatment was stopped, benefit continued without additional thymic factor treatment at least for a time. However, patients with lymphoproliferative features associated with ataxia telangiectasia and histiocytosis X showed clinical progression. Humoral immune defects (hypo- or hyper-) were not resolved.

Of all the described congenital immune defects in which thymic deficiency might suggest the potential benefit of direct replacement by thymic factors, thymic hypoplasia associated with the DiGeorge syndrome has provided the strongest rationale. This anomaly arises from abnormal development of the third and fourth pharyngeal pouches and can affect the first to sixth branchial pouches. Thymic absence, hypoparathyroidisin with attendant hypocalcemia, congenital heart defects involving the aortic arch and conotruncal abnormalities, midline defects producing typical focus hypoplastic mandible, short philtrum, hypertelorism, and low set ears are the principal features.[38] Initially a very high degree of fatality was associated with this syndrome, much of which was attributed to thymic absence. With improved surgical and anesthesia methods, two cardiovascular defects, interrupted aortic arch and truncus arteriosus, became manageable and the extent of the immunodeficiency associated with thymic absence could be accurately assessed. In subsequent studies it became clear that a significant number of infants with classical DiGeorge anomaly showed gradual improvement in immune function and appeared to develop normally. This tendency towards spontaneous remission was originally reported by Sieber *et al.*[39] However, some infants did develop intractable infections which were ultimately fatal.

Recently Bastian *et al.*[40] found that a subgroup of patients who had persistently low CD4$^+$ T-cell numbers did not do well. These investigators stressed the importance of finding a way to identify patients with persistent immune abnormalities before these deficiencies lead to morbidity and mortality.

DiGeorge syndrome is now considered to be a developmental field defect that may have more than one cause. Several chromosomal abnormalities, including monosomy 22_q 11 and monosomy 10_p 13, single gene defects, have been described. In some cases, teratogenic exposure has been suggested. As a result of this range of defects it has become customary to refer to infants with essentially total thymic and parathyroid aplasia and conotruncal defects as having "complete" DiGeorge syndrome. Greenberg[41] noted that the variable immune function in DiGeorge syndrome is paralled by variable expression of parathyroid dysfunction which may also resolve without continued treatment in some patients but not in others. This uncertainty about what constitutes DiGeorge syndrome has been reflected in a general lack of consensus which could lead to the establishment of minimal diagnostic criteria for the syndrome.

In patients with DiGeorge syndrome immunologic reconstitution was achieved with fetal thymus transplantation, thymic epithelial transplants, and injections of thymic factors.[37,42] There has been no comprehensive review of these patients that could provide long-term assessment of outcome. However, Goldsobel *et al.*[43] in a

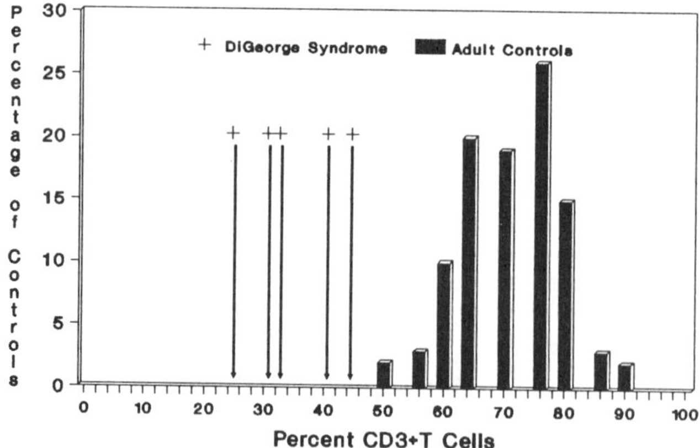

FIGURE 1. Data for the percentage of CD3[+] T cells of patients with DiGeorge syndrome in peripheral blood, as shown by the *arrows*, in comparison with adult CD3[+] T-cell percentages ($n = 88$) arranged to show percentile distribution. Data were obtained by flow cytometry.

review of 26 previously reported cases by correspondence revealed that only 8 remained alive. Three died from immunologically related causes, two from cardiac defects, and one from unknown causes. This information may indicate that the concept of sustained spontaneous resolution in DiGeorge syndrome needs revision.

Occasionally B-cell defects are observed in patients with DiGeorge syndrome. In a case reported by Goldsobel *et al.*,[43] successful reconstitution was achieved with bone marrow transplantation. This case is apparently paradoxical because it might have been assumed that in the absence of the thymus the T-cell system could not develop. However, it suggests that in some cases, minimal thymic influence is needed to provide an active differentiating signal to postthymic T cells in the donor graft. This study further suggests that effects at different levels may affect outcome.

IMMUNE MANIFESTATIONS OF THYMIC DEFICIENCY IN DiGEORGE SYNDROME

In light of the Bastian study suggesting that susceptibility to infections may not resolve spontaneously in DiGeorge syndrome, we undertook immune assessment to establish criteria that might identify infants according to the level of risk. In studies presented here, we restricted the definition of DiGeorge syndrome to infants with thymic hypoplasia, midline defects, and either a typical cardiac defect or hypoparathyroidism. In these studies we generally confirmed the studies of Bastian *et al.* of a distinct subset of infants with persistent immune defects.

Over a 2-year period we studied five cases of DiGeorge syndrome, four in infants and one in an older child. Four patients had conotruncal cardiac defects and midline defects. Hypoparathyroidism was evident in four. One infant had generally normal calcium levels with occasional stress-related depletion. All of the infants lacked thymic tissue as noted by x-ray. The older child has partial thymic absence.

As shown in FIGURE 1, in comparison with normal adult controls, arranged according to percentile distribution of CD3[+] T cells, all children showed a reduced

TABLE 1. Longitudinal Evaluation of Immune Response in DiGeorge Syndrome

	Lymphocyte Subsets[a]			Proliferative Response			
Age	CD3	CD4	CD8	PHA	*C. albicans*	*S. aureus*	PWM
1 mo	23.5	19.1	42.8	18,000	2,96	198	3,404
3 mo	31.8	20.8	31.5	22,909	4,079	1,188	8,518
1 yr	32.4	25.8	17.5	18,407	7,470	184	7,803
2 yr	32.5	16.0	27.0	20,300	ND	ND	3,936

[a]Normal values for T-cell subsets (n = 88): CD3, X = 69.8% (SD = 8.0); CD4, X = 44.9% (SD = 9.0); CD8, X = 29.7%.

[b]Proliferative response normal values (n = 88): phytohemogglutinin (PHA), X = 34,600 (19,770-46,660, SD = 6297); *C. albicans*, X = 10,950 (SD = 5,309); *S. aureus*, X = 3,439 (SD = 1,054); pokeweed mitogen (PWM), X = 8,741 (5,466-14,390, SD = 8,741).

percentage of CD3$^+$ T cells by flow cytometry of whole blood. The relative percentage of CD4$^+$ T cells was also strikingly reduced in most (4 of 5), but CD8$^+$ T cells were characteristically normal or even elevated, which was associated with an inverted CD4/CD8 ratio as shown in FIGURE 2. This imbalance between T-cell subsets had some bearing on susceptibility to infections, because those infants with greater CD4$^+$ T-cell deficiency had more frequent and more severe infections requiring hospitalization. Two infants died of overwhelming sepsis during the first 2 months of life.

At first evaluation of lymphocyte response to activators *in vitro,* all infants showed a normal proliferative response to the T-cell mitogen phytohemagglutinin, but a low response to microbial activators. All except the older child, who had partial thymic absence, had evidence of growth failure. Improvement in the immune response to microbial activators during the first months of life was observed in one infant in association with an increased percentage of CD4$^+$ T cells (TABLE 1). Before this

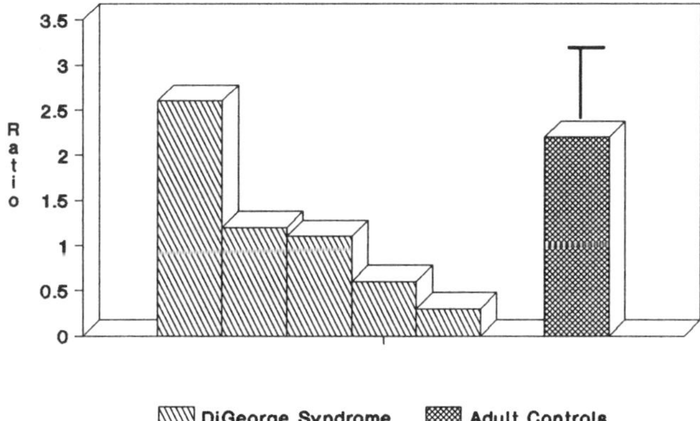

FIGURE 2. CD4/CD8 ratio for each patient with DiGeorge syndrome in comparison with the mean CD4/CD8 ratio in 59 adult controls.

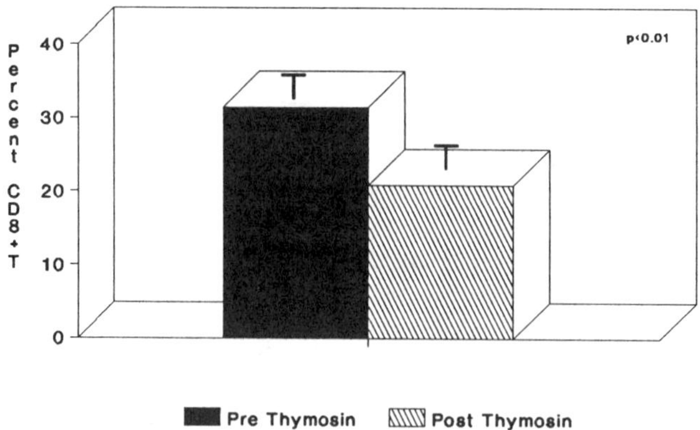

FIGURE 3. Effect of thymosin fraction 5 (TF-5) treatment on CD8[+] T-cell percentage in patients with DiGeorge syndrome.

improvement occurred, the infant had had candidiasis and diarrhea. These clinically significant infections gradually resolved, and this improvement was accompanied by the development of an immune response *in vitro.* At 2 years of age, however, this child began to have recurrent infections and also showed a reduced percentage of CD4[+] T cells as well as a diminished response to pokeweed mitogen.

TREATMENT OF DiGEORGE SYNDROME WITH THYMOSIN FRACTION 5

One of the remaining two infants with DiGeorge syndrome just described did not have evidence of spontaneous improvement. This child had recurrent infections, pneumonia, and otitis media, requiring almost continuous hospitalizations and failing to grow. After unsuccessful treatment of a fever for 1 month, reconstitution of immune function was attempted using TF-5 by twice weekly subcutaneous injection at 1.5 mg/kg. Initial immune studies showing a normal response to phytohemagglutinin and almost no response to microbial activators and an inverted CD4/CD8 ratio had not changed significantly during the first year of life (CD3 = 24.5%, CD4 = 13.2%, and CD8 = 30.0%). The absolute CD4[+] T-cell level was 470. In a very dramatic response to TF-5 therapy, the clinical condition resolved within a week and the child was discharged. During the next 2 years this patient continued to develop normally, with dose escalations as needed for weight gain. Infections noted on several occasions before weight adjustment suggested a continued need for thymic factor replacement.

Immune evaluation in this case before TF-5 therapy and during treatment has shown two principal features: (1) a decline in CD8[+] T-cell percentage and (2) an increased response to IL-2. A decline in CD8[+] T-cell percentage was analyzed statistically using two pretreatment baseline values *versus* 13 posttreatment determinations, and the difference was significant (p <0.01) (FIG. 3). In addition, the response to IL-2 was significantly improved. As a result of the decreasing percentage of CD8[+]

T-cells, the CD4/CD8 ratio normalized for some months, but not completely consistently. It seems probable that survival of the patient was directly related to TF-5.

THYMIC FACTOR THERAPY IN IDIOPATHIC CD4⁺ T-CELL DEFICIENCY

Recently there have been reports of an AIDS-like CD4⁺ T-cell lymphopenia of unknown cause[44] with a fatal outcome in some cases. There appears to be no single underlying link, and in fact there may be multiple causes and no successful treatment. In evaluating immune deficiency in a young child we evaluated and ultimately treated a potentially related case. A 2-month-old girl developed respiratory syncytial virus infection, and despite extensive treatment with antiviral, antifungal, and antimicrobial medications continued to be febrile and in serious condition. Previous history included herpes stomatitis, herpes encephalitis, and chronic dermal and fungal infections. Although HIV testing of both parents and child gave persistently negative results, this child had a CD4⁺ T-cell percentage of less than 25%, which in the context of persistent lymphopenia was associated with an absolute CD4⁺ T-cell level of about 200. Percentages of CD3⁺ and CD8⁺ T cells were normal.

Evaluation of immune deficiency in this case revealed chronic susceptibility to viral and fungal infections, anergy to intradermal skin testing, consistent reduction of CD4⁺ T cells, and pan hypogammaglobulinemia. Adenosine deaminase and nucleoside phosphorylase activities were normal. The primary defect involved the T-cell system. B-cell percentages were normal, and the natural killer cell system was intact in terms of both the number of CD56⁺ lymphocytes and the level of killing of K562 target cells *in vitro*. Response to pokeweed mitogen *in vitro* was normal. As the condition of this child worsened, she was intubated and ventilated. Ultimately, following multiple pneumothoraces she required two bronchoscopies to drain and attempt reexpansion of the right upper lobe. An attempt to reconstitute her immune system in the context of essentially refractory pneumonia was undertaken as a last resort, and TF-5 was given. Clinical improvement was gradual but steady over a 2-month period. As we had observed previously with TF-5 treatment in the DiGeorge syndrome, the percentage of CD4$_4$⁺ T cells increased. Lymphopenia lessened in severity and remained improved, as shown in FIGURE 4. Skin test responsiveness was normal after 5 months of treatment, and immunoglobulin levels normalized. Although residual reactive airway disease continued with chronic pulmonary fibrosis and recurrent but treatable oral thrush, the child grew well on TF-5. The immune response *in vitro* has not yet fully normalized, supporting the hypothesis of an intrinsic T-cell defect possibly related to increased apoptosis *in vitro* (data not shown). Response to IL-2, as shown in FIGURE 5, improved markedly however. It is evident that TF-5 had a reconstituting effect and directly affected T-cell function in this case.

SUMMARY AND CONCLUSIONS

Current knowledge on the role of thymic factors in the immune response is inadequate and remains relatively primitive when compared with present technical possibilities for assessing lymphocyte subsets or cytokine interaction. New studies

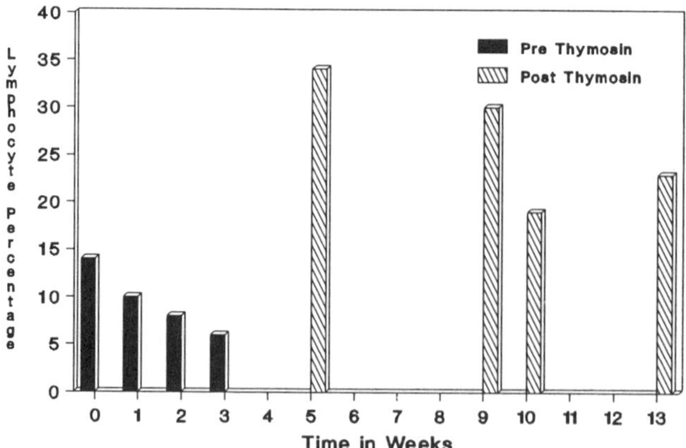

FIGURE 4. Effect of thymosin fraction 5 (TF-5) treatment on percentage of lymphocytes in idiopathic CD4+ T-cell deficiency.

support the potential importance of thymic factors as regulators of immune interactions. Indirect evidence supports the concept that thymic factors may work at the level of IL-2. The functional identity of cells responsive to thymic factors and the relation of observed effects to cytokine network interactions need to be established. The use of thymic factors in the future will depend on the development of criteria to identify appropriate settings in which to use such factors and the implementation of appropriate measures of immune functional response.

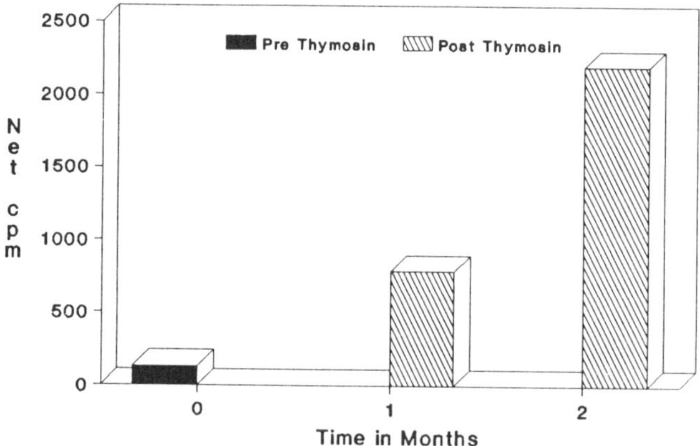

FIGURE 5. Data representing response to interleukin-2 (IL-2) before and after TF-5 therapy. Data are presented as cpm of proliferative response *in vitro* of isolated peripheral blood mononuclear cells.

ACKNOWLEDGMENTS

The authors acknowledge the expert technical assistance of Cindy (X) Chen, MD, Desiree Ehleiter, Theresa Manalo, Carola Poggenberg, Fotini Halkias, Sang-Hyun Kim, and Daphne Liu.

REFERENCES

1. DiGeorge, A. M. 1968. Congenital absence of the thymus and its immunological consequences: Concurrence with congenital hypoparathyroidism. *In* Immunological Deficiency in Man. Birth Defects. D. Bergsma & R. A. Good, eds. Original Article Series IV, p. 116.

2. Harrington, H. 1829. (Letter to the Editor.) London Med. Gaz. **3:** 314.

3. Ammann, A. J., D. W. Wara, S. Salman, & H. Perkins. 1973. Thymus transplantation: Permanent reconstitution of cellular immunity in a patient with sex linked combined immunodeficiency. N. Engl. J. Med. **289:** 5-9.

4. Ammann, A. J., D. W. Wara, N. E. Doyle, & M. S. Golbus. 1975. Thymus transplantation in patients with thymic hypoplasia and abnormal immunoglobulin synthesis. Transplantation **20:** 457-466.

5. Barrett, D. B., D. W. Wara, A. J. Ammann, & M. J. Cowan. 1980. Thymosin therapy in DiGeorge syndrome. J. Pediatr. **97:** 66-71.

6. Steele, R. W., C. Lenias, G. B. Thurman, M. Schuelein, H. Bauer, & J. A. Bellanti. 1977. Familial thymic aplasia: Attempted reconstitution with fetal thymus in a millipore diffusion chamber. N. Engl. J. Med. **287:** 787-791.

7. Miller, J. F. A. P. 1961. Immunological function of the thymus. Lancet **2:** 748-749.

8. Good, R. A., A. P. Dalmasso, G. Martinez, O. K. Archer, J. C. Pierre, & B. W. Papermaster. 1962. The role of the thymus in development of immunologic capacity in rabbits and mice. J. Exp. Med. **116:** 773-778.

9. Osoba, D. & J. F. A. Miller. 1963. Evidence for a humoral thymus factor responsible for the maturation of immunological faculty. Nature **199:** 653-658.

10. Schulof, R. S. & A. L. Goldstein. 1983. Clinical applications of thymosin and other thymic hormone. *In* Recent Advances in Clinical Immunology. N.A. Thompson & N.R. Rose, eds.: 243-285. Churchill Livingstone. New York.

11. Stutman, O., E. J. Yunis & R. A. Good. 1970. Studies on thymus function. I. Cooperative effect of thymic function and lymphopoietic cells in restoration of neonatally thymectomized mice. J. Exp. Med. **132:** 583-600.

12. Stutman, O. 1975. The post thymic precursor cell. *In* The Biological Activity of Thymic Hormones. D.W. Van Bekkum, ed.: 87-94. Kooyker Sci. Pub. Rotterdam.

13. Incefy, G. S., N. Flomenberg, G. Heller, N. A. Kernan, J. Brochstein, D. Kirkpatrick, N. Kapoor, S. Groshen, & R. J. O'Reilly. 1990. Evidence that appearance of thymulin in plasma follows lymphoid chimerism and precedes development of immunity in patients with lethal combined immunodeficiency transplanted with T cell-depleted haploidentical marrow. Transplantation **50:** 55-61.

14. Miller, J. F. A. P. 1962. Immunological significance of the thymus of the adult mouse. Nature (Lond) **195:** 1318-1319.

15. Steinman, G. G., B. Klaus, & H.-K. Muller-Hermelink. 1985. The involution of the aging human thymic epithelium is independent of puberty. Scand. J. Immunol. **22:** 563-575.

16. Clarke, A. G. & K. A. MacLennan. 1986. The many facets of thymic involution. Immunol. Today **7:** 204-205.

17. DARDENNE, M., P. A. KELLY, J. F. BACH, & W. SAVINO. 1991. Identification and functional activity of prolactin receptors in thymic epithelial cells. Proc. Natl. Acad. Sci. USA **88:** 9700–9704.

18. BESCHORNER, W. E., J. DIVIC, H. PULIDO, X. YAO, P. KENWORTHY & G. BRUCE. 1991. Enhancement of thymic recovery after cyclosporine by recombinant human growth hormone and insulin-like growth faction. Transplantation **53:** 879–884.

19. IWATA, T., G. S. INCEFY, S. CUNNINGHAM-RUNDLES, C. CUNNINGHAM-RUNDLES, E. SMITHWICK, N. GELLER, P. J. O-REALLY & R. A. GOOD. 1981. Circulating thymic hormone activity (FTS) in patients with primary and secondary immunodeficiency diseases. Am. J. Med. **71:** 385–394.

20. GRAVENSTEIN, S., E. H. DUTHIE, B. A. MILLER, E. ROECKER, P. DRINKA, K. PRATHIPATI & W. B. ERSHLER. 1989. Augmentation of influenza antibody response in elderly men by thymosin α_1. A double blind placebo controlled clinical study. J. Am. Geriatr. Soc. **37:** 1–8.

21. GOLDSTEIN, A. L., ED. 1984. Thymic Hormone and Lymphokines; Basic Chemistry and Clinical Applications. Plenum Press. New York.

22. HAYNES, B. F., S. M. DENNING, P. T. LE & K. H. SINGER. 1990. Human intrathymic T cell differentiation. Semin. Immunol. **2:** 67–77.

23. CHEN, W. F., W. FAN, L. X. CAO & P. X. ZHANG. 1992. Multiple types of cytokines constituitively produced by an established murine thymic epithelial cell line. Eur. Cytokine Netw. **3:** 43–52.

24. DEMAN, J., M. T. MARTIN, P. DELVENNE, C. HUMBLET, J. DONIVER & M. P. DEFRESNE. 1992. Analysis by *in situ* hybridization of cells expressing mRNA for tumor necrosis factor in the developing thymus of mice. Dev. Immunol. **3:** 103–109.

25. GIROIR, B. P., T. BROWN & B. BEULLER. 1992. Constitutive synthesis of tumor necrosis factor in the thymus. Proc. Natl. Acad. Sci. USA **89:** 4864–4868.

26. DARDENNE, M. & J. F. BACH. 1993. Rationale for mechanism of zinc interaction in the immune system. *In* Nutrient Modulation of Immune Response. S. Cunningham-Rundles, ed.: 501–510 Marcel Dekker. Inc. New York.

27. DARDENNE, M., N. BOUKAIBA, M. C. GAGNERAULT, F. HOMO-DELARCHE, P. CHAPPUIS, D. LEMONNIER & W. SAVINO. 1993. Restoration of the thymus in aging mice by *in vivo* zinc supplementation. Clin. Immunol. Immunopathol. **66:** 127–135.

28. COTO, J. A., E. M. HADDEN, M. SAURO, N. ZORN & J. W. HADDEN. Interleukin 1 regulates secretion of zinc-thymulin by human thymic epithelial cells and its action on T-lymphocyte proliferation and nuclear protein kinase C. Transplant **50:** 55–61.

29. MURPHY, M., D. S. FRIEND, L. PIKE-NOBILE & L. B. EPSTEIN. 1992. Tumor necrosis factor-α and IFN γ expression in human thymus. Localization and over expression in Down syndrome (trisomy 21). J. Immunol. **149:** 2506–2512.

30. PESCARMONA, E, A. PISACANE, E. PIGNATELLI & C. D. BARONI. 1993. Expression of epidermal and nerve growth factor receptors in human thymus and thymomas. Histopathology **23:** 39–44.

31. ANTONIO, M., C. FAVALLI, S. GRELLI, F. INNOCENTI & E. GARACI. 1991. Thymosin α 1 potentitiates interleukin 2-induced cytotoxic activity in mice. Cell Immunol. **133:** 196–205.

32. MASTINO, A., C. FAVALLI, S. GRELLI, G. RASI, F. PICA, A. L. GOLDSTEIN & E. GARACI. 1992. Combination therapy with thymosin α_1 potentiates the anti-tumor activity of interleukin-2 with cyclophosphamide in the treatment of the Lewis lung carcinoma in mice. J. Cancer **50:** 493–499.

33. SERRATE, S., R. SCHULOF, M. B. LEONDARIDIS, A. L. GOLDSTEIN & M. B. SZTEIN. 1987. Modulation of human natural killer cell cytotoxic activity lymphokine production and interleukin 2 receptor expression by thymic hormones. J. Immunol. **139:** 2338–2343.

34. LIN, C. Y., Y. C. KUO, C. C. LIN & B. R. OU. 1988. Enhancement of interleukin-2 and γ-interferon production *in vitro* on cord blood lymphocytes and *in vivo* on primary cellular immunodeficiency patients with thymic extract (thymostimulin). J. Clin. Immunol. **8:** 103-107.

35. MUTCHNICK, M. G., H. D. APPELMAN, H. T. CHUNG, E. ARAGONA, T. P. GUPTA, G. D. CUMMINGS, J. G. WAGGONER, J. H. HOOFNAGLE & D. A. SHAFRITZ. 1991. Thymosin treatment of chronic hepatitis B: A placebo-controlled pilot trial. Hepatology **14:** 409-415.

36. ROILIDES, E., M. CLERICI, C. DEPALMA, M. RUBIN, P. A. PIZZO & G. M. SHEARER. 1991. Helper T cell response in children infected with human immunodeficiency virus type-1. J. Pediatr. **118:** 724-729.

37. WARA, D. W., A. L. GOLDSTEIN, N. E. DOYLE & A. J. AMMANN. 1975. Thymosin activity in patients with cellular immunodeficiency. N. Engl. J. Med. **292:** 70-74.

38. CONELY, M. C., J. B. BECKWITH, J. F. K. MANCIE & L. J. TENCKHOFF & H. W. J. LISHNER. 1979. The spectrum of the DiGeorge syndrome. Pediatrics **94:** 883.

39. SIEBER, O., B. G. DURIE, B. G. HATTLER, S. E. SALMON & V. A. FULGINITI. 1974. Spontaneous evolution of immune competence in DiGeorge syndrome (Abstr.). Pediatr. Res. **8:** 144.

40. BASTIAN, J., S. LAW, L. VOGLER, A. LAUTAN, H. HERROD, S. ANDERSON, S. HEROWITZ & R. HONG. 1989. Prediction of persistent immunodeficiency in the DiGeorge anomaly. J. Pediatr. **115:** 391.

41. GREENBERG, F. 1989. What defines DiGeorge anomaly? J. Pediatr. **115:** 412-413.

42. CLEVELAND, W. W., B. D. FOGEL, W. T. BROWN & H. E. M. KAY. 1968. Foetal thymic transplant in a case of DiGeorge's syndrome. Lancet **2:** 1211.

43. GOLDSOBEL, A. B., A. HAAS & E. R. STIEHM. 1987. Bone marrow transplantation in DiGeorge syndrome. J. Pediatr. **111:** 40-44.

44. HO., D. D., Y. COO, T. ZHU, C. FORTHING, N. WANG, G. GU., R. T. SCHOOLEY & Z. S. DAAR. Idiopathic CD4$^+$ T lymphocytopenia immunodeficiency without evidence of HIV infection. N. Engl. J. Med. **328:** 429-431.

Interaction between the Innate and the Acquired Immune System following Infection of Different Mouse Strains with *Leishmania major*[a]

PHILLIP SCOTT AND TANYA SCHARTON

Department of Pathobiology
School of Veterinary Medicine
University of Pennsylvania
3800 Spruce Street
Philadelphia, Pennsylvania 19104

Leishmania are intracellular parasites of macrophages that cause a diverse range of diseases, from nonapparent infections to fatal visceral disease. Whether infected individuals heal depends on attributes of both the host and the species or strain of *Leishmania*. Murine models of cutaneous leishmaniasis have been studied extensively over the last decade in order to identify some of these host and parasite factors.[1] One of the principal findings is that the nature of the CD4[+] Th cell subset that develops determines if mice are able to heal or control their infections.[2] CD4[+] Th1 cells, which mediate cell-mediated immunity, are the primary cell type associated with protection. Thus, C3H/HeN and C57BL/6 mice infected with *L. major* develop a dominant Th1 response characterized by high levels of gamma interferon (IFN-γ) and little or no interleukin-4 (IL-4), and cutaneous lesions in these mice eventually heal.[3,4] In contrast, infection with *L. major* in BALB/c mice is associated with a predominant CD4[+] Th2 response characterized by the production of IL-4, and the disease is ultimately fatal. The inability of mice to heal, however, is not always associated with a dominant Th2 response, but it can in some cases be associated with the absence of a sufficient Th1 response. For example, *L. amazonensis* infection in C57BL/10 mice fails to heal, whereas *L. major* infections in the same mouse strain resolve.[5] The cytokine response in the *L. amazonensis*-infected B10 mice is characterized by low levels of both IFN-γ and IL-4, whereas cells from B10 mice infected with *L. major* produce high levels of IFN-γ.[5]

One of the most important issues in this field is to identify what determines if mice develop a protective Th1 response. In several systems including experimental leishmaniasis, it has been shown that cytokines influence which T-cell subsets predominate. Thus, when the normally susceptible BALB/c mouse strain is treated with anti-IL-4 antibody prior to *L. major* infection, the mice fail to develop CD4[+] Th2 cells

[a]This work was supported by National Institutes of Health grant AI-30073.

and control the parasite, whereas administration of anti-IFN-γ monoclonal antibodies in healing strains, such as C3H/HeN, inhibits Th1 cell, and promotes Th2 cell, development, and the disease is progressive.[4,6 8] The most elegant *in vitro* model designed to elucidate the mechanisms involved in Th cell subset differentiation used T cells from T-cell receptor transgenic mice, where naive T cells with a particular antigen specificity can be primed with antigen under various conditions.[9-11] As predicted from the leishmanial studies, the conclusions from these studies indicate that a major influence on whether cells become IFN-γ- producing T cells (Th1) or IL-4-producing T cells (Th2) are the levels of certain cytokines present during the primary stimulation. Thus, when IL-4 is included in the primary culture, T cells develop that produce IL-4, but little IFN-γ, when restimulated.[9,10] In contrast, if IL-12 is included in the primary stimulation, cells that produce IFN-γ, but little IL-4, develop.[11] IFN-γ itself does not initiate Th1 cell development, but the capacity of IL-12 to induce IFN-γ-producing T cells appears to depend on the presence of IFN-γ.[12] These studies show that cytokines present at the initial stages of infection may be critical in determining which Th subset predominates, indicating that the environment in which T cells are first exposed to antigen can influence how those T cells subsequently develop. A logical extension of these observations is that the innate immune response occurring during the first several days of infection, during which time *Leishmania*-specific T cells are being primed, could influence the nature of the acquired immune response.[13,14] For this reason, we have been interested in defining the immunologic events occurring during the first several days of *Leishmania* infection. This paper compares the early immunologic responses associated with *L. major* infection in highly resistant (C3H/HeN), relatively resistant (C57BL/6), and susceptible (BALB/c) mice.

MATERIALS AND METHODS

Animals. Female BALB/cAnNCr, C57BL/6NCr, and C3H/HeNCr mice (6 weeks old) were obtained from the National Cancer Institute (Bethesda, MD). Animals were maintained in a pathogen-free environment. Footpad lesion development in *L. major*-infected mice was measured in groups of five mice by monitoring the increase in footpad thickness using a dial micrometer (L. S. Starrett C., Athol, MA) and calculating the difference against the contralateral uninfected footpad measurements.

Parasites and Antigens. A clone of *L. major* (WHO MHOM/IL/80/Friedlin) was used in these studies. Parasites were grown and metacyclic organisms obtained as previously described.[15] Soluble leishmanial antigen was obtained from promastigotes.[16]

Production and Analysis of Cytokines. Single-cell suspensions were prepared from popliteal LNs at various times after infection. Cells were adjusted to a final concentration of 5×10^6 cells/ml in DMEM containing 4.5 mg of glucose per milliliter (Gibco Laboratories, Grand Island, NY), 10% fetal bovine serum, 2 mM glutamine, 100 U/ml penicillin-6-potassium, 100 μg/ml streptomycin sulfate, 25 mM Hepes, and 5×10^{-5} 2-ME. IFN-γ was measured in a two-site ELISA.[17]

Analysis of Natural Killer Cell Activity. Specific cytotoxic activity of the LN was measured against ^{51}Cr-labeled YAC-1 targets in a standard 4-hour chromium release assay.[15]

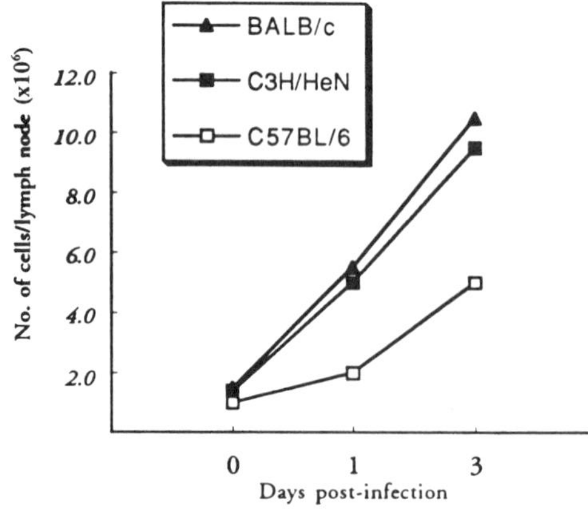

FIGURE 1. LN size following infection with *L. major*. Normal animals or mice infected with 10⁶ *L. major* metacyclic promastigotes were sacrificed after 1 or 3 days, and the popliteal LNs removed and the number of cells quantitated. The data are representative of more than five experiments.

RESULTS

Early Immune Response to L. major *Infection*

BALB/c, C57BL/6, and C3H/HeN mice were infected with 10^6 parasites in the footpad. Normal controls and infected animals were sacrificed at days 1, 2, and 3, and the popliteal lymph node draining the site of infection was removed. LN cells were assayed for their capacity to proliferate and produce IFN-γ. The most apparent difference in the response to infection between these strains was the size of the draining LN (FIG. 1). In all strains an increase in LN size was noticeable as early as day 1 and peaked by day 3. However, the size of the LNs from C3H/HeN and BALB/c mice was significantly different from that of C57BL/6 mice. Consistently, the LNs from C57BL/6 mice were much smaller than those from the two other strains. Furthermore, when the proliferative capacity of these cells was assessed, cells from both BALB/c and C3H/HeN mice responded much better than did cells from C57BL/6 mice to stimulation with soluble leishmanial antigen (FIG. 2). In no case

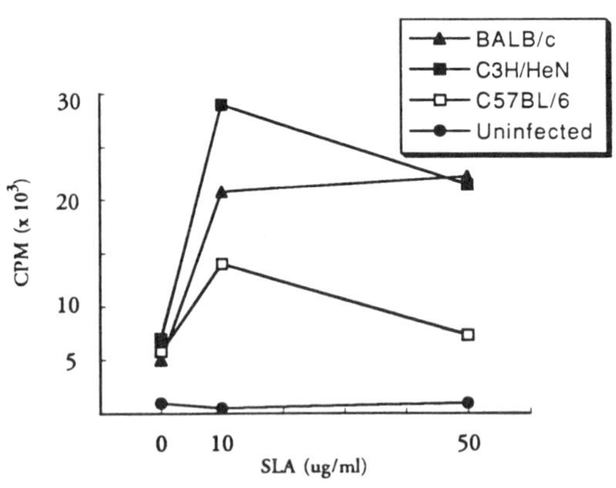

FIGURE 2. The proliferative response of LN cells from normal or *L. major*-infected mice. Mice were infected as described in FIGURE 1 and the popliteal LNs harvested after 3 days. Cells were cultured in the presence or absence of soluble leishmanial antigen (SLA), pulsed with (³H)thymidine on day 3, and harvested on day 4. LN cells from uninfected BALB/c, C3H/HeN, and C57BL/6 all failed to proliferate in response to SLA. (Only the data from uninfected C3H/HeN mice are shown, because identical data were obtained in all three strains.)

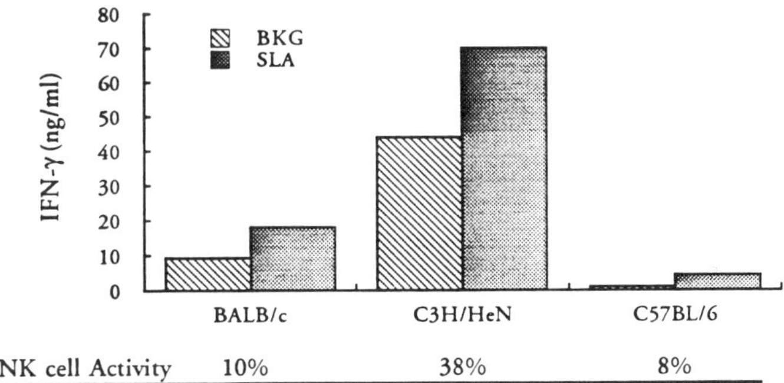

FIGURE 3. IFN-γ production and NK cell activity of LN cells from *L. major*-infected mice. IFN-γ levels were assessed by culturing LN cells harvested 3 days after *L. major* infection without or with soluble leishmanial antigen (SLA) (50 μg/ml) for 72 hours. Supernatants were then collected, and IFN-γ was measured by ELISA. Specific cytotoxic activity of LNs from mice infected for 2 days was measured as previously described.[15] The data shown are from a 100 : 1 effector to target ratio.

was there any response to soluble leishmanial antigen by popliteal LN cells from uninfected mice. These results suggest that while C3H/HeN and BALB/c mice exhibit a rapid and relatively large response to infection, C57BL/6 mice may be delayed in their response.

During the first 2-4 days of infection, differences in cytokine responses were previously observed between BALB/c and C3H/HeN mice. Thus, LN cells from C3H/HeN mice produce high levels of IFN-γ and no detectable IL-4, whereas cells from BALB/c mice produce lower levels of IFN-γ and IL-4.[4,8] To characterize the cytokine response of C57BL/ 6 mice, cells were cultured in the presence or absence of soluble leishmanial antigen and the supernatants assayed for cytokines. Similar to previous results, BALB/c mice produced IL-4 and lower levels of IFN-γ than did C3H/HeN mice (only IFN-γ levels are shown in FIGURE 3). Interestingly, however, cells from C57BL/6 mice produced less IFN-γ than did BALB/c mice. In fact, when adjusted for LN size, the difference was even more dramatic. In unstimulated cultures, BALB/c and C3H/HeN mice produced 19 and 84 ng/LN, respectively, whereas C57BL/6 mice produced 1 ng/LN of IFN-γ. In contrast to C3H/HeN mice in which IL-4 is not detected, IL-4 was produced by cells from C57BL/6 mice, but the presence of IL-4 was variable between experiments. Furthermore, the amount of IL-4 produced when adjusted for the size of the LN was relatively low in these mice compared to BALB/c mice.

Natural Killer Cell Activity in **L. major**-*Infected Mice*

The major source of IFN-γ besides T cells are natural killer (NK) cells. Therefore, we assayed whether the high levels of IFN-γ observed in C3H/HeN mice following *L. major* infection were associated with the induction of an NK cell response. As shown in FIGURE 3, only infection in C3H/HeN mice was associated with a significant

NK cell cytotoxic response. We also found that treatment of mice with an anti-asialo GM1 antiserum abrogated more than 70% of the IFN-γ response associated with *L. major* infection in C3H/HeN mice.[15]

L. major *Infection in C3H/HeN and C57BL/6 Mice*

Inasmuch as the initial response to infection was dramatically different in C3H/HeN and C57BL/6 mice, we tested whether differences in the course of infection between these two resistant strains could be detected. Mice were infected in the footpad with several doses of parasites. As seen in FIGURE 4, for each dose a large difference was noted between the lesion sizes of C3H/HeN and those of C57BL/6 mice. Moreover, while almost all of the C3H/HeN mice had healed infection by 6 weeks regardless of the initial dose, none of the C57BL/6 mice had resolved lesions by this time.

DISCUSSION

Efforts to define the factors responsible for the induction of distinct Th subsets have accelerated over the last year. It is now recognized that components of the innate immune response can signal the adaptive immune response to appropriately react to infection.[13,14] In experimental leishmaniasis we identified three patterns of early responsiveness to *L. major* infection. These include high responders associated with an NK cell response (C3H/ HeN), high responders not associated with an NK cell response (BALB/c), and low responders (C57BL/6). At present, the factors determining which of these responses develops are undefined. Nevertheless, the data demonstrate that infection with this protozoan, at least in BALB/c and C3H/HeN mice, does not go unnoticed by the immune system and suggest that differences in the patterns of early responsiveness may contribute to the type of disease that develops in these mice.

We proposed that the ability to activate NK cells is a major factor involved in the early development of a protective CD4+ Th1 cell response in C3H/HeN mice.[15] In fact, depletion of NK cells in C3H/HeN mice resulted in delayed Th1 cell development as well as increased susceptibility to infection.[15] The ability to develop an early NK cell response may be an important characteristic of infections associated with cell-mediated immunity. At present, determination of the factors involved in NK cell activation (and the absence of such activation) in leishmaniasis is an active area of investigation in this laboratory. However, the ability of mice to eventually develop a Th1 response, or to heal a *L. major* infection, is not absolutely dependent upon an early NK cell response. Thus, C57BL/6 mice failed to exhibit a significant cytokine or NK cell response during the first several days of infection, but their lesions eventually healed. Although the eventual dominance of Th1 cells in C57BL/6 mice does not depend on an early NK cell response, it still depends on IFN-γ, because anti-IFN-γ treatment renders this strain susceptible to *L. major*.[7] We postulated that a delayed mechanism exists for the generation of Th1 cells in these animals.[15] How such a mechanism functions is unclear. However, it has been postulated that the slow development of an immune response favors cell-mediated immunity,[18] which might

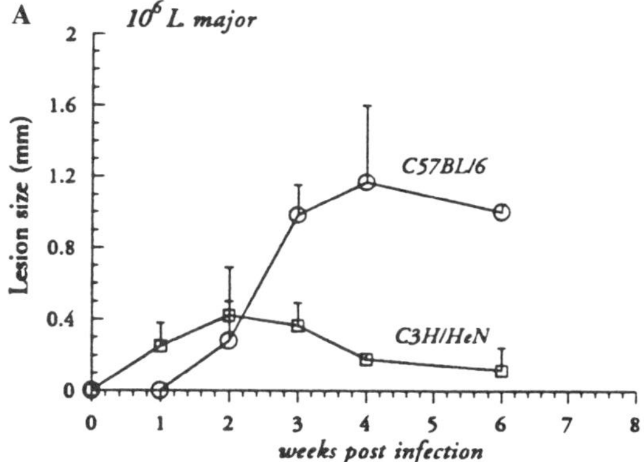

FIGURE 4. Course of *L. major* infection in C3H/HeN and C57BL/6 mice. Five mice were infected in the right hind footpad with either 10^6 (**A**), 10^7(**B**), or 10^8 (**C**) metacyclic promastigotes, and the lesion size was assessed by comparing infected and uninfected hind feet. The data represent the mean ± SD of five mice. The *asterisk* in **B** indicates that one mouse, which had a lesion greater than 3 mm in size, was excluded from this measurement.

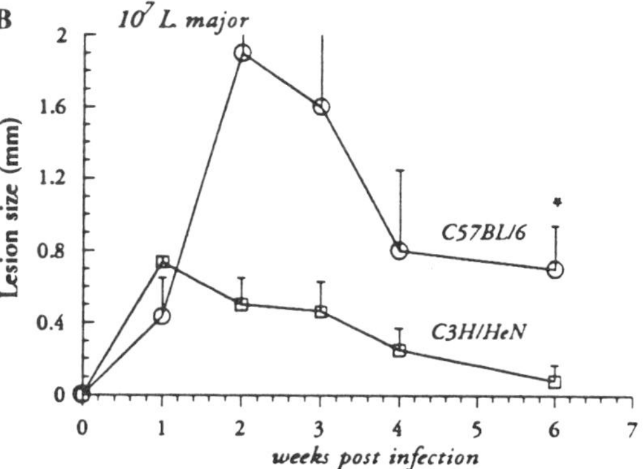

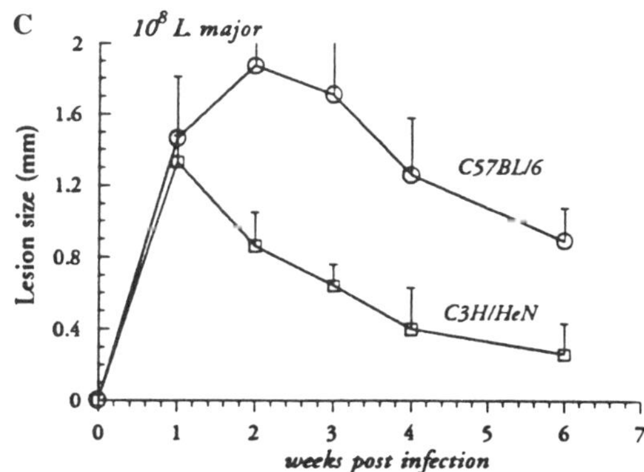

explain the ability of C57BL/6 mice to eventually develop a protective Th1 response. In support of this idea, a variety of immunosuppressive treatments, such as depletion of CD4[+] T cells[19] or low level irradiation,[20] which are expected to suppress the early immune response, promote resistance to *L. major* in the normally susceptible BALB/ c mouse. Similarly, transfer of low numbers of T cells from normal BALB/c mice into BALB/c nude or *SCID* mice leads to enhanced resistance, whereas transfer of larger numbers of cells promotes susceptibility.[21,22] One hypothesis to explain these observations is that an early strong immune response leads to increased levels of IL-4 that initiate CD4[+] Th2 cell development. However, if NK cells are a component of this early response, as occurs in C3H/HeN mice, IL-4 production is suppressed. On the other hand, if no rapid immune response develops that can substantially augment IL-4 levels, CD4[+] Th1 cells develop over time as the "default pathway" for CD4[+] Th cell development.

For the most part, mice have been classified as either resistant or susceptible to *L. major*. However, all mice are susceptible to infection, and even following healing they maintain low numbers of parasites either at the initial infection site or in the draining lymph node (authors' observations). Thus, susceptible mice are those in which the lesions do not heal. The best example are BALB/c mice, in which an infection with greater than 10^4 parasites routinely causes a disease characterized by a progressive increase in lesion size, metastasis of the parasites, and eventual death of the mice. Interestingly, even these "susceptible" mice may develop resistance if infected with very low numbers of parasites.[23] In contrast, resistant strains of mice develop lesions that eventually resolve. However, within the category of resistant mice are strains that develop minimal lesions and rapidly resolve, whereas others develop much larger lesions that take longer to heal. For example, although C3H/ HeN and C57BL/6 mice developed lesions that eventually healed, the severity of these lesions was different. Thus, at all parasite doses tested, C3H/ HeN exhibited transient lesions that healed within 6 weeks, whereas C57BL/6 mice developed lesions that were two- to threefold larger than those of C3H/HeN mice and were delayed in healing. We postulate that the difference in the course of infection between C3H/ HeN and C57BL/6 mice is related to the absence of an early NK cell response.[15]

Many questions concerning the nature of the early immune response to *L. major* infection have yet to be answered. For example, is the proliferative response of cells taken from infected mice at 3 days antigen specific, which cells are proliferating during this early phase of infection, what determines whether NK cells are activated, and why do C57BL/6 mice exhibit a minimal early response. The answers to these questions will be important both for further understanding the factors responsible for susceptibility to *L. major* as well as for defining the factors that contribute to CD4[+] Th cell subset development *in vivo*.

ACKNOWLEDGMENTS

The authors thank Drs. L. C. C. Afonso and L. Q. Vieira for helpful comments and Leslie Taylor for technical assistance.

REFERENCES

1. LIEW, F. Y. & C. A. O'DONNELL. 1993. Immunology of leishmaniasis. Adv. Parasitol. **32:** 161–259.

2. LOCKSLEY, R. M. & P. SCOTT. 1991. Helper T-cell subsets in mouse leishmaniasis: Induction, expansion and effector function. Immunol. Today **12:** A58–A61.

3. HEINZEL, F. P., M. D. SADICK, S. S. MUTHA & R. M. LOCKSLEY. 1991. Production of IFN-g, IL-2, IL-4 and IL-10 by CD4+ lymphocytes *in vivo* during healing and progressive murine leishmaniasis. Proc. Natl. Acad. Sci. USA **88:** 7011–7016.

4. SCOTT, P. 1991. IFN-gamma modulates the early development of Th1 and Th2 responses in a murine model of cutaneous leishmaniasis. J. Immunol. **147:** 3149–3155.

5. AFONSO, L. C. C. & P. SCOTT. 1993. Immune responses associated with the susceptibility of C57BL/10 mice to *Leishmania amazonensis.* Infect. Immunol. **61:** 2952–2959.

6. BELOSEVIC, M., D. S. FINBLOOM, P. H. VAN DER MEIDE, M. V. SLAYTER & C. A. NACY. 1989. Administration of monoclonal anti-IFN-gamma antibodies *in vivo* abrogates natural resistance of C3H/HeN mice to infection with *Leishmania major.* J. Immunol. **143:** 266–274.

7. SADICK, M. D., F. P. HEINZEL, B. J. HOLADAY, R. T. PU, R. S. DAWKINS & R. M. LOCKSLEY. 1990. Cure of murine leishmaniasis with anti-interleukin 4 monoclonal antibody. Evidence for a T cell-dependent, interferon gamma-independent mechanism. J. Exp. Med. **171:** 115–127.

8. CHATELAIN, R., K. VARKILA & R. L. COFFMAN. 1992. IL-4 induces a Th2 response in *Leishmania major*-infected mice. J. Immunol. **148:** 1182–1187.

9. HSIEH, C.-S., A. B. HEIMBERGER, J. S. GOLD, A. O'GARRA & K. M. MURPHY. 1992. Differential regulation of T helper phenotype development by interleukins 4 and 10 in an α,β T-cell-receptor transgenic system. Proc. Natl. Acad. Sci. USA **89:** 6065–6069.

10. SEDER, R. A., W. E. PAUL, M. M. DAVIS & B. FAZEKAS DE ST. GROTH. 1992. The presence of interleukin 4 during *in vitro* priming determines the lymphokine-producing potential of CD4+ T cells from T cell receptor transgenic mice. J. Exp. Med. **176:** 1091–1098.

11. HSIEH, C.-S., S. E. MACATONIA, C. S. TRIPP, S. F. WOLF, A. O'GARRA & K. M. MURPHY. 1993. Development of Th1 CD4+ T cells through IL-12 produced by *Listeria*-induced macrophages. Science **260:** 547–549.

12. MACATONIA, S. E., C.-S. HSIEH, K. M. MURPHY & A. O'GARRA. 1993. Dendritic cells and macrophages are required for Th1 development of CD4+ T cells from ab-TCR transgenic mice: IL-12 can substitute for macrophages to stimulate IFN-g production. Int. Immunol. **5:** 1119–1128.

13. ROMAGNANI, S. 1992. Induction of Th1 and Th2 responses: A key role for the 'natural' immune response? Immunol. Today **13:** 379–383.

14. JANEWAY, C. A., JR. 1992. The immune system evolved to discriminate infectious nonself from noninfectious self. Immunol. Today **13:** 11–16.

15. SCHARTON, T. M. & P. SCOTT. 1993. Natural killer cells are a source of IFN-g that drives differentiation of CD4$^+$ T cell subsets and induces early resistance to *Leishmania major* in mice. J. Exp. Med. **178:** 567–577.

16. SCOTT, P., E. PEARCE, P. NATOVITZ & A. SHER. 1987. Vaccination against cutaneous leishmaniasis in a murine model. I. Induction of protective immunity with a soluble extract of promastigotes. J. Immunol. **139:** 221–227.

17. MOSMANN, T. R. & T. A. T. FONG. 1989. Specific assays for cytokine production by T cells. J. Immunol. Methods **116:** 151–155.

18. BRETSCHER, P. A. 1992. An hypothesis to explain why cell-mediated immunity alone can contain infections by certain intracellular parasites and how immune class regulation of the response against such parasites can be subverted. Immunol. Cell Biol. **70:** 343–351.

19. TITUS, R. G., R. CEREDIG, J. C. CEROTTINI & J. A. LOUIS. 1985. Therapeutic effect of anti-L3T4 monoclonal antibody GK1.5 on cutaneous leishmaniasis in genetically-susceptible BALB/c mice. J. Immunol. **135:** 2108–2114.

20. HOWARD, J. G., C. HALE & F. Y. LIEW. 1981. Immunologic regulation of experimental cutaneous leishmaniasis. IV. Prophylactic effect of sublethal irradiation as a result of abrogation of suppressor T cell generation in mice genetically susceptible to *Leishmania tropica.* J. Exp. Med. **153:** 557–568.

21. MITCHELL, G. F., J. M. CURTIS, R. G. SCOLLAY & E. HANDMAN. 1981. Resistance and abrogation of resistance to cutaneous leishmaniasis in reconstituted BALB/c nude mice. Aust. J. Exp. Med. Biol. Sci. **59:** 539–554.

22. VARKILA, K., R. CHATELAIN, L. M. C. C. LEAL & R. L. COFFMAN. 1993. Reconstitution of C.B-17 *scid* mice with BALB/c T cells initiates a T helper type-1 response and renders them capable of healing *Leishmania major* infection. Eur. J. Immunol. **23:** 262–268.

23. BRETSCHER, P. A., G. WEI, J. N. MENON & H. BIELEFELDT-OHMANN. 1992. Establishment of stable, cell-mediated immunity that makes "susceptible" mice resistant to *Leishmania major.* Science **257:** 539–542.

Modification of Amphotericin B's Therapeutic Index by Increasing Its Association with Serum High-Density Lipoproteins[a]

KISHOR M. WASAN [b-d] AND
GABRIEL LOPEZ-BERESTEIN [e,f]

[b]Department of Cell Biology
Cleveland Clinic Foundation
Research Institute
Cleveland, Ohio 44195

[c]Department of Thoracic, Head and Neck Medical Oncology
and
[e]Section of Immunobiology and Drug Carriers
Department of Clinical Investigations
The University of Texas M.D. Anderson Cancer Center
Houston, Texas 77030

Amphotericin B (AmpB) remains one of the most effective and widely used agents in the treatment of systemic fungal infections (ie, *Candida albicans, Histoplasma capsulatum,* and *Aspergillosis niger*).[1] Its clinical use, however, is limited by dose-dependent renal toxicity that can result in a twofold decrease in the glomerular filtration rate and renal plasma flow, followed by renal potassium and magnesium wasting.[2,3] AmpB's antifungal activity is related to its amphiphilic structure, which facilitates binding to cell membrane sterols causing a disruption in membrane integrity and specifically to its preferential binding to ergosterol in fungal membranes rather than to cholesterol in mammalian membranes.[4] Several approaches have been developed to modify the therapeutic index of AmpB.

One approach is to reduce the nephrotoxicity associated with the administration of AmpB without altering its antifungal activity by incorporating AmpB into liposomes. Liposomes are nontoxic lipid particles that are taken up predominantly by the mononuclear phagocyte system.[5] When AmpB was incorporated into liposomes (L-AmpB) composed of dimyristoyl phosphatidylcholine (DMPC) and dimyristoyl phosphatidylglycerol (DMPG) (7:3 w/w), it was shown to be more active in experimental fungal

[a]This work was supported in part by Core grant CA 16672.

[d]Fellow of the American Society of Pharmacology and Experimental Therapeutics.

[f]Address for correspondence: Gabriel Lopez-Berestein, MD, Section of Immunobiology and Drug Carriers, Box 60, The University of Texas M.D. Anderson Cancer Center, 1515 Holcombe Blvd., Houston, TX 77030.

infections, well tolerated in doses up to 5 mg per kg of body weight, and effective when conventional AmpB therapy had failed.[6-9] When L-AmpB was administered, an increased concentration of AmpB occurred in the kidney without the associated renal toxicity of free AmpB, suggesting that AmpB's incorporation into a lipid carrier altered the drug's interaction with renal tissue.[9] Previous studies demonstrated a decrease of AmpB cytotoxicity when the agent was delivered as L-AmpB to LLC PK1 pig renal cells[10,11] and to primary cultures of rabbit proximal tubular cells.[12] To date, the mechanisms that result in the decreased renal cytotoxic effects of L-AmpB are not fully understood. Krause and Juliano[11] suggested that the decreased toxicity of L-AmpB compared with that of AmpB is related to a selective transfer of the drug from liposomes to fungal membranes, but membranes of mammalian cells.

When AmpB-free liposomes composed of DMPC and DMPG in a 7:3 w/w ratio were injected into the bloodstream of humans, a large volume of distribution (V_d) and a long terminal half-life ($t_{1/2\beta}$) resulted.[1,3] The large V_d of AmpB in humans (4 L/kg) seems to be a result of its high accumulation in the kidney, liver, and lung tissues.[1,3] Furthermore, pharmacokinetic studies in humans have shown AmpB to have a long $t_{1/2\beta}$ (15 days) and a very short distribution half-life ($t_{1/2\alpha}$). When AmpB was injected intravenously into mice, only 15% of the original dose could be accounted for: 10% in the lung and 5% in the liver.[7] AmpB injected intravenously into animals infected with *C. albicans* resulted in the slow release of the drug from tissue sites.[2,13,14]

We further demonstrated a lower area under the serum AmpB concentration time-curve (AUC), a greater V_d, and a systemic clearance of AmpB in an induced-diabetic rat model, a direct result of the rat's hyperlipidemia and hyperlipoproteinemia.[9] Lower distribution of AmpB to the kidney and liver and fewer nephrotoxic effects of AmpB were further observed in diabetic rats; however, the pharmacokinetics, tissue distribution, and extent of nephrotoxic effects of L-AmpB were unchanged.[9]

The interaction of a number of lipophilic compounds including cyclosporine[15] and AmpB[13] with serum lipoproteins may explain the pharmacokinetics and tissue distribution of these compounds. Lipoproteins, important in the homeostasis of cholesterol in the systemic circulation, are spherical particles ranging from 7 to 25 nm in size, that contain a nonaqueous core.[16] Recent studies have shown that high-density lipoproteins (HDL) target cholesterol to the liver from peripheral tissues, whereas low-density lipoproteins (LDL) target cholesterol to a variety of other tissues besides the liver (ie, kidney, skeletal muscle, and spleen).[17]

Brajtburg and coworkers demonstrated that AmpB was equally distributed among HDL and LDL after 1 hour of incubation at 25°C[18] and that AmpB-induced cytotoxic effects on mammalian red blood cells but not on *C. albicans* fungal cells, decreased in the presence of either HDL or LDL.[19] Further work by Koldin and coworkers[20] observed that a dose level of AmpB considered to be nontoxic (1.0 mg/kg) given to rabbits in a mixture with LDL was more toxic than was AmpB administered alone. The authors attributed the differences to the modified tissue distribution of AmpB; however, no studies were performed to confirm their hypothesis. Investigators have further reported that a formulation of an emulsion of AmpB and Intralipid® (20%) used to treat fungal infections in neutropenic patients[21] and systemic murine candidasis[22] reduced acute AmpB toxicity without altering its antifungal activity.

This review describes a series of experiments designed to further explain the enhanced therapeutic index reported following the administration of L-AmpB.

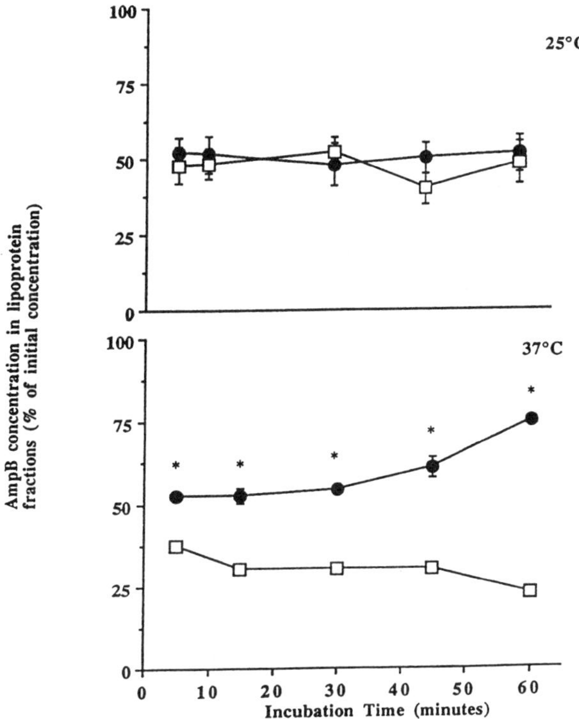

FIGURE 1. AmpB (Fungizone) concentrations in the high-density lipoproteins (●) and low-density lipoproteins (□) fractions when 20 μg/ml of AmpB were incubated at different time intervals in pooled human sera 25 °C and 37 °C. (Mean ± standard deviation, $n = 3$; $p^{(*)} <$ 0.05 *vs* AmpB concentration in low-density lipoprotein fraction.)

INFLUENCE OF TEMPERATURE AND LIPOSOMAL-LIPID CHARGE ON THE DISTRIBUTION OF AMPB INTO SERUM LIPOPROTEINS

We first examined the effects of changes in temperature on the distribution of AmpB into serum lipoproteins.[13] When AmpB (20 μg/mL) was incubated in pooled human sera for 5 through 60 minutes at 25°C, an equal distribution of AmpB between HDL and LDL fractions was observed at the different time-point studies (FIG. 1). However, following 5 through 45 minutes of incubation at 37°C, 54% to 61% of the initial AmpB concentration was recovered in the HDL fraction. After 60 minutes of incubation, more than 75% of the initial AmpB concentration was recovered in the HDL fraction (FIG. 1). The change in distribution of AmpB into serum lipoproteins at 37°C may be related to the transition temperature of lipoproteins, which is between 27°C and 34°C.[23] During the transition, cholesteryl esters within the lipoprotein core that interact with AmpB in serum[23] exist as an isotropic solution, whereas below this temperature the cholesteryl esters form disordered liquid crystals.[23] The core of HDL becomes more ordered at the higher temperature, thus making it easier for the AmpB molecule to associate with it.

Next we examined the role of liposomal charge on the distribution of AmpB into serum lipoproteins.[13] When AmpB was incorporated into negatively charged liposomes composed of DMPC and DMPG (7:3 w/w) at 37 °C, 87% to 92% of the initial AmpB concentration was recovered in the HDL fraction following 5 through 60 minutes of incubation (FIG. 2A). With neutral liposomes composed of DMPC alone, 59% to 79% of the initial AmpB concentration was recovered in the HDL fraction (FIG. 2B). When L-AmpB composed of DMPG alone was studied, 60% to 80% of AmpB was recovered in the HDL fraction (FIG. 2C). With positively charged liposomes of DMPC and stearylamine (SA) (7:1 w/w), 75% to 88% of the initial AmpB concentration was recovered in the HDL fraction (FIG. 2D). The increased distribution of AmpB to HDL when it was incorporated into DMPC:stearylamine (positively charged) and DMPC:DMPG (negatively charged) liposomes may be explained in part by the influence of surface charge on lipid transfer among lipoproteins. Surewicz and coworkers[24] suggested the formation of thermally stable complexes between anionic phospholipids such as DMPG and apolipoprotein A-I, which is one of the major protein components associated with HDL.

We further investigated whether the drug alone transfers to lipoproteins or whether liposomal-lipid transfer is required.[13] Because DMPG is an exogenous anionic phospholipid, its distribution into HDL as opposed to LDL may be responsible for the concurrent transport of AmpB to HDL. When L-AmpB (DMPG:AmpB at a 4:1 molar ratio) composed of DMPC and DMPG (7:3 w/w) was incubated in pooled human sera for 60 minutes at 37°C, 90% and 80% of the initial concentrations of AmpB and DMPG, respectively, were found in a 3:1 molar ratio of DMPG:AmpB in the HDL fraction (TABLE 1). The presence of a surface negative charge appears to be responsible in the altered distribution patterns of AmpB into lipoproteins. In addition, the DMPG:AmpB molar ratio found in the HDL fraction is similar to the initial molar ratio of the liposomes prior to incubation, suggesting that the drug-lipid complex remains intact as it travels to HDL.[13]

INFLUENCE OF LIPOPROTEIN-ASSOCIATED AmpB AND L-AmpB ON THE DRUG'S RENAL TOXICITY AND ANTIFUNGAL ACTIVITY

We next examined the therapeutic importance of a lower AmpB distribution into LDL by determining the influence of AmpB's association with HDL and LDL on its cytotoxic effects to *C. albicans* fungal cells[25] and to further understand the decrease in renal cell toxicity that results when AmpB associates with lipoproteins on LLC PK1 renal cells.[25] For *C. albicans,* the minimum inhibitory concentrations of AmpB and L-AmpB after 18 hours of incubation in the presence or absence of HDL and LDL were not significantly different (FIG. 3). Similar results were obtained for *Aspergillus niger* (data not shown). HDL alone, LDL alone, deoxycholate alone, and empty DMPC plus DMPG containing liposomes did not inhibit fungal growth (data not shown). L-AmpB was significantly less toxic than Fungizone® (AmpB plus Deoxycholate provided by Bristol-Myers Squibb) at 20 μg/ml of AmpB (81.3% ±

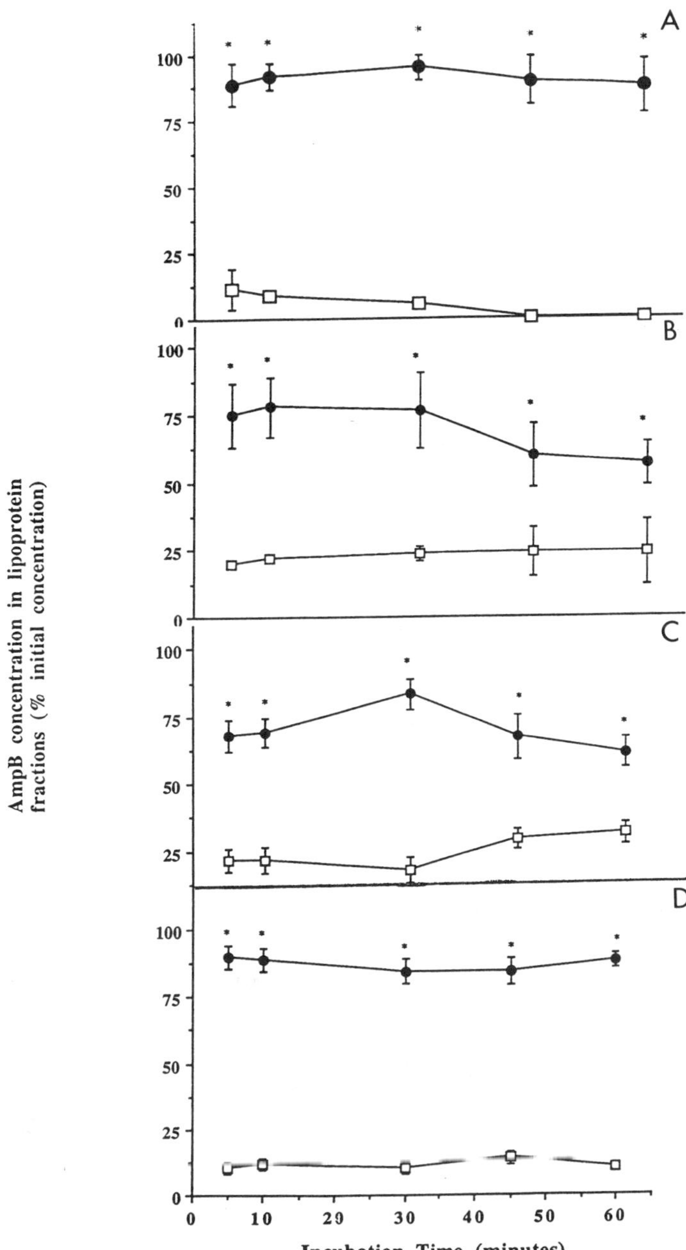

FIGURE 2. AmpB concentrations in the high-density (●) and low-density lipoprotein (□) fractions when 20 µg/ml of L-AmpB composed of **(A)** DMPC:DMPG 7:3 w/w, **(B)** DMPC:AmpB, 10:1 w/ w, **(C)** DMPG:AmpB 10:1 w/w, and **(D)** DMPC:stearylamine, 7:1 w/ w were incubated at different time intervals in pooled human sera at 37°C. (Mean ± standard deviation, $n = 5$; $p^{(*)} < 0.05$ *vs* AmpB concentration in low-density lipoprotein fraction.)

TABLE 1. Distribution of Dimyristoyl Phosphatidylglycerol (DMPG) and Amphotericin B into Serum Lipoproteins after One Incubation at 37°C of Liposomal Amphotericin B

| | DMPG:AmpB Average (Range) | | |
| | Experiment Number | | |
Fraction	1	2	3
Drug-lipid complex	4.17 (0.02):1	4.10 (0.2):1	4.12 (0.02):1
High-density lipoprotein fraction	2.78 (0.75):1	3.15 (0.32):1	3.70 (0.52):1
Low-density lipoprotein fraction	6.25 (1.38):1	5.04 (1.24):1	7.79 (2.76):1

3.6% *vs* 48.3% ± 1.5% cytotoxicity). HDL-associated AmpB, HDL-associated L-AmpB, and LDL-associated L-AmpB were less toxic to LLC PK1 cells than was AmpB (53.0% ± 2.5%, 25.5% ± 2.2%, and 52.2% ± 2.5% *vs* 81.3% ± 3.6% cytotoxicity, respectively), whereas AmpB and LDL-associated AmpB were equally toxic (FIG. 4).

DETERMINATION OF LDL AND apo A-I RECEPTORS ON LLC PK1 CELL CULTURE

To further understand why HDL-associated AmpB causes reduced renal cell toxicity, we next examined LLC PK1 renal cells for the presence of HDL and LDL

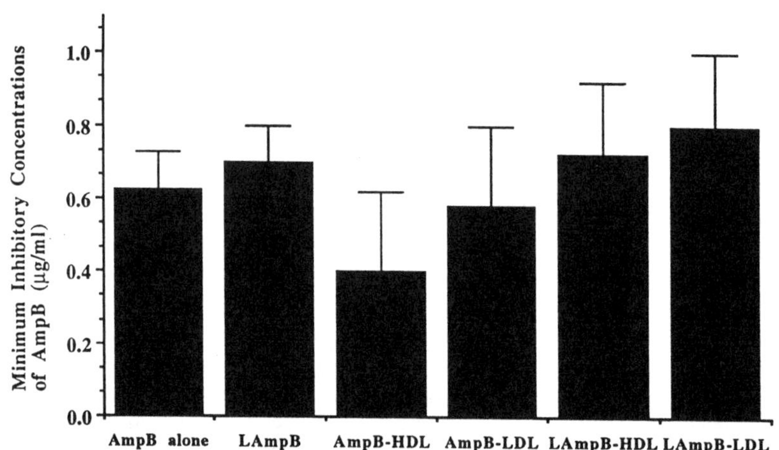

FIGURE 3. Influence of serum lipoprotein-associated AmpB and L-AmpB on *in vitro* antifungal activity of *C. albicans*. Minimal inhibitory concentration of various treatments: AmpB, L-AmpB, mixtures of AmpB with high-density lipoproteins (0.5 mg protein/ml) (AmpB-HDL) or low-density lipoproteins (0.5 mg protein/ml) (AmpB-LDL), and mixtures containing L-AmpB with high-density (L-AmpB-HDL) or low-density lipoproteins (L-AmpB-LDL). (Mean ± standard deviation; $n = 6$; $p^{(*)} < 0.05$ *vs* AmpB alone.)

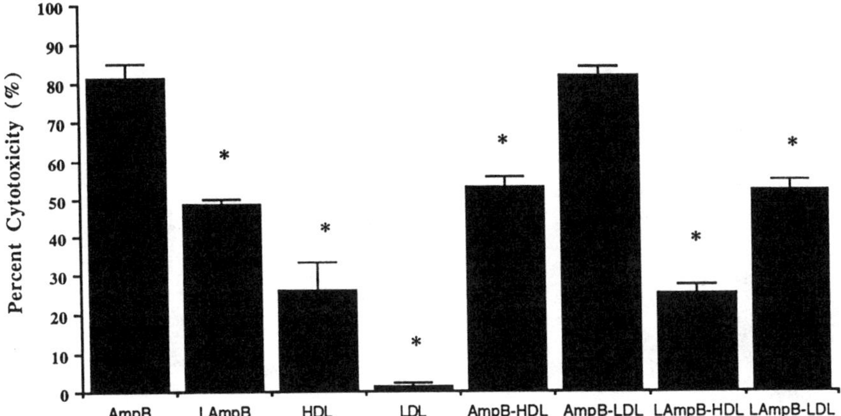

FIGURE 4. Influence of serum lipoprotein-associated AmpB and L-AmpB on the drug's toxicity to LLC PK1 renal cells. Percent cytotoxicity of LLC PK1 cells in serum-free medium at 37°C containing various treatments: AmpB (20 μg/ml), L-AmpB (20 μg/ml of AmpB), high-density lipoproteins (0.5 mg protein/ml), low-density lipoproteins (0.5 mg/ml), mixtures of AmpB (20 μg/ ml) with high-density lipoproteins (AmpB-HDL) or low-density lipoproteins (AmpB-LDL), and mixtures of L-AmpB (20 μg/ml) with high-density lipoproteins (L-AmpB-HDL) or low-density lipoproteins (L-AmpB-LDL). (Mean ± standard deviation; $n = 3$; $p^{(*)}$ <0.05 *vs* AmpB.)

receptors.[25] LLC PK1 renal cells expressed high-affinity ($K_d = 0.054$ ng/ml; 96,000 sites/cell) and low-affinity ($K_d = 222.22$ ng/ml; 77 sites/cell) LDL receptors but only a low-affinity ($K_d = 71.43$ ng/ml; 2 sites/cell) apo A-I receptor (TABLE 2). When the cells were treated with 10% trypsin for 10 minutes, only the high-affinity LDL receptors were not detected. Incubating cells with trypsin did not alter the expression of the low-affinity LDL receptors or the apo A-I receptor (TABLE 2).

INFLUENCE OF REDUCED LDL RECEPTOR EXPRESSION ON HDL- AND LDL-ASSOCIATED AmpB TOXICITY TO LLC PK1 RENAL CELLS

Following incubation with trypsin, HDL- and LDL-associated AmpB was less toxic to the cells than was AmpB (46.6% ± 10.9% and 16.8% ± 15.98% *vs* 74.7% ± 7.7% cytotoxicity, respectively). HDL- and LDL-associated L-AmpB was also less toxic to the cells than was AmpB (20.4% ± 6.2% and 13.5% ± 8.6% *vs* 74.7% ± 7.7% cytotoxicity, respectively) (FIG. 5). The reduced toxicity of HDL-associated AmpB may be explained by the low level of expression of HDL receptors in LLC PK1 cells. The sustained toxicity observed with AmpB alone in trypsinized cells may be related to a direct effect within the cell membrane. However, when AmpB is associated with LDL, the toxicity is maintained, suggesting that both direct membrane-related and nonmembrane-related toxicity may occur (FIG. 6).

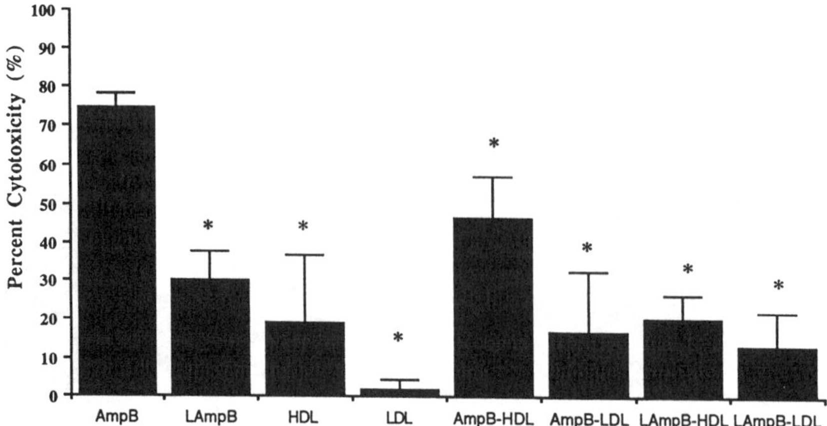

FIGURE 5. Influence of reduced low-density lipoprotein receptor expression on high-density and low-density lipoprotein-associated AmpB toxicity of LLC PK1 renal cells. Percent cytotoxicity of LLC PK1 cells in serum-free medium at 37 °C after trypsin wash containing same treatments as in FIGURE 4. (Mean ± standard deviation; $n = 3$; $p^{(*)} < 0.05$ *vs* AmpB.)

Lipoprotein-associated AmpB and L-AmpB were equally toxic to fungal cells, suggesting that the presence of lipoproteins does not alter the antifungal activity of AmpB and L-AmpB. Such effects may be related to the liberation by fungal lipases of monomeric AmpB from AmpB and L-AmpB independent of its association with lipoproteins.[26,27] The low concentrations of unbound and water-soluble monomeric AmpB present in L-AmpB[28–30] may be sufficient for fungal toxicity but not adequate

TABLE 2. Equilibrium Binding of ^{125}I-Labeled LDL and ^{125}I-Labeled apo A-I (HDL) to LLC PK1 Renal Cells before and after Treatment with Trypsin in Serum-Free Media Using Scatchard Analysis

Lipoprotein Fraction	Surface-Binding Sites (sites/cell)	K_d (ng/ml)
[125]I-apo A-I		
Before trypsin wash	2	71.43
After trypsin wash	17	70.49
^{125}I-LDL (low affinity)		
Before trypsin wash	77	222.22
After trypsin wash	69	198.23
^{125}I-LDL (high affinity)		
Before trypsin wash	96,000	0.0538
After trypsin wash	—	—

ABBREVIATIONS: LDL = low-density lipoproteins; HDL = high-density lipoproteins.

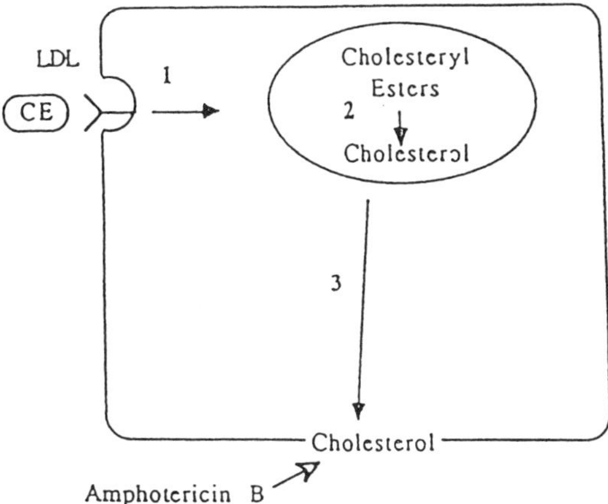

FIGURE 6. Schematic diagram of low-density lipoprotein-associated AmpB's direct membrane and nonmembrane (through endocytosis by the low-density lipoprotein receptor) interaction with renal cells.

for forming AmpB aggregates that are toxic to mammalian cells.[28,30] AmpB-induced mammalian cell toxic effects are reduced when AmpB is in a complex with lipids rather than in its monomeric form.[26,27] The relative distribution of AmpB among serum lipoproteins seems to be a major factor influencing the enhanced therapeutic index of L-AmpB.

PHARMACOKINETICS AND TISSUE DISTRIBUTION OF AmpB AND L-AmpB IN RATS RECEIVING CONTINUOUS INFUSION OF INTRALIPID

The dose level of Intralipid administered as a nutritional supplement in debilitated patients is regulated to prevent the development of severe hypertriglyceridemia but may increase plasma HDL levels.[14,31] Several investigators demonstrated that intravenous fat emulsions are rapidly hydrolyzed by lipoprotein lipase and the exogenously supplied phospholipids and cholesterols accumulate primarily into LDL.[32–35] We demonstrated that a continuous infusion of 5% Intralipid administered to rats for 6 days results in an increase in total serum cholesterol and HDL cholesterol without altering LDL cholesterol (TABLE 3).[36]

AmpB mixed with Intralipid reduced renal toxicity in neutropenic patients without altering total sodium intake.[21] Kirsh and coworkers[22] further reported that the formulation of an emulsion of AmpB and 20% Intralipid used for treating systemic murine candidiasis reduced acute AmpB toxicity without altering its antifungal activity. We examined the influence of concurrent Intralipid infusion on the pharmacokinetics and tissue distribution of AmpB and L-AmpB in rats.[37] The administration of AmpB resulted in a higher AUC and reduced volume of distribution of the central compartment and systemic clearance of AmpB (TABLE 4) without altering AmpB's tissue

TABLE 3. Total Serum Cholesterol, HDL Cholesterol, and LDL Cholesterol Levels in Rats Receiving Continuous Infusion of 0.45% Normal Saline Solution or 5% Intralipid for 6 Days at a Flow Rate of 1.2 ml/Hour

	0.45% Normal Saline Infusion	5% Intralipid Infusion
Total serum cholesterol (mg/dl)	34.3 ± 4.2	68.7 ± 7.1^a
HDL cholesterol (mg/dl)	13.1 ± 2.8	25.7 ± 1.9^a
LDL cholesterol (mg/dl)	8.1 ± 4.2	11.9 ± 1.0
HDL cholesterol:LDL cholesterol	1.62 ± 0.7	2.16 ± 0.5

ABBREVIATIONS: HDL = high-density lipoproteins; LDL = low-density lipoproteins.
NOTE: Data are mean $\pm$ standard deviation ($n = 7$).
[a] p <0.05 *versus* 0.45% normal saline infusion.

distribution in animals receiving Intralipid *versus* 0.45% normal saline infusion (TABLE 5), suggesting that AmpB remains longer in the systemic circulation. The administration of Intraplipid appears not to alter the elimination rate of apolipoprotein A-I and HDL from the bloodstream,[38] but it increases serum HDL,[35] partly as a result of an increase in hepatic protein synthesis of apolipoprotein A-I and A-II.[39] Because the administration of Intralipid may increase lecithin:cholesterol acyltransferase activity,[33] an enzyme that converts free cholesterol into cholesteryl esters within HDL, the increased HDL cholesterol and HDL cholesterol:LDL cholesterol ratio may be caused

TABLE 4. Pharmacokinetic Parameters after a Single Intravenous Dose of AmpB or L-AmpB (1.0 mg/kg) in Rats Receiving Continuous Infusion of 0.45% Normal Saline Solution or 5% Intralipid for 7 Days

		AmpB		L-AmpB	
		0.45% Normal Saline Solution	5% Intralipid	0.45% Normal Saline Solution	5% Intralipid
AUC	ng × min/ml	$75{,}422 \pm 13{,}992$	$157{,}487 \pm 11{,}453^a$	$119{,}000 \pm 57{,}000$	$159{,}000 \pm 65{,}000^a$
k_α	min^{-1}	0.0082 ± 0.002	0.015 ± 0.002^a	0.0105 ± 0.004	0.0094 ± 0.002
k_γ	min^{-1}	0.57 ± 0.45	0.98 ± 1.03	0.504 ± 0.392	0.574 ± 0.568
$t_{1/2\alpha}$	min	165.85 ± 11.46	51.33 ± 18.11^a	73.2 ± 26.9^a	76.0 ± 16.7^a
$t_{1/2\gamma}$	min	1.95 ± 1.53	0.945 ± 0.58	2.43 ± 2.04	4.15 ± 1.41
Cl_s	ml/min/kg	13.55 ± 2.35	5.51 ± 1.58^a	10.14 ± 5.46	7.28 ± 3.72^a
V_c	ml/kg	200.6 ± 61.2	81.75 ± 15.4^a	281.8 ± 212	245.4 ± 234.2

ABBREVIATIONS: AUC = area under the concentration curve for AmpB; k_α = distribution rate constant from systemic circulation; k_γ = distribution rate constant within systemic circulation; $t_{1/2\alpha}$ = α phase half-life; $t_{1/2\gamma}$ = γ phase half-life; Cl_s = systemic clearance of AmpB; V_c = volume of distribution of the central compartment.
NOTE: Data are mean $\pm$ standard deviation ($n = 3$).
[a] p <0.05 *versus* AmpB + 0.45% normal saline solution.

by this increase in lecithin:cholesterol acyltransferase activity and by the absence in the rat of lipid transfer protein, an enzyme responsible for the transfer of cholesteryl esters between HDL and LDL.[40] The increase in HDL cholesterol without the alteration in LDL cholesterol may increase the interaction of AmpB with the cholesterol and cholesteryl esters of HDL and may contribute to the observed decrease in the clearance of AmpB from the bloodstream. However, because the half-life of HDL cholesteryl esters in the rat from the bloodstream is 4 hours,[41] measuring AmpB tissue concentrations 4 hours after intravenous administration of AmpB may not be enough time to see changes in the tissue distribution of AmpB.

Animals given L-AmpB had lower AmpB concentrations in the kidney and lung but higher AmpB concentrations in the spleen when administered Intralipid than when given 0.45% normal saline solution (TABLE 5). Animals receiving infusions of 0.45% normal saline solution had lower concentrations of AmpB in the kidney when given L-AmpB than when given AmpB. Inasmuch as L-AmpB predominantly associates with HDL,[13] the reduced AmpB concentration in the kidney of animals receiving Intralipid or 0.45% normal saline infusion may be a result of the low expression of HDL receptors in the kidney.[25]

These results suggest that AmpB's association with HDL may be responsible for the decreased clearance of the drug from the blood. Increasing AmpB's association with HDL by incorporating the drug into negatively charged liposomes (L-AmpB) further reduced the amount of AmpB found in the kidney (TABLE 5) and may be responsible for the decreased renal toxicity associated with the intravenous administration of L-AmpB.

SUMMARY

AmpB remains one of the drugs of choice in the treatment of systemic fungal infection; however, its therapy is limited by the development of renal toxicity. When AmpB was incorporated into negatively charged liposomes composed of DMPC and

TABLE 5. Tissue Distribution of AmpB or L-AmpB (1.0 mg/kg) in Rats Receiving Continuous Infusion of 0.45% Normal Saline Solution or 5% Intralipid® for 7 Days

| Tissue | AmpB | | L-AmpB | |
	0.45% Normal Saline Solution	5% Intralipid	0.45% Normal Saline Solution	5% Intralipid
Kidney	735.1 ± 285.6	657.8 ± 210	298.2 ± 96.2[a]	155.9 ± 56.3[a,b]
Liver	468.2 ± 169.2	587 ± 305.5	398 ± 280.4	667.9 ± 665.3
Lung	1,906.4 ± 1,526.8	1,799 ± 1,605	695.3 ± 250.2	160.1 ± 46.2[a,b]
Spleen	2,112.9 ± 403.4	2,242.5 ± 1,445	906.6 ± 52.6[a]	1,489 ± 419.9[b]

NOTE: Data are mean ± standard deviation ($n = 3$); ng of AmpB/g of tissue.
[a] $p < 0.05$ *versus* AmpB + 5% Intralipid.
[b] $p < 0.05$ *versus* L-AmpB + 0.45% normal saline solution.

DMPG (L-AmpB), it was less toxic but as effective as free AmpB. However, the mechanism of L-AmpB's enhanced therapeutic index remains unknown.

We have demonstrated that AmpB predominantly associates with HDL when incorporated into positively and negatively charged liposomes. To further understand the therapeutic importance of AmpB predominantly associating with HDL, we next examined the influence of lipoproteins on the antifungal activity and renal cytotoxicity of AmpB. The antifungal activity of AmpB and L-AmpB was not altered in the presence of HDL or LDL. The reduced nephrotoxicity associated with the use of L-AmpB, however, was related to a decreased uptake of AmpB by renal cells when AmpB was associated with HDL, and it may be a result of the low expression of HDL receptors in the LLC PK1 renal cells.

REFERENCES

1. CIPOLLE, R. T. & J. S. SOLOMKIN. 1986. Amphotericin B. *In* W. T. Taylor, M. H. Diers-Caviness, Eds.: 321–328. A Textbook for the Clinical Application of Therapeutic Drug Monitoring. Abbot. Irving, TX.
2. TOLINS, J. P. & L. RAIJ. 1988. Adverse effect of amphotericin B administration on renal hemodynamics in the rat neurohumoral mechanisms and influence of calcium channel blocker. J. Pharmacol. Exp. Ther. **245:** 594–599.
3. CABOR, G. G., R. PAZDUR, F. A. VALERIOTE & L. H. H. BAKER. 1989. Pharmacokinetics and toxicity of continuous infusion of amphotericin B in cancer patients. J. Pharm. Sci. **78:** 307– 310.
4. ANDREOLI, T. E. 1973. On the anatomy of amphotericin B-cholesterol pores in liquid bilayer membranes. Kidney Int. **4:** 337–345.
5. JULIANO, R. L. & J. LAYTON. 1980. *In* Drug Delivery Systems: Characteristics and Biomedical Applications. R. L. Juliano, Ed.: 189–206. Oxford University Press. London.
6. LOPEZ-BERESTEIN, G., R. MEHTA, R. L. HOPER, K. MILLS, L. KASI, K. MEHTA, V. FAINSTEIN, M. LUNA, E. M. HERSH & R. L. JULIANO. 1983. Treatment and prophylaxis of disseminated infection due to *Candida albicans* in mice with liposome-encapsulated amphotericin B. J. Infect. Dis. **147:** 939–945.
7. LOPEZ-BERESTEIN, G., M. G. ROSENBLUM & R. MEHTA. 1984. Altered tissue distribution of amphotericin B by liposomal encapsulation: Comparison of normal mice to mice infected with *Candida albicans.* Cancer Drug Delivery **1:** 199–205.
8. LOPEZ-BERESTEIN, G. 1988. Liposomes as carriers of antifungal drugs. Ann. N.Y. Acad. Sci. **544:** 590–597.
9. WASAN, K. M., K. VADIEI, G. LOPEZ-BERESTEIN & D. R. LUKE. 1990. Pharmacokinetics, tissue distribution, and toxicity of free and liposomal amphotericin B in diabetic rats. J. Infect. Dis. **161:** 562–566.
10. JULIANO, R. L., C. W. M. GRANT, K. R. BARBER & M. A. KALP. 1987. Mechanism of the selective toxicity of amphotericin B incorporated into liposomes. Mol. Pharmacol. **31:** 1– 11.
11. KRAUSE, H. J. & R. L. JULIANO. 1988. Interactions of liposome-incorporated amphotericin B with kidney epithelial cells. Mol. Pharmacol. **34:** 286–297.
12. JOLY, V., S. J. LINE, C. CARBON & P. YENI. 1990. Interactions of free and liposomal amphotericin B with renal proximal tubular cells in primary culture. J. Pharmacol. Exp. Ther. **255:** 17– 22.
13. WASAN, K. M., G. A. BRAZEAU, A. KEYHANI, A. C. HAYMAN & G. LOPEZ-BERESTEIN. 1993. Role of liposome composition and temperature on the distribution of amphotericin B in serum lipoproteins. Antimicrob. Agents Chemoth. **37:** 246–250.

14. GOLDBERG, I. J., W. B. BLANER & T. VANNI. 1990. Role of lipoprotein lipase in the regulation of high density lipoprotein apolipoprotein metabolism. J. Clin. Invest. **86:** 463-473.

15. VADIEI, K., G. LOPEZ-BERESTEIN, R. PEREZ-SOLER & D. R. LUKE. 1989. Efficacy and toxicity of liposomal cyclosporine. Int. J. Pharm. **57:** 125-131.

16. SHAW, J. M., K. V. SHAW, S. YANOVICH, M. IWANIK, W. S. FUTCH, A. ROSOWSKY & L. B. SCHOOK. 1987. Delivery of lipophilic drugs using lipoproteins. Ann. N.Y. Acad. Sci. **81:** 507- 527.

17. MILLER, G. J. & N. E. MILLER. 1975. Serum lipoproteins analysis. Lancet **1:** 16-19.

18. BRAJTBURG, J., S ELBERG, J. BOLARD & G. MEDOFF. 1984. Interaction of plasma proteins and lipoproteins with amphotericin B. J. Infect Dis. **149:** 986-997.

19. BRAJTBURG, J., S. ELBERG, G. S. KOBAYASHI & G. MEDOFF. 1986. Effects of serum lipoproteins on damage to erythrocytes and *Candida albicans* cells by polyene antibiotics. J. Infect. Dis. **153:** 623-626.

20. KOLDIN, M. H., G. S. KOBAYASHI, J. BRAJTBURG & G. MEDOFF. 1985. Effects of elevation of serum cholesterol and administration of amphotericin B complexed to lipoproteins on amphotericin B-induced toxicity in rabbits. Antimicrob. Agents Chemother. **28:** 144-145.

21. MOREAU, P., N. MILPIED, N. FAYETTE, J. F. RAMEE & J. L. HAROUSSEAU. 1992. Reduced renal toxicity and improved clinical tolerance of amphotericin B mixed with Intralipid compared with conventional amphotericin B in neutropenic patients. J. Antimicrob. Chemother. **30:** 535-541.

22. KIRSH, R., R. GOLDSTEIN, J. TARLOFF, D. PARRIS, J. HOOK & N. HANNA. 1988. An emulsion formulation of amphotericin B improves the therapeutic index when treating systemic murine candidiasis. J. Infect. Dis. **158:** 1065-1070.

23. CUSHLEY, R. J., W. D. TRELEAVEN, Y. I. PARMAR, R. S. CHANA & D. B. FENSKE. 1987. Surface diffusion in human serum lipoproteins. Biochem. Biophys. Res. Commun. **146:** 1139-1145.

24. SUREWICZ, W. K., R. M. EPAND, H. J. POWNALL & S. W. HUI. 1986. Human apolipoprotein A-I forms thermally stable complexes with anionic but not with zwitterionic phospholipids. J. Biol. Chem. **261:** 16191-16197.

25. WASAN, K. M., M. G. ROSENBLUM, L. CHEUNG & G. LOPEZ-BERESTEIN. 1994. Influence of lipoprotein-associated amphotericin B on its renal cytotoxicity and antifungal activity. Antimicrob. Agents Chemother. **38:** 223-227.

26. JANOFF, A. S., L. T. BONI, M. C. POPESCU, S. R. MINCHEY, P. R. CULLIS, T. D. MADDEN, T. TARASCHI, S. M. GRUNER, E. SHYAMSUNDER, M. W. TATE, R. MENDELSOHN & D. BONNER. 1988. Unusual lipid structures selectively reduce the toxicity of amphotericin B. Proc. Natl. Acad. Sci. USA **85:** 6122-6126.

27. PERKINS, W. R., S. R. MINCHEY, L. T. BONI, C. E. SWENSON, M. C. POPESCU, R. F. PASTERNACK & A. S. JANOFF. 1992. Amphotericin B-phospholipid interactions responsible for reduced mammalian cell toxicity. Biochim. Biophys. Acta **1107:** 271-282.

28. BOLARD, J., J. LEGRAND, F. HEITZ & B. CYBULSKA. 1991. One-sided action of amphotericin B on cholesterol-containing membranes is determined by its self-association in the medium. Biochemistry **30:** 5707-5715.

29. JULLIEN, S., A. VERTUT-CROQUIN, J. BRAJTBURG & J. BOLARD. 1988. Circular dichroism for the determination of amphotericin B binding to liposomes. Anal. Biochem. **1972:** 197-202.

30. JULLIEN, S., J. BRAJTBURG & J. BOLARD. 1990. Affinity of amphotericin B for phosphatidylcholine vesicles as a determinant of the *in vitro* cellular toxicity of liposomal preparations. Biochim. Biophys. Acta **1021:** 39-45.

31. TASKINEN, M. R., E. A. NIKKILA, T. KUUSI & I. TULILOURA. 1983. Changes of high density lipoprotein subfraction concentration and composition by Intralipid *in vivo* and by lipolysis of Intralipid *in vitro*. Arteriosclerosis **3:** 607–615.

32. GRIFFIN, E., W. C. BRECKENRIDGE, A. KUKSIS, M. H. BRYAN & A. ANGEL. 1979. Appearance and characterization of lipoprotein X during continuous Intralipid infusions in the neonate. J. Clin. Invest. **64:** 1703–1712.

33. BRECKENRIDGE, W. C., G. KAKIS & A. KUKSIS. 1979. Identification of lipoprotein X-like particles in rat plasma following Intralipid infusion. Canad. J. Biochem. **57:** 72–82.

34. UNTRACHT, S. H. 1982. Intravascular metabolism of an artificial transporter of triacylglycerols. Biochim. Biophys. Acta **711:** 176–192.

35. TASHIRO, T., Y. MASHIMA, H. YAMAMORI, K. HORIBE, M. NISHIZAWA, M. SANADA & K. OKUI. 1986. Alteration of lipoprotein profile during total parenteral nutrition with Intralipid 10%. J. Parenter. Enteral. Nutr. **10:** 622–626.

36. WASAN, K. M., V. B. GROSSIE, JR. & G. LOPEZ-BERESTEIN. 1994. Effects of Intralipid infusion on rat serum lipoproteins. Lab. Anim. **28:** 1–5.

37. WASAN, K. M., V. B. GROSSIE, JR. & G. LOPEZ-BERESTEIN. 1994. Serum concentration and tissue distribution of free and liposomal amphotericin B in rats on continuous Intralipid infusion. Antimicrob. Agents Chemother., in press.

38. GOLDBERG, I. J., T. M. VANNI & R. RAMAKRISHNAN. 1992. Effects of Intralipid-induced hypertriglycemia on plasma high-density lipoprotein metabolism in the cynomolgus monkey. Metabolism **41:** 1176–1184.

39. FORTE, T. M. & O. GANZEL-BOROVICZENY. 1989. Effect of total parenteral nutrition with intravenous fat on lipid and high density lipoprotein heterogeneity in neonates. J. Parenter. Enteral. Nutr. **13:** 490–500.

40. MORTON, R. E. 1990. Interaction of lipid transfer protein with plasma lipoproteins and cell membranes. Experientia **46:** 552–560.

41. PITTMAN, R. C., C. K. GLASS, D. ATKINSON & D. M. SMALL. 1987. Synthetic high density lipoprotein particles: Application to studies of the apoprotein specificity for selective uptake of cholesterol esters. J. Biol. Chem. **262:** 2435–2442.

Induction of Protective Immunity Using Minigenes[a]

J. LINDSAY WHITTON

Department of Neuropharmacology
The Scripps Research Institute
10666 N Torrey Pines Rd
La Jolla, California 92037

Antiviral vaccination has been remarkably successful, at least in "developed" countries, in protecting against several viral diseases. Smallpox has been eradicated, and the incidences of paralytic poliomyelitis, measles, and mumps have been markedly reduced. The clinical efficacy of antiviral vaccination was demonstrated at a relatively early stage, and perhaps in part because of this success, research to identify the component(s) of the vaccine-induced immune response that actually conferred the protection has been limited. For at least four reasons, however, complacency should be discouraged, and a full understanding of vaccine-induced immunity should be pursued. Firstly, new approaches may be necessary to cope with certain pathogenic organisms such as HIV. Secondly, new synthetic vaccines are being suggested to augment and/or supplant the vaccines that have been used successfully over the past four decades; before discarding or supplementing these highly successful reagents, we must ensure that their substitutes can induce immune responses capable of combatting subsequent exposure to the pathogenic viruses. Thirdly, "inappropriate" vaccination can be harmful to the vaccinee; killed measles[1] and respiratory syncytial virus[2] vaccines given to children in the late 1960s induced good antiviral antibody levels, but led to greater morbidity and mortality than those of unvaccinated individuals on subsequent exposure to the wild-type pathogen. Fourthly, changes in successful vaccine programs may have unforeseen consequences. Measles vaccination in Africa has radically reduced the incidence of disease; much of the remaining morbidity and mortality occurs in young children. To further improve vaccine efficacy, a high-titer vaccine was adopted and given to children of 6 months. Unexpectedly, an increase in mortality (cause unknown) was noted within 3 years postvaccination, particularly in females, and use of this vaccine is no longer recommended. Current recommendations have reverted to the previous protocol.

In this brief review, the new generation of vaccines currently being tested cannot all be discussed at length. Vaccines have historically been classified as "live" or "killed," but in terms of their interactions with the antigen presentation system they may better be respectively distinguished as "producing proteins within the host" or "administering preformed proteins to the host." The former type of vaccine can

[a] This work was supported by PHS grants AG-04342 and AI-27028. The author is a Harry Weaver Scholar of the National Multiple Sclerosis Society (NMSS JF2037-A-1). This is manuscript number 8098-NP from the Research Institute of Scripps Clinic.

generally induce good antibody and cytotoxic T-lymphocyte (CTL) responses, whereas the latter type induces mainly antibody responses. Synthetic peptide vaccines, which belong to the latter type, rely on the inoculation of short (often 9–20 mer) peptides, and these may induce marked antibody responses. Synthetic peptide vaccines, although potentially effective in protecting against foot and mouth disease virus,[3–5] have proven less effective against other pathogens, and at present no synthetic peptide vaccine is licensed for human or veterinary use. Several adjuvants have been developed to improve the immunogenicity of these and other soluble-protein vaccines. Recombinant viral vaccines (for example, those that use vaccinia or adenovirus as the vector system) belong to the former vaccine type and have the advantage of replication *in vivo;* this optimizes the chance that both CTL and antibody responses to the foreign antigen will be induced. Nevertheless, these recombinant viral vectors have certain disadvantages: they may themselves be pathogenic; their production requires growth in eukaryotic cell lines and therefore the preparations risk being contaminated with adventitious agents; and these recombinant vectors have a limited capacity for foreign DNA—even vaccinia virus, which has a large capacity in comparison to most other viral vectors, may carry only 25 kb of foreign material.

Antibody levels have been used as the measure of immunogenicity of most licensed vaccines, and for most vaccines a good correlation exists between these levels and protection against pathogenic challenge. This correlation does not prove that the antibodies are the source of protection; a different component of the vaccine-induced immune response may confer protection, and the antibodies may simply reflect the overall level of the vaccine-induced immune response. Without doubt, antiviral antibodies can and do have significant effects in controlling many viral infections. Nevertheless, experiments of nature suggest that antiviral antibody responses are nonessential; persons with agammaglobulinemia or with deficiencies in the complement cascade appear capable of controlling most viral infections but are unable to control many suppurative bacterial infections.[6–9] The control of many primary viral infections depends on CTL. In attempting to build an ideal "new-generation" vaccine, we wished to determine the relative roles of antibody and CTL in protective immunity. By identifying all of the potentially protective components, we diminished the risk of omitting factors from the vaccine that would induce a biologically relevant immune response. Our initial approach was to establish whether induction of CTL alone in the absence of antiviral antibodies would confer sufficient advantage on the host to protect it from a subsequent lethal-dose viral challenge.

In this manuscript, I wish to establish two principles. First, CTL can play a decisive role in vaccine-induced protection. Induction of CTL in the absence of antiviral antibody can confer sufficient advantage on the host to result in 100% protection against a lethal-dose virus challenge and confers protection against the establishment of persistent infection by an immunosuppressive strain of lymphocytic choriomeningitis virus. Second, the effective coding capacity of recombinant viral vectors can be increased 25- to 30-fold, using a novel technique which "distills" the immunologically relevant wheat and disregards the chaff. This technique relies on the identification of the immunologically significant sequences in a pathogen, the expression of such important short sequences in "minigenes," and the linkage of several minigenes, resulting in a vaccine which we have termed a "string-of-beads."

We use as our model system the *arenavirus* family. Arenaviruses, named for their "sandy" appearance on electron microscopy, are a group of enveloped viruses usually harbored in rodent populations, causing little apparent disease therein, but on transmission to man several of the agents are highly pathogenic[10]; Lassa virus is the etiologic agent of Lassa fever, Junin virus is the cause of Argentinian hemorrhagic fever, and Bolivian hemorrhagic fever is caused by Machupo virus. A fourth virus, lymphocytic choriomeningitis virus (LCMV), is by far the most studied of the arenaviruses; although its natural host is the mouse, *Mus musculis,* it can infect humans, causing hydrocephalus[11] and sometimes even death.[12]

LCMV is the prototype of the family and has a bisegmented single-stranded RNA genome. The short (S) segment, which has been sequenced,[13] encodes two proteins, glycoprotein-C (GP-C), a 498-amino acid precursor which undergoes posttranslational cleavage to yield the two mature virus polypeptides GP-1 and GP-2,[14] and a 558-residue nucleoprotein (NP); the long (L) segment also encodes two proteins, the large L protein, the putative viral polymerase,[15] and the Z protein, a zinc-containing protein of undefined function.[16] The S segment is *ambisense*[17]; it encodes GP-C in the positive sense and NP in the negative.

LCMV is an excellent model in which to delineate the effects of CTL; the interaction between host and virus revolves around CTL. Peripheral administration of the virus to an immunocompetent adult induces a brisk $CD8^+$ CTL response, easily measurable *in vitro* without any secondary *in vitro* stimulation. These CTL are responsible for viral clearance, and in the absence of CTL a lifelong persistent infection ensues. CTL are not always protective, however; if the virus is administered intracerebrally to an immunocompetent adult, the resultant CTL response causes immunopathology and death.

MATERIALS AND METHODS

Mouse Strains Used. Mouse strains (C57BL/6 [H2b] and BALB/c [H2d]) were obtained from the breeding colony at Scripps Research Institute. Mice were used at 6–12 weeks of age.

Cell Lines and Viruses. BALB C17 (H2d) and MC57 (H2b) cell lines are maintained in continuous culture in the laboratory. Both lines are maintained in RPMI supplemented with 7% fetal calf serum, ɪ-glutamine, and penicillin/streptomycin. Viruses used were LCMV (Armstrong strain) and recombinant vaccinia viruses as outlined below.

Construction of Recombinant Vaccinia Viruses. Recombinant vaccinia viruses carrying minigenes were constructed as follows: minigene sequences were designed and synthesized as complementary synthetic oligonucleotides, and the double-stranded DNA was cloned into a vaccinia transfer vector and subsequently introduced into the virus by homologous recombination, as described previously.[18] In all cases the recombinant plasmids were sequenced to ensure the correct sequence and orientation of the minigenes. Furthermore, to ensure that recombination had occurred faithfully, the appropriate region of the recombinant vaccinia virus DNA was amplified by polymerase chain reaction (PCR), and the resulting DNA was sequenced.[19]

Cloning Procedures and DNA Sequencing. All cloning procedures were carried out according to the manufacturer's recommendations, and DNA sequencing was done using the dideoxy chain termination method with double-stranded template DNA and Sequenase version 2 (United States Biochemical Corporation, Cleveland, Ohio).

In Vitro *Cytotoxicity Assays.* These assays were carried out as previously described.[18] Effector cells were either day 7 primary splenocytes or CTL clones of previously defined specificity. Target cells were infected appropriately with virus, labeled with Cr51, washed, and incubated for 5 hours with effector cells at the indicated effector-to-target (E : T) ratio. Supernatant was harvested, and specific Cr51 release calculated using the formula ([sample release − spontaneous release] × 100) ÷ (total release − spontaneous release).

In Vivo *Protection Studies.* Mice (6-12 weeks of age) were inoculated with either a single intraperitoneal (ip) dose of 2×10^7 plaque-forming units (PFU) of recombinant vaccinia virus; a single dose of LCMV ARM (2×10^5 PFU ip) as positive control; or 200 ml of medium ip as a negative control. Six weeks later the animals were challenged with a potentially lethal dose (20 LD_{50}) of LCMV administered intracranially. Mice were observed daily, and all recorded deaths occurred between days 6 and 12 following lethal dose LCMV challenge.

RESULTS

LCMV CTL Epitopes and Their Expression as Minigenes in Recombinant Vaccinia Viruses. To induce CTL but not antibody responses, it was necessary first to identify the precise regions of the virus against which CTL responses were directed. These CTL epitopes were identified by a combination of three technologies.[18,20,21] First, CTL clones were obtained which were specific for individual LCMV epitopes. Second, recombinant vaccinia viruses were made which encoded and expressed serially deleted fragments of LCMV proteins. Applied together, these techniques allowed epitopes to be approximately located in the LCMV proteins. Third, the epitopes were more precisely located using synthetic peptide techniques; peptides were synthesized and used to sensitize uninfected target cells against CTL killing, and those peptides that sensitized were known to contain the desired epitopes. Using these three techniques we obtained a CTL epitope map of LCMV on several MHC backgrounds. In TABLE 1 the CTL epitopes that were identified on the H2b (C57BL/6) and H2d (BALB/c) backgrounds are shown, as are the amino acid sequences of each epitope. We attempted to capitalize on this knowledge by immunizing animals with the epitope sequences and thus inducing CTL in the absence of antibodies. Initial attempts to induce CTL activity by inoculating the host with appropriate synthetic peptides failed. Therefore we designed a different system of short open reading frames, each of which encoded a single CTL epitope. These open reading frames varied in length between 10 and 14 amino acids and were termed by us "minigenes."[22] In all cases a translational initiation codon (ATG) was placed 5′ of the CTL epitope sequence which then was followed by translation termination codons in all reading frames. The designations of the recombinant vaccinia viruses expressing these short LCMV CTL epitopes are shown in TABLE 1. With the exception of VVMG6, these recombinant viruses are recognized by LCMV-specific CTL in an MHC-dependent manner (not

TABLE 1. LCMV CTL Epitopes[a]

Mouse Strain	MHC Molecule	LCMV Protein	Amino Acid Sequence	Expressed as Minigene in:
BALB/c	Ld	GP	KAVYNFATCG	VVMG3, VVMG34
BALB/c	Ld	NP	RPQASGVYMG	VVMG4, VVMG34
C57BL/6	Db	GP	KAVYNFATCG	VVMG3, VVMG34
C57BL/6	Db	GP	SGVENPGGYCL	VVMG7
C57BL/6	Db	NP	FQPQNGQFI	VVMG6

[a] Location on the LCMV S segment of the five MHC class I restricted CTL epitopes identified on the H2d (BALB/c) and H2b (C57BL/6) haplotypes along with their amino acid sequences. The recombinant vaccinia viruses in which these epitopes are expressed as minigenes also are shown.

shown), indicating that the short products of the minigenes are being correctly processed within the infected cell and transported to the cell surface with class I MHC.

Minigene Vaccination Protects against Challenge with a Normally Lethal Virus Dose. As just stated, intracranial inoculation of LCMV into a naive mouse results in CTL-mediated immunopathology and death. If the mouse was previously infected by peripheral inoculation of LCMV, from which it recovered uneventfully, then it is protected against the normally lethal effects of subsequent intracranial virus challenge. This demonstrates that vaccination is possible in the LCMV system, but the immune components that conferred protection have not been previously identified. We wished to determine the protective effect of a vaccine that would induce CTL in the absence of antiviral antibody. We have shown that our recombinant vaccinia viruses can induce anti-LCMV CTL responses in the absence of anti-LCMV antibodies[23,24]; can these responses confer protection against a CTL-mediated disease? VVMG3 and VVMG4 were used to vaccinate H2b and H2d mice. VVMG3 expresses a CTL epitope from the LCMV glycoprotein which is presented by the Db molecule in H2b mice; VVMG4 expresses an epitope from the LCMV nucleoprotein which is presented by the Ld molecule in H2d mice. Six weeks postvaccination, animals were challenged by the intracranial administration of 10 LD$_{50}$ of LCMV. As shown in FIGURE 1, vaccination of H2d mice with VVMG4 confers almost complete protection against subsequent challenge with LCMV. In stark contrast, the same vaccine administered to H2b mice confers no protection whatever; all LCMV-challenged mice die. These results show that, first, a single administration of a recombinant vaccine expressing as few as 14 LCMV residues can confer complete protection in the absence of an antibody response, and second, they underline a risk of using subunit vaccines, because one strain of mouse is fully protected, but another strain remains entirely unprotected. We have shown that protection requires the appropriate class I MHC locus, and the protective effect is clearly CTL mediated.[23]

VVMG3 gives similar but distinct results. As expected, this recombinant vaccine, which contains only 10 LCMV residues which include a CTL epitope recognized by H2b mice, protects mice of this strain efficiently (85% of mice protected; FIG. 1). Surprisingly, however, a certain percentage of H2d mice also are protected by

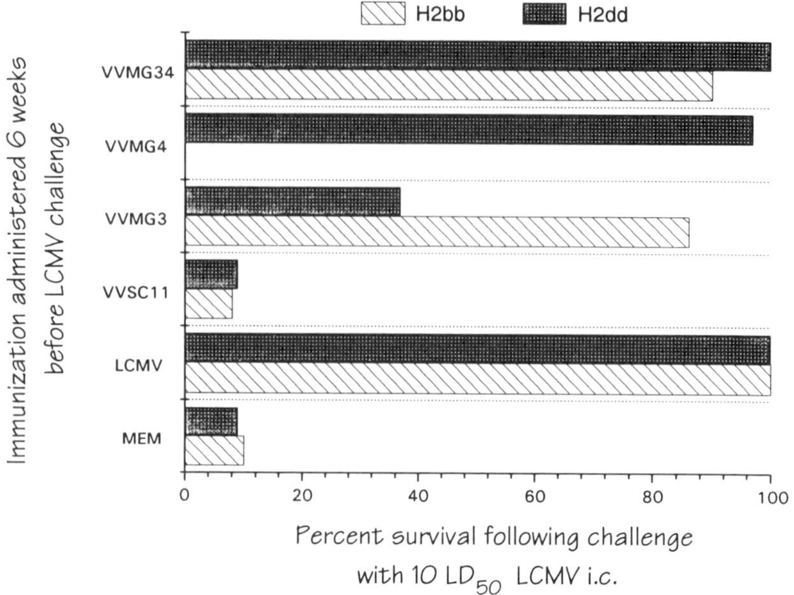

FIGURE 1. Minigene vaccines confer protection, and a string-of-beads vaccine overcomes the problem of nonresponder vaccinees. Animals of the indicated MHC haplotype (*hatched:* H2b; *solid:* H2d) were immunized with either minimal essential medium (MEM; negative control), LCMV (2×10^5 PFU ip), VVSC11 (a control recombinant vaccinia virus that contains no LCMV sequences), VVMG3, VVMG4, or VVMG34. (For LCMV sequences encoded, see FIG. 2.) All vaccinia viruses were administered as 2×10^7 PFU ip. Six weeks following immunization, all animals were challenged with 10 LD$_{50}$ of LCMV intracerebrally and thereafter were monitored daily for 21 days. All deaths occurred between 7 and 14 days postchallenge.

VVMG3 (38%). Although a CTL epitope has not been positively identified in this location in H2d mice, we have unpublished results which show that LCMV-infected H2d mice produce low levels of CTL activity directed against GP 1-60; we consider it probable, therefore, that VVMG3 contains an epitope for H2d mice which was not precisely identified by our previous epitope mapping, but whose activity is unveiled by our vaccination/protection study.

Nonresponder Vaccine Failure Prevented by a String-of-Beads Vaccine. For two reasons we wished to link two isolated CTL epitopes in close apposition and to determine the biological efficacy of such a construct. First, we wished to determine whether close apposition of two CTL epitopes would result in interference with MHC presentation or with their individual biological efficacy. Second, such a construct, if effective, would overcome the nonresponder problem seen in vaccination of the "wrong" haplotype (for example, VVMG4 in H2b mice). Consequently, a vaccine VVMG34 was made in which the H2b and H2d epitopes were linked together. This recombinant vaccine was recognized by CTL from both H2b and H2d LCMV-infected mice. Most importantly a single administration of this recombinant virus to either

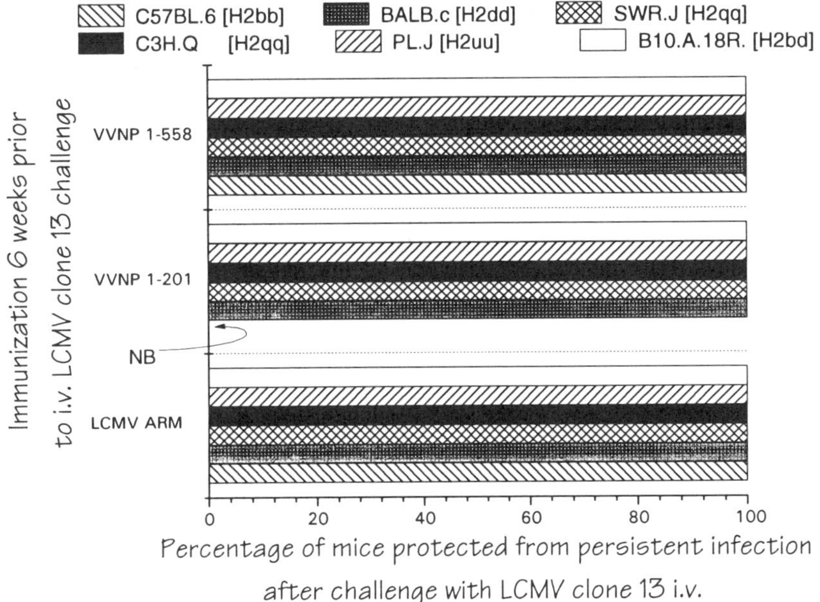

FIGURE 2. Establishment of persistent infection by an immunosuppressive virus is prevented by CTL vaccination. Six different mouse strains were vaccinated as shown and 6 weeks later were challenged intravenously with LCMV clone 13. Fifteen days following infection, serum was harvested and titrated for the presence of LCMV. Virus is present in 100% of unvaccinated animals (not shown above) and indicates the establishment of persistent infection.

H2b or H2d mice resulted in a high level of protection against subsequent lethal-dose LCMV challenge (FIG. 1).

CTL Vaccination Can Protect against Persistent Infection by an Immunosuppressive Virus. We also tested the role of CTL in protective acquired immunity against LCMV clone 13. This virus is a variant, plaque-purified from the spleen of an infected mouse; when administered intravenously to an immunocompetent adult mouse, this variant does not induce a detectable CTL response and established a lifelong persistent infection.[25] LCMV clone 13 challenge leads to persistence in 100% of unimmunized mice of all strains (not shown in FIG. 2). Could preexisting CTL, induced by vaccination with the recombinant vaccinia viruses, protect against a virus which appears to evade the CTL response? We used as vaccine in this experiment a recombinant vaccinia virus expressing LCMV NP residues 1-201; this fragment of NP contains the sequence RPQASGVYMG (a CTL epitope in H2dd [BALB/c] mice; TABLE 1), but the vaccine lacks the sequence presented by H2bb (C57BL/6) mice. FIGURE 2 shows that (1) several recombinant vaccinia viruses can protect against the establishment of persistent infection by LCMV clone 13 and (2) this protection maps with the presence of a CTL epitope along with its presenting molecule; the VVNP 1-201 fails to protect H2bb mice (arrow with NB opposite), but it protects B10.A(18)R

(H2bd) as well as several other strains, including mice of the H2uu and H2qq haplotypes, which present the RPQASGVYMG epitope.[26]

DISCUSSION

These studies show the importance of CTL in vaccine-induced immunity. Clearly, induction of antiviral CTL alone in the absence of induction of any antiviral antibody can confer a sufficient advantage on the host that subsequent lethal-dose challenge results not in death but instead in virus clearance and host recovery. The ability of CTL to protect against a CTL-mediated disease may at first appear paradoxical; one might have predicted that the priming of anti-LCMV CTL would have resulted in more rapid onset of CTL-mediated immunopathology on subsequent intracranial challenge. That the opposite is the case most probably reflects the kinetics of the situation. Presumably, intracerebral challenge of a naive host results in LCMV replication in the choriomeninges. The virus replicates and disseminates before the host immune response (CTL) has been fully activated, and by the time the host CTL response has developed, the virus has spread within the CNS, and the immune response is therefore targeted to many sites of infection; death ensues. In contrast, challenge of an immunized mouse results in rapid influx of primed LCMV-specific CTL into the CNS, with consequently rapid control of infection and limitation of viral spread. This scenario, which demonstrates the delicate balance between immunity and immunopathology, is a comment on the remarkable speed and specificity of the antiviral CTL response and a measure of the benefit accrued by the host from the ability of CTL to recognize infected cells early after infection. Note, however, that the balance can tip in the other direction, and in some instances vaccination results in exacerbation rather than amelioration of disease.[27]

Observations in humans suggest that our findings of the importance of CTL in postimmunization immunity are not specific to the LCMV system. Agammaglobulinemic children infected with measles virus most often have an apparently normal course of infection, with a rash (which is T-cell mediated), typical symptoms, and eventual viral clearance, most likely attributable to the antiviral T-cell response. Notably, however, such children, when subsequently reexposed to measles (against which, remember, they have produced no antiviral antibodies during the primary infection), do not develop any signs or symptoms of disease. This indicates that the antiviral immunity induced by primary infection (most probably a T-cell immunity) is sufficient to confer protection against disease from subsequent reexposure and is as close as one can get, in the human system, to our mouse model findings. Therefore, we strongly argue that any new generation antiviral vaccine must induce **both** antibody **and** CTL antiviral responses. This strategy may allow broad, cross-reactive, and long-lasting protection against these organisms.

Several delivery systems have been explored for new generation vaccines. As outlined in the introduction, some workers, driven by the limited capacity of recombinant viral vector systems for foreign DNA, have evaluated synthetic delivery vehicles (such as ISCOMs[28–30]), while others have employed microbes with a larger capacity for foreign material (eg, bacteria[31]). Our solution to this problem has been to demonstrate that CTL epitopes can be made as very short open reading frames and that these can be expressed in recombinant vaccinia viruses in a manner recognizable to antiviral cytotoxic T lymphocytes. These short viral sequences, expressed from recombinant vectors, confer complete protection against normally lethal virus challenge and against persistence following infection by an immunosuppressive viral variant. Furthermore, epitopes can be linked in a string-of-beads manner to protect more than one mouse strain. Thus, this technique allows us to concentrate the immunologically relevant sequences and to exclude the immunologically irrelevant sequences from our recombinant viral vaccines. The precise compression ratio will depend on a variety of factors; for LCMV, however, we have shown that the NP epitope expressed as a decamer (RPQASGVYMG) can protect H2d, H2q, and H2u mice.[26] Furthermore, the three epitopes on H2b mice have been fully mapped. It would therefore be possible to accommodate all four CTL epitopes in a polypeptide of approximately 40 amino acids; in contrast, expression of full-length LCMV GP and NP would require 1,056 amino acids. We therefore achieve an approximately 26-fold concentration using our minigene technique.

In the future we shall include MHC class II-restricted (mainly T_{helper}) epitopes and B-cell (antibody) epitopes in minigene cassettes to determine whether these sequences too can be incorporated into our technology. We shall further expand our studies by incorporating epitopes from other murine pathogens, to define whether a single recombinant vaccine can be made that will simultaneously confer protection against multiple pathogens.

ACKNOWLEDGMENTS

I thank my collaborators for their great help in these vaccine studies, in particular Michael Oldstone, in whose lab many of these studies were done, Tom McKee, and Linda Klavinskis. I am grateful to Terry Calhoun for skilled secretarial assistance.

REFERENCES

1. FULGINITI, V. A., J. J. ELLER, A. W. DOWNIE & C. H. KEMPE. 1967. Atypical measles in children previously immunized with inactivated measles virus vaccine. JAMA **202:** 1075–1080.
2. KAPIKIAN, A. Z., R. H. MITCHELL, R. M. CHANOCK, R. A. SHVEDOFF & C. E. STEWART. 1969. An epidemiologic study of altered clinical reactivity to respiratory syncitial (RS) virus infection in children previously vaccinated with an inactivated RS vaccine. Am. J. Epidemiol. **89:** 404–421.
3. BITTLE, J. L., R. A. HOUGHTEN, H. ALEXANDER, T. M. SHINNICK, J. G. SUTCLIFFE, R. A. LERNER, D. J. ROWLANDS & F. BROWN. 1982. Protection against foot-and-mouth disease by immunization with a chemically synthesized peptide predicted from the viral nucleotide sequence. Nature **298:** 30–33.
4. BROWN, F. 1988. Use of peptides for immunization against foot-and-mouth disease. Vaccine **6:** 180–182.
5. BROWN, F. 1992. New approaches to vaccination against foot-and-mouth disease. Vaccine **10:** 1022–1026.
6. GOOD, R. A. 1991. Experiments of nature in the development of modern immunology. Immunol. Today **12:** 283–286.

7. MCWHINNEY, P. H., P. LANGHORNE, W. C. LOVE & K. WHALEY. 1991. Disseminated gonococcal infection associated with deficiency of the second component of complement. Postgrad. Med. J. **67:** 297–298.
8. BERGER, M. 1990. Complement deficiency and neutrophil dysfunction as risk factors for bacterial infection in newborns and the role of granulocyte transfusion in therapy. Rev. Infect. Dis. **12**(Suppl 4): S401–S409.
9. GOOD, R. A. & S. J. ZAK. 1956. Disturbance in gamma-globulin synthesis as "experiments of nature." Pediatrics **18:** 109–149.
10. MCCORMICK, J. B. 1990. Arenaviruses. *In* Fields Virology, 2nd Ed. B. N. Fields and D. M. Knipe, eds. Vol 1: Chapt 44: 1245–1267. Raven Press. New York.
11. LARSEN, P. D., S. A. CHARTRAND, K. M. TOMASHEK, L. G. HAUSER & T. G. KSIAZEK. 1993. Hydrocephalus complicating lymphocytic choriomeningitis virus infection. Pediatr. Infect. Dis. J. **12:** 528–531.
12. WARKEL, R. L., D. F. RINALDI, W. H. BANCROFT, R. D. CARDIFF, G. E. HOLMES & R. E. WILSNACK. 1973. Fatal acute meningoencephalitis due to lymphocyte choriomeningitis virus. Neurology **23:** 198–203.
13. SALVATO, M. S., E. SHIMOMAYE, P. SOUTHERN & M. B. A. OLDSTONE. 1988. Virus-lymphocyte interactions. IV. Molecular characterization of LCMV Armstrong CTL-positive small genomic segment and that of its variant clone 13 CTL-negative. Virology **164:** 517–522.
14. BUCHMEIER, M. J. & M. B. A. OLDSTONE. 1979. Protein structure of lymphocytic choriomeningitis virus: Evidence for a cell associated precursor of the virion glycopeptides. Virology **99:** 111– 120.
15. SALVATO, M. S., E. SHIMOMAYE & M. B. A. OLDSTONE. 1989. The primary structure of the lymphocytic choriomeningitis virus L gene encodes a putative RNA polymerase. Virology **169:** 377–384.
16. SALVATO, M. S. & E. M. SHIMOMAYE. 1989. The completed sequence of lymphocytic choriomeningitis virus reveals a unique RNA structure and a gene for a zinc finger protein. Virology **173:** 1–10.
17. BISHOP, D. H. L. & D. D. AUPERIN. 1987. Arenavirus gene structure and organization. *In* Current Topics in Microbiology and Immunology, M. B. A. Oldstone, ed. **133:** 5–17. Springer-Verlag. New York.
18. WHITTON, J. L., P. J. SOUTHERN & M. B. A. OLDSTONE. 1988. Analyses of the cytotoxic T lymphocyte responses to glycoprotein and nucleoprotein components of lymphocytic choriomeningitis virus. Virology **162:** 321–327.
19. SHENG, N., J. ZHANG, T. A. MCKEE & J. L. WHITTON. 1993. A rapid and simple method for determining the DNA sequences of fragments inserted into recombinant vaccinia viruses. Biotechniques **14:** 781–784.
20. OLDSTONE, M. B. A., J. L. WHITTON, H. LEWICKI & A. TISHON. 1988. Fine dissection of a nine amino acid glycoprotein epitope a major determinant recognized by lymphocytic choriomeningitis virus-specific class I-restricted H-2D^b cytotoxic T lymphocytes. J. Exp. Med **168:** 559– 570.
21. WHITTON, J. L., A. TISHON, H. LEWICKI, J. R. GEBHARD, T. COOK, M. S. SALVATO, E. JOLY & M. B. A. OLDSTONE. 1989. Molecular analyses of a five-amino-acid cytotoxic T-lymphocyte (CTL) epitope: An immunodominant region which induces nonreciprocal CTL cross-reactivity. J. Virol. **63:** 4303–4310.
22. WHITTON, J. L. & M. B. A. OLDSTONE. 1989. Class I MHC can present an endogenous peptide to cytotoxic T lymphocytes. J. Exp. Med. **170:** 1033–1038.
23. KLAVINSKIS, L. S., J. L. WHITTON & M. B. A. OLDSTONE. 1989. Molecularly engineered vaccine which expresses an immunodominant T-cell epitope induces cytotoxic T lymphocytes that confer protection from lethal virus infection. J. Virol. **63:** 4311–4316.

24. KLAVINSKIS, L. S., M. B. A. OLDSTONE & J. L. WHITTON. 1989. Designing vaccines to induce cytotoxic T lymphocytes: Protection from lethal viral infection. *In* Vaccines 89. Modern Approaches to New Vaccines Including Prevention of AIDS. F. Brown, R. Chanock, H. Ginsberg & R. Lerner, eds.: 485–489. Cold Spring Harbor Laboratory. Cold Spring Harbor, NY.

25. AHMED, R., A. SALMI, L. D. BUTLER, J. M. CHILLER & M. B. A. OLDSTONE. 1984. Selection of genetic variants of lymphocytic choriomeningitis virus in spleens of persistently infected mice: Role in suppression of cytotoxic T lymphocyte response and viral persistence. J. Exp. Med. **160:** 521–540.

26. OLDSTONE, M. B., A. TISHON, R. GECKELER, H. LEWICKI & J. L. WHITTON. 1992. A common antiviral cytotoxic T-lymphocyte epitope for diverse major histocompatibility complex haplotypes: Implications for vaccination. Proc. Natl. Acad. Sci. USA **89:** 2752–2755.

27. OEHEN, S., H. HENGARTNER & R. M. ZINKERNAGEL. 1991. Vaccination for disease. Science **251:** 195–198.

28. MOWAT, A. M. & A. M DONACHIE. 1991. ISCOMS—a novel strategy for mucosal immunization? Immunol. Today **12:** 383–385.

29. FEKADU, M., J. H. SHADDOCK, J. EKSTROM, A. OSTERHAUS, D. W. SANDERLIN, B. SUNDQUIST & B. MOREIN. 1992. An immune stimulating complex (ISCOM) subunit rabies vaccine protects dogs and mice against street rabies challenge. Vaccine **10:** 192–197.

30. MOREIN, B. 1990. The ISCOM: An immunostimulating system. Immunol. Lett. **25:** 281–283.

31. JACOBS, W. R. J., S. B. SNAPPER, L. LUGOSI & B. R. BLOOM. 1990. Development of BCG as a recombinant vaccine vehicle. Curr. Top. Microbiol. Immunol. **155:** 153–160.

An Evolutionary and Functional Approach to the TNF Receptor/Ligand Family

BRUCE BEUTLER AND CHRISTOPHE VAN HUFFEL

Howard Hughes Medical Institute
5323 Harry Hines Blvd.
Dallas, Texas 75235-9050

Hormones undergo pronounced structural change in the course of evolution, yet each one retains its affinity for a specific receptor. Receptors also undergo change over time. How is it that structural changes in one member of a receptor/ligand pair are "anticipated" by changes in the structure of its partner? On an evolutionary scale, such changes may be very rapid. Hence, murine gamma interferon has but little affinity for the human gamma interferon receptor, and *vice versa*, although within each of these two species, the affinity between gamma interferon and its receptor has remained strong. Moreover, present-day functions of a given hormone may bear little semblance to the functions that its molecular ancestor served one billion years ago. How, then, were changes in function tolerated?

The molecular cloning of several dozen proteins, somewhat arbitrarily lumped together as "interleukins," "colony-stimulating factors," "chemokines," and "tumor necrosis factors" has permitted very detailed consideration of this issue. Not only the structure, but also the function of phylogenetically related molecules may be applied toward construction of a hypothesis as to how coevolution of hormones and their receptors may occur.

Inasmuch as understanding of function is usually best advanced by analysis of the failure of function, much effort has been spent on the identification of defects of cytokine production or activity. Certain diseases can now be attributed to discrete mutations of genes encoding cytokines[1-3] or their receptors,[4,5] and when nature has not provided such mutations, attempts have been made to introduce them artificially.[6-11] As a result, the essential actions of cytokines have become somewhat clearer than they were a few years ago.

In the present review, we offer a detailed description of the TNF ligand and receptor families and speculate as to their evolutionary and functional origins.

TUMOR NECROSIS FACTOR AND ITS RELATIVES

For nearly a decade, it has been suspected that tumor necrosis factor (TNF or TNF-α) mediates the shock state induced by bacterial endotoxin[12,13] and the wasting diathesis produced by many types of chronic disease.[14] It has also been believed that TNF-α somehow checks the spread of infections, particularly those caused by intracellular pathogens.[15,16] These deductions grew from studies in which TNF-α was directly administered to experimental animals or blocked in its action by the administration of anti-TNF-α antibodies. Concurrently, it became clear that TNF-α was but one member of a family of cytokines with varying degrees of structural homology. First lymphotoxin (LT or LT-α)[17] and, in turn, the ligands for CD40,[18] CD27,[19] 4-1BB,[20] and Fas[3] were shown to be structurally related. The recently discovered protein known as lymphotoxin-β (LT-β), a ligand still in search of a receptor, is part of the same group.[21] It is believed that the ligands for CD30 and OX40 are as well. This cytokine family, in turn, engages a set of homologous receptors, activating them by a common mechanism (aggregation) and in some cases transducing similar effects.

The solubility of protein hormones, once a characteristic that was taken for granted, is now known to be incidental to their function, at least in some instances. This point is illustrated by the TNF family of molecules, some of which do, indeed, exist as soluble factors secreted from the cells that produce them, whereas others are type II plasma membrane proteins, acting to trigger a biological response on adjacent cells while tethered to the membrane of the cell of origin.

Although TNF-α and LT-α are largely secreted, the former protein can also exist in a membrane-associated form. So far as is known at present, LT-β is entirely membrane associated and may act to maintain LT-α in close proximity with the cell membrane by forming an [LT-α]₂[LT-β] or [LT-α] [LT-β]₂ heterotrimer. The ligands for the Fas antigen and for CD27, CD30, CD40, OX40, and 4-1BB are believed to be strictly membrane associated and to work their effects through intercellular contact.

All members of the TNF ligand family are believed to be trimeric proteins or to participate in trimer formation. The case has been proven crystallographically for TNF-α and LT-α,[22-25] and extended to other members of the group on the basis of structural modeling or biochemical analyses. Each TNF has three sites capable of engaging the TNF receptors. These sites are formed by the interface between adjacent subunits. In binding to the TNF receptors, TNFs cause receptor aggregation or changes in receptor conformation in such a way that a signal is generated.[26] The majority of the effects elicited by TNF-α and LT-α are identical, but certain discrepancies have been reported.[27,28] The major difference between these cytokines, at a functional level, is seen at the level of their production; the two proteins are produced in response to different stimuli and, often, by different types of cells. TNF-α is produced largely by macrophages as well as by lymphocytes and certain extrahematopoietic cell types. LT-α is expressed almost exclusively by lymphocytes.[29] Thus, it seems that a common biological activity may be produced at different sites in response to different inducing agents.

Although its receptor bears homology to the TNF family of receptors, nerve growth factor (NGF) is not sufficiently similar to the TNFs and their homologues to be classified as a member of the TNF ligand family. It might therefore be said that a family of receptors existing *ab initio*, coopted two-gene families encoding ligands and directed their development as regulated "triggers" of a biological response.

The separate members of the TNF gene family have been diverging for a long time. The "tree" shown in FIGURE 1 gives some indication of the evolutionary relationship that defines this protein family. Even the TNF proteins themselves must be separated by several hundred million years of evolution. As such, TNF-α, LT-α,

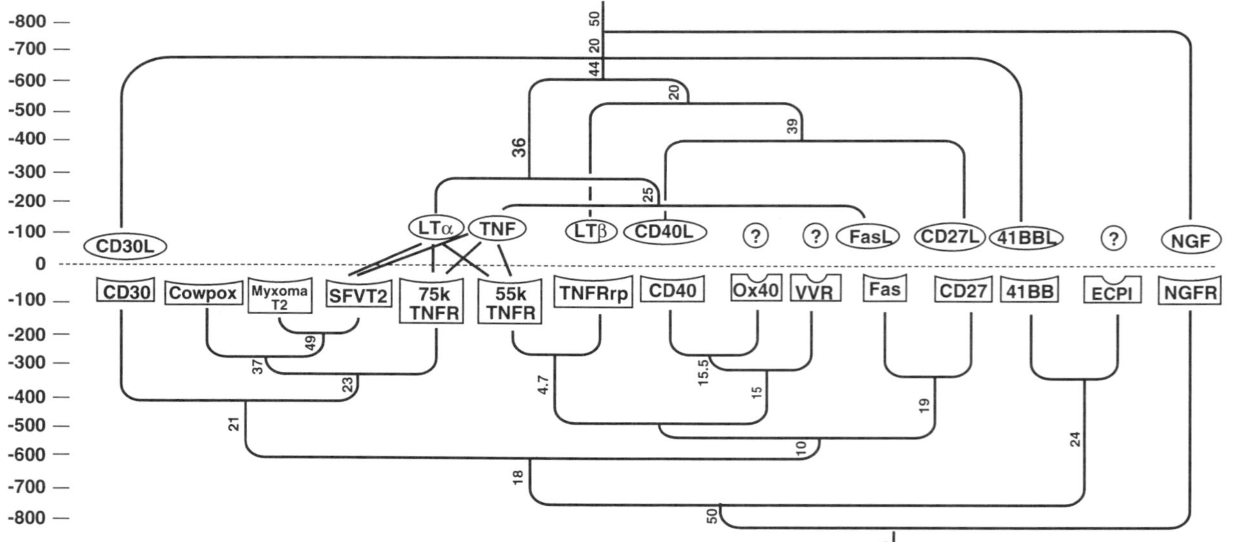

FIGURE 1. The phylogenetic origin of the TNF/NGF ligand and receptor families. Two phylogenetic trees were generated using a maximum parsimony method (PROTPARS) of the PHYLIP program package.[72] The upper part tree is based on the alignment of the sequences of the processed ligands (lacking transmembrane and secretion signal domains), and the lower part tree on the two first cysteine repeats of the extracellular domains of the receptor family members (except for ECP1 which contains only one repeat). PROTPARS assumes that the simplest path in evolution is the one followed and thus attempts to find the branching topology requiring the fewest possible mutations to get from a single unknown ancestral sequence to the present array. The multiple alignments needed as input into PROTPARS were generated by the ClustalV package.[73] Confidence intervals were estimated by the technique of bootstrap resampling:[74] the SEQBOOT program of the PHYLIP package was used to create multiple ($n = 50$) randomly sampled datasets from the original alignment. PROTPARS was then run on these datasets, and the resulting phylogenetic trees were then compared by the CONSENSE program of the PHYLIP package to give a measure of robustness of the data producing the various nodes. The numbers at the forks indicate the number of times the group consisting of the genes that are following occurred among 50 trees. A distance matrix method[75] was also used to confirm the organization of the trees. Sequences were retrieved from the GenBank data library: The TNFRrp has accession number L04270; ECP1 is a fungal tomato pathogen receptor-like protein (Z14023). Cowpox CrnB (L08906), MyxomaT2 (M95181), VVSalF19R (M58054), and SFVT2 are viral proteins. The connections between ligand and receptor family members indicate direct physical interaction between the molecules. "?" implies that the sequence of the respective ligand is not available at present. The time scale is approximate and should be taken only to indicate that, with the exception of some very closely related proteins, the point of phylogenetic divergence is very ancient.

and LT-β exhibit only about 30% identity to one another at the protein level. Four of the nine known ligand family members (TNF-α, LT-α, LT-β, and the 4-1BB ligand) are MHC linked, suggesting that the original ligand gene might have arisen in this genomic context.

THE TNF/NGF FAMILY OF RECEPTORS

The TNF/NGF family of receptors now has 14 representatives, including those of viral origin, and is defined by polypeptide chains composed of repeated cysteine-rich motifs, present in six copies (the CD30 molecule), four copies (the TNF receptors, the NGF receptor, the TNF receptor-related protein [TNFRrp],[30] the CD40 molecule, and the soluble TNF receptors [encoded by the Shope fibroma, cowpox, and the myxoma viruses][31-34]), three copies (the Fas antigen, the 4-1BB molecule, the CD27 molecule, and the OX40 protein), two copies (the soluble TNF receptor putatively expressed by vaccinia viruses), and one copy (the fungal ECP1 protein).[35] It is possible that none of the molecules exists in a truly monomeric form on the plasma membrane. At minimum, they may be present as dimers, which undergo conformational change following interaction with their respective ligands. The CD27 molecules are, in fact, maintained as disulfide-linked dimers on the cell surface.[36]

One of the most striking effects of TNF-α, LT-α, and the Fas ligand is their ability to trigger the programmed death (apoptosis) of certain susceptible cells *in vitro*. Although it remains a matter of some controversy, either one[37] or both[38,39] types of TNF receptor, as well as the Fas antigen,[40-43] act to transduce an apoptotic signal when activated by aggregation. CD40[44,45] and the 75-kD NGF receptor[46] seem capable of triggering a cytotoxic response when *not* engaged by their respective ligands. Other receptor/ligand couples have growth-stimulatory effects. For example, the 75-kD TNF receptor,[47] CD27,[19] and 4-1BB[20] molecules trigger cell proliferation when activated. Thus, the diversity of cytoplasmic domain structure has permitted the development of distinct responses to ligands which, to initial appearances, have very similar structures, cell surface targets, and mechanisms of receptor activation.

A homologous motif is observed on comparison of the cytoplasmic domain of the 55-kD TNF receptor, the Fas antigen, and the CD40 protein.[42] Termed the ''death domain''[48] in the former two proteins, this region is perhaps responsible for transduction of an apoptotic signal, insofar as mutations within the domain are known to abolish the cytolytic effect of the activated receptors. However, it is not clear that all of the signaling pathways activated by these receptors are identical, and indeed, evidence to the contrary has been adduced.[48]

COEVOLUTION OF THE TNF RECEPTORS AND THEIR LIGANDS

It must be considered that receptors antedate hormones in most evolutionary processes, because the receptor is the ''business end'' of a ligand/receptor couple. Although it is possible to imagine the exertion of a biological effect that is enhanced by the presence of a hormone, it is not possible to envision the exertion of that effect by the hormone acting alone, given that the hormone lacks any cytoplasmic domain and any semblance of structures required for signal transduction. On this basis, it may be assumed that the primordial TNF receptor arose prior to the primordial TNF. Molecules bearing a structure similar to the repeating unit that defines the TNF receptor family have been identified in fungi that act as plant pathogens,[35] and indeed, this may imply the existence of defensive molecules that resemble TNFs or NGF in plants. As the basic structural unit of the receptor seems to exist in lower eukaryotes, we assume that the evolution of this ligand receptor family began long ago, even prior to the division of plant and animal kingdoms.

Repeated duplication of the receptor genes[49] may then have occurred, with subsequent modification of cytoplasmic domains. In the modern receptor family, clear evidence of such duplications is preserved, in that the extracellular domains of all family members are modular in their design and relatively similar, whereas most of the cytoplasmic domains have become highly divergent. It is to be imagined that in some instances, modification of the cytoplasmic domains may have occurred rather drastically, through such events as exon shuffling, rather than by a gradual mutational process. Because many hormone receptors are activated through dimerization, the modified receptors might be expected to function immediately. This would lead to the immediate adoption of new signals initiated by the same ligand and immediately broaden the function of a given ligand. Subsequently, duplication of the ligand gene might provide an opportunity for a true split to occur, that is, for the broader function to be subserved by two separate hormones rather than one. Thus, a finer degree of control might be exercised. This sequence of events, which may underlie the coevolution of most hormones and their receptors, is depicted in FIGURE 2.

Such an evolutionary mechanism, with certain qualifications (noted below), may be seen with the TNF receptors; here, the extracellular domains are sufficiently similar to permit engagement of both TNF-α and LT-α by both types of receptor. However, the receptor extracellular domains are slightly more divergent than are TNF-α and LT-α themselves, and the receptor genes have become unlinked from one another, consistent with the notion that duplication of the receptor genes anticipates duplication of the ligand genes. Moreover, the cytoplasmic domains encoded by the two TNF receptors are very different and appear to transduce entirely different signals. It may be imagined that a primordial receptor gene underwent duplication, which was followed by extensive modification of the region encoding the cytoplasmic domain, but that the products of the duplicated locus still managed to engage the precursor of modern TNF-α and LT-α.

Given an existing duplication of the ancestral TNF receptor gene, duplication of the ancestral TNF locus, with gradual accumulation of the mutations that distinguish TNF-α and LT-α, may well have occurred thereafter. TNF-α and LT-α still exert similar or identical effects on the cell; however, the different regulatory mechanisms that govern their synthesis have already permitted refinements of hormone action that would not be possible if a single ligand gene were present instead of two genes. Furthermore, LT-α is distinguished from TNF-α by its ability to form heterotrimers with LT-β.[21] These LT-α/ LT-β heterotrimers are thought to be engaged by a receptor that is incapable of binding the homotrimeric TNF species. The signals that it transduces remain mysterious. Ultimately, further duplications and structural modifications may permit complete functional separation of TNF-α and LT-α, as separation from CD27L, CD30L, and CD40L has already occurred.

Sequence-based analysis of the evolution of ligand and receptor molecules (FIG. 1) allows certain other conclusions concerning the origins of some family members, though mutation has strained the limits of confidence with which assignments of ancestry can be made. The genes encoding both ligand and receptor families almost certainly originated more than one billion years ago, antedating the split between plant and animal kingdoms. Thus, divergence has occurred over a time frame at least 10 times greater than that allowed for the divergence of mammalian species.

With regard to the receptor family, the first and most obvious conclusion to be drawn is that three of the viral representatives are closely related to one another. One might infer that the cowpox virus, the myxoma virus, and the Shope fibroma virus each independently captured the genes encoding the larger rather than the smaller of the two TNF receptors. The reasons for this are a matter of conjecture. The gene captured by vaccinia virus was perhaps a host CD40 or OX40 gene; indeed, it is not clear that the vaccinia product is expressed or that it can engage TNFs.

The two TNF receptors are surprisingly divergent in view of the fact that they are functionally related by their ability to bind the two TNFs. Indeed, they are more divergent than the TNF ligands, and the genes encoding the receptors, unlike the genes encoding the ligands, have undergone physical separation from one another as the result of translocation. Although the molecules share an obvious common ancestry and must originally have arisen from a single locus, convergent evolutionary processes might also have come into play, and it is possible that at one stage in its evolution, the 75-kD receptor (or its ancestor) transiently lost its ability to engage TNFs.

The Fas antigen and the 55-kD TNF receptor, which are functionally related to one another, are clearly close relatives, and it may be assumed that the genes encoding them split more recently than did the genes encoding the two TNF receptors. Also closely related to Fas and the 55-kD receptor is the gene encoding TNFRrp.

SACRIFICES ATTEND THE ACQUISITION OF NEW FUNCTIONS AND THE RETENTION OF EXISTING FUNCTIONS

It is difficult to argue that shock is beneficial to either the host or the kindred of which he is a part. The obvious propensity of cytokines to cause shock must therefore be viewed as a deleterious consequence of the protective effects that they offer. The TNF receptor/ligand system, as noted, may well have evolved before circulatory shock was an issue to be dealt with. The protection that it offered may have been sufficiently indispensable that it was retained despite the dangers it posed to the integrity of the advanced metazoan structures that subsequently emerged. Precisely what advantages are these?

Deletion of TNF receptor genes or functional impairment of TNF activity *in vivo* leads to a state of enhanced susceptibility to facultative intracellular pathogens such as listeria and mycobacteria. A similar increase in susceptibility is observed with the deletion of genes encoding gamma interferon or its receptor. It is likely that this is not coincidental, but that the TNFs and gamma interferon are cooperative in their protective effects or that one mediator acts to promote the induction of the other.[50] TNF-α is also known to offer protection against viral infections,[51] and certain viruses have evolved to produce specific proteins that either neutralize the TNFs[31,52] or abolish the intracellular signals that the TNFs initiate,[53,54] thus furthering their pathogenicity. Whatever the mechanism, it is clear that TNF-α (and, by implication, LT-α) offers protection against microbial invaders, and this in itself could be sufficient explanation for the persistence of the TNFs in evolution.

PHENOTYPIC EFFECTS OF LIGAND AND RECEPTOR MUTATIONS

The function of several members of the TNF and TNF/NGF receptor families has been illuminated by mutations that affect the expression or structure of these proteins. *Gld* (generalized lymphoproliferative disease) and *Lpr* (lymphoproliferation) are recessive mutations in mice that lead to the accumulation of CD4⁻, CD8⁻ T cells in the peripheral lymph nodes and spleen of homozygous animals. It is now known that the *Gld* mutation leads to functional deletion of the Fas ligand, whereas the *Lpr* mutation represents a rearrangement of the Fas antigen gene caused by retroposon insertion.[55] A different allele of *Lpr,* known as *Lpr^cg*, leads to the expression of Fas antigens that are defective in their ability to signal. Hence, an *Lpr^cg/+*; *Gld/+* genotype specifies the development of lymphoproliferation, the diminished number of active receptors, the presence of ''decoy'' receptors, and the diminished quantity of available ligand yielding disease.[56]

Because defects of the Fas antigen or its ligand contribute to the excessive proliferation of a certain unusual class of T lymphocytes and ultimately to the development of a lupus-like autoimmune disease, it is probable that the Fas system normally serves to regulate an apoptotic process responsible for the removal of these cells. By analogy, it might be expected that the TNFs and their 55-kD receptor, which transduces a signal similar to that of the Fas antigen, might do something very similar.

Knockout mutations of the 55-kD TNF receptor revealed no such function, however. Animals lacking the 55-kD receptor are, to outward appearances, healthy and normally developed. However, they are unusually susceptible to infection by facultative intracellular pathogens such as *Listeria monocytogenes* and are also partially resistant to the lethal effect of lipopolysaccharides (LPS) in galactosamine-sensitized animals.[10,11] A still more subtle phenotype (resistance to LPS in the absence of galactosamine sensitization and lack of dermal scab formation in response to repeated intradermal TNF injection) is observed in animals lacking a 75-kD TNF receptor (Goeddel, personal communication).

FIGURE 2. Model of coevolution of receptor/ligand pair recognition driven by duplication and shuffling of the receptor genes. Mutations affecting the receptor gene and the ligand gene are depicted as *crossshades* and *solid crosses,* respectively. The model illustrates how gene duplication and cumulative mutations ''reshape'' the receptor A/ligand A pair into a receptor B/ligand B pair. EC = exons encoding the receptor extracellular domain; Cytopl. = exons encoding the receptor cytoplasmic domain.

Gene
Protein
Ligand A
Receptor A
EC domain
Cytopl. domain
Signal
A
1 Receptor Gene Duplication
Signal
A
2 Receptor Gene Mutation and Exon Shuffling
Signal
A
Signal
B
3 Ligand Gene Duplication
Signal
A
Signal
B
4 Ligand Gene Mutation
Ligand A
Ligand B
Receptor A
Receptor B
Signal
A
Signal
B

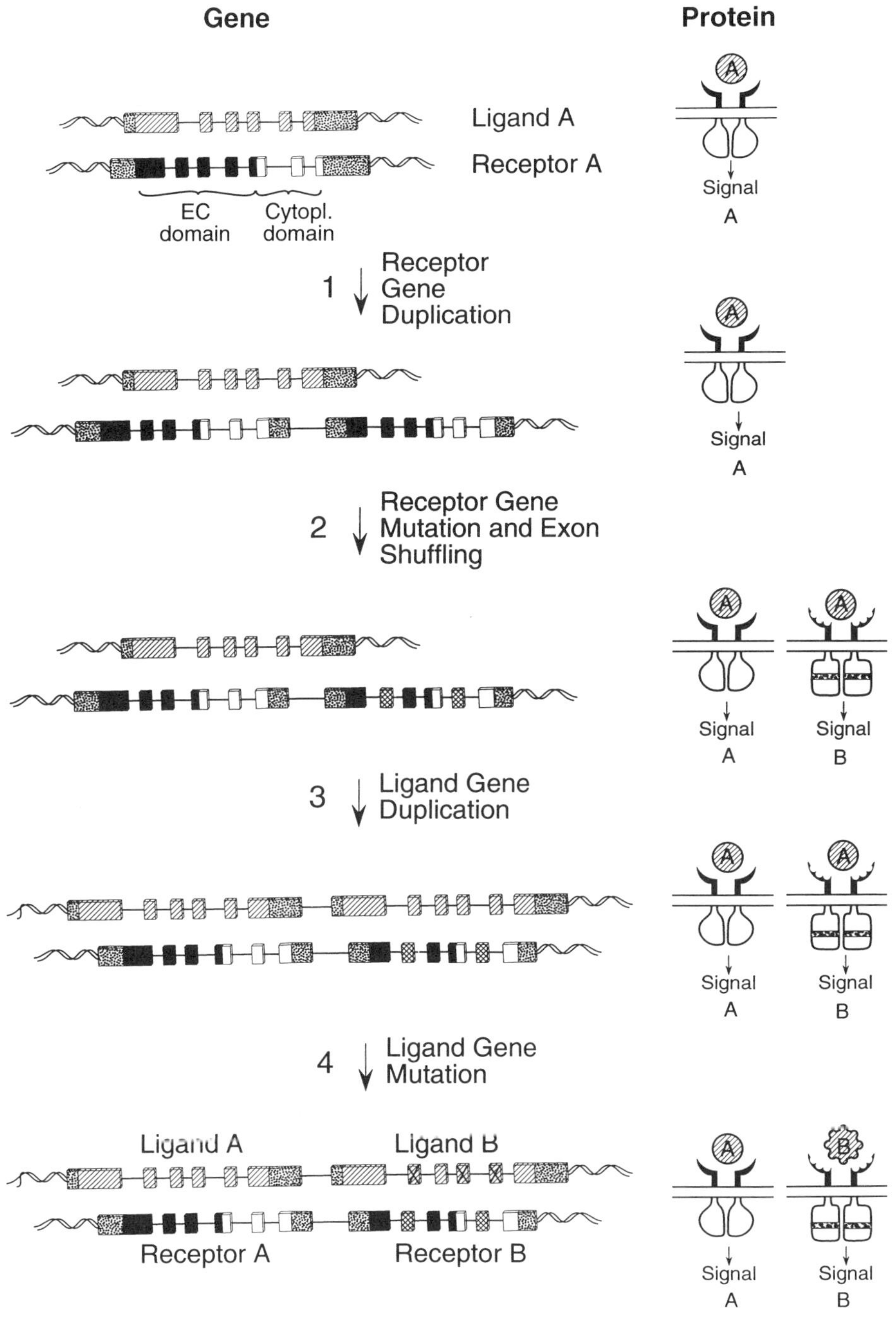

FIGURE 2.

If either or both of the TNFs normally serve to remove a class of T cell, the cell has yet to be identified. However, certain lines of experimental evidence do suggest that TNFs may be involved in the development of tolerance and/or autoimmunity through a mechanism that is not yet clear (see below).

Mutations affecting the CD40 ligand have been observed in humans and result in a rare form of X-linked immunodeficiency, characterized by a normal or elevated level of circulating IgM and diminished or absent circulating IgG, IgA, and IgE.[1,2,57–60] The CD40 ligand, represented on the surface of T cells, is believed to be required for initiation of signals leading to the immunoglobulin heavy chain "switch" that occurs in the course of the immune response. No mutations of the CD40 molecule itself have yet been observed; however, a similar phenotype would be anticipated.

DO MUTATIONS AFFECTING TNF PRODUCTION CONTRIBUTE TO AUTOIMMUNITY?

Jacob et al.[61] as well as Satoh et al.[62] observed that nonobese diabetic (NOD) mice, normally destined to develop autoimmune insulitis and diabetes, were protected as a result of administration of small doses of TNF-α during adult life. Satoh and coworkers extended the observation to encompass autoimmune diabetes in BB rats, using not only TNF-α,[63] but also LT-α as well.[64] More recently, McDevitt and colleagues showed that precisely the opposite is true in young NOD mice; if TNF-α administration is initiated during the neonatal period of life, the development of diabetes is encouraged. Conversely, the administration of antibodies against TNF-α to neonatal NOD mice leads to absolute protection against insulitis and diabetes (H.O. McDevitt, personal communication).

A similar observation was made in NZW/NZB F1 hybrid mice, which normally develop a syndrome similar to systemic lupus erythematosus. When treated with TNF-α, the F1 hybrid mice were substantially protected against the development of autoimmune disease.[65]

These findings strongly suggest that TNF-α is somehow involved in the development of autoimmune diseases, particularly those with an MHC-linked component. Since TNF-α is an MHC-linked gene, questions have been raised as to whether *cis*-acting mutations of the TNF-α gene are primarily responsible for the development of autoimmunity. In this context, it is interesting that both the NOD and NZW strains, which carry MHC-linked mutations required for the development of autoimmunity, underexpress TNF-α relative to most other strains, when their macrophages are exposed to LPS.

Do *cis*-acting mutations that interfere with TNF-α synthesis lead to the development of autoimmune disease?

To answer this question, Bazzoni and Beutler[66] made use of mutations within the 3'-untranslated region (UTR) of the mouse TNF-α gene, previously identified by direct sequencing studies.[67] A suspect TNF-α gene in its normal chromosomal context was placed together with a control TNF-α gene by crossing NZW with NZB mice or NOD with BALB/c mice. The relative contribution of each allele to the total pool of TNF-α mRNA could then be assessed by reverse transcription and polymerase chain reaction. In both types of hybrid, the two alleles contributed equally to the pool of mRNA, proving that at all pretranslational levels, the NOD and NZW TNF-α genes are normally expressed. Other studies, utilizing reporter constructs, suggest that translational activation of the NZW TNF-α mRNA is also normal (unpublished data).

It therefore appears that *cis*-acting mutations affecting "output" from the TNF-α genes are not primarily responsible for the observed differences in responsiveness of TNF-α genes to endotoxin and presumably are not primarily responsible for the development of autoimmunity, at least in the models examined. On the other hand, *trans*-acting mutations of MHC-linked genes, the products of which are involved in TNF-α synthesis, may indeed be responsible for autoimmune syndromes. One candidate gene is that encoding NF-κB. The NF-κB gene is closely linked to the TNF gene cluster, residing within the class III region of the MHC. It might be allowed that mutations affecting expression of NF-κB could impact on the expression of a variety of cytokines operating in *trans*.

A DOMINANT NEGATIVE APPROACH TO THE FUNCTIONAL DELETION OF TNF GENES

Although gene knockout experiments offer the most definitive approach to the understanding of gene function, the approach is problematic in several respects. First, it is not conditional. For example, while mutation of the IL-2Rγ chain creates a severe combined immunodeficiency state in humans,[4] this fact says little about the effects that interleukin-2 (IL-2) exerts on mature T cells. Second, knockouts are species- and strain-specific, and therefore are somewhat inflexible as tools for the study of cytokine effects in diverse conditions. Finally, given the redundancy of function within cytokine families, the knockout of a single family member may not provide conclusive results. For example, the knockout of TNF-α alone would leave LT-α intact, and the latter might, to some extent, compensate for a deficiency of the former. The knockout of LT-α alone would remove both the LT-α homotrimer and the LT-α/LT-β heterotrimer, but leave TNF-α intact, again permitting compensation for the loss of the LT-α homotrimer.

To circumvent these problems, it may be advantageous to employ a dominant-negative approach that permits the functional deletion of whole classes of cytokines, as defined by their ability to bind specific receptors, both alone or in conjunction with one another and in a variety of different species or strains. This has been accomplished through the development of recombinant cytokine-binding proteins, consisting of the extracellular domain of a cytokine receptor spliced (at a genetic level) to an IgG heavy chain. Such proteins can be expressed at high levels *in vivo*, are non-antigenic, and are relatively long-lived.[68–70] Through transduction with the inhibitor gene, animals may be rendered blind to any TNFs that they might produce.[71]

The functional ablation of TNF-α and LT-α that is achieved by this means mimics deletion of the 55-kD TNF receptor.[10,11] Animals that lose the ability to respond to TNFs develop normally, but are demonstrably immunodeficient insofar as they cannot clear infections by *Listeria monocytogenes* (and presumably other intracellular pathogens). Ongoing studies employing mutant animals and other inhibitory molecules may help to define essential interactions and functional duplications among different cytokines and their receptors.

CONCLUSIONS: DISSECTION OF CYTOKINE ANCESTRY AND FUNCTION

Characteristically, the most essential functions served by a protein are retained in perpetuity, whereas new functions only emerge as permitted by gene duplication. The coevolution of cytokines and their receptors provides a notable case in point. Most cytokine receptors seem to be activated by multimerization, occurring in the presence of a specific ligand. This is true not only of members of the TNF receptor/ligand family, but also of members of the larger hematopoietin/receptor family as well. As such, cytokines may be considered "missing subunits" of enzymes that act to initiate signals. The modular design of these enzymes, and in particular, the principle that activation depends on multimer formation, whatever its cause, has permitted rapid diversification of responses to external signals in the course of evolution.

Redundancy of cytokine function should be viewed in light of this principle. It stems partly from the fact that mutations, particularly those affecting the ligands, have not yet been sufficient to permit a complete separation of receptor binding. Thus, numerous chemokines engage a common receptor; IL-1α, IL-1β, and the IL-1ra engage a common receptor; and interferons-α and -β engage a common receptor, just as TNF-α and LT-α do. At the receptor level, it stems from the fact that mutations affecting cytoplasmic domains have not yet caused diversification of signals: witness the signals transduced by the Fas antigen and the 55-kD TNF receptor.

Certain gaps in our understanding of cytokine function may be filled in the future, as genes similar to the ancestors of those encoding modern cytokines are cloned and as a clear understanding of functional overlap among different cytokine family members becomes more highly developed. Many vertebrate species, "frozen in time" morphologically, might carry genes that are but little changed from those borne by our own distant ancestors. To this end, the isolation of cytokine genes from more primitive species and the determination of their function would seem a worthwhile task.

REFERENCES

1. KORTHÄUUER, U., D. GRAF, H. W. MAGES, F. BRIERE, M. PADAYACHEE, S. MALCOLM, A. G. UGAZIO, L. D. NOTARANGELO, R. J. LEVINSKY & R. A. KROCZEK. 1993. Defective expression of T-cell CD40 ligand causes X-linked immunodeficiency with hyper-IgM. Nature **361**: 539-541.
2. ALLEN, R. C., R. J. ARMITAGE, M. E. CONLEY, H. ROSENBLATT, N. A. JENKINS, N. G. COPELAND, M. A. BEDELL, S. EDELHOFF, C. M. DISTECHE, D. K. SIMONEAUX, W. C. FANSLOW, J. BELMONT & M. K. SPRIGGS. 1993. CD40 ligand gene defects responsible for X-linked hyper-IgM syndrome. Science **259**: 990-993.
3. SUDA, T., T. TAKAHASHI, P. GOLSTEIN & S. NAGATA. 1993. Molecular cloning and expression of the Fas ligand, a novel member of the tumor necrosis factor family. Cell **75**: 1169-1178.
4. NOGUCHI, M., H. YI, H. M. ROSENBLATT, A. H. FILIPOVICH, S. ADELSTEIN, W. S. MODI, O. W. McBRIDE & W. J. LEONARD. 1993. Interleukin-2 receptor gamma chain mutation results in X-linked severe combined immunodeficiency in humans. Cell **73**: 147-157.

5. WATANABE-FUKUNAGA, R., C. I. BRANNAN, N. G. COPELAND, N. A. JENKINS & S. NAGATA. 1992. Lymphoproliferation disorder in mice explained by defects in Fas antigen that mediates apoptosis. Nature **356:** 314-317.

6. DALTON, D. K., S. PITTS-MEEK, S. KESHAV, I. S. FIGARI, A. BRADLEY & T. A. STEWART. 1993. Multiple defects of immune cell function in mice with disrupted interferon-gamma genes. Science **259:** 1739-1742.

7. HUANG, S., W. HENDRIKS, A. ALTHAGE, S. HEMMI, H. BLUETHMANN, R. KAMIJO, J. VILCEK, R. M. ZINKERNAGEL & M. AGUET. 1993. Immune response in mice that lack the interferon-gamma receptor. Science **259:** 1742-1745.

8. SCHORLE, H., T. HOLTSCHKE, T. HÜNIG, A. SCHIMPL & I. HORAK. 1991. Development and function of T cells in mice rendered interleukin-2 deficient by gene targeting. Nature **352:** 621-624.

9. KUHN, R., K. RAJEWSKY & W. MULLER. 1991. Generation and analysis of interleukin-4 deficient mice. Science **254:** 707-710.

10. PFEFFER, K., T. MATSUYAMA, T. M. KÜNIG, A. WAKEHAM, K. KISHIHARA, A. SHAHINIAN, K. WIEGMANN, P. S. OHASHI, M. KRONKE & T. W. MAK. 1993. Mice deficient for the 55 kd tumor necrosis factor receptor are resistant to endotoxic shock, yet succumb to *L. monocytogenes* infection. Cell **73:** 457-467.

11. ROTHE, J., W. LESSLAUER, H. LOTSCHER, Y. LANG, P. KOEBEL, F. KONTGEN, A. ALTHAGE, R. ZINKERNAGEL, M. STEINMETZ & H. BLUETHMANN. 1993. Mice lacking the tumour necrosis factor receptor 1 are resistant to TNF-mediated toxicity but highly susceptible to infection by *Listeria monocytogenes.* Nature **364:** 798-802.

12. BEUTLER, B., I. W. MILSARK & A. CERAMI. 1985. Passive immunization against cachectin/tumor necrosis factor (TNF) protects mice from the lethal effect of endotoxin. Science **229:** 869-871.

13. TRACEY, K. J., B. BEUTLER, S. F. LOWRY, J. MERRYWEATHER, S. WOLPE, I. W. MILSARK, R. J. HARIRI, T. J. FAHEY, III, A. ZENTELLA, J. D. ALBERT, G. T. SHIRES & A. CERAMI. 1986. Shock and tissue injury induced by recombinant human cachectin. Science **234:** 470-474.

14. BEUTLER, B. & A. CERAMI. 1986. Cachectin and tumor necrosis factor as two sides of the same biological coin. Nature **320:** 584-588.

15. KINDLER, V., A.-P. SAPPINO, G. E. GRAU, P.-F. PIGUET & P. VASSALLI. 1989. The inducing role of tumor necrosis factor in the development of bactericidal granulomas during BCG infection. Cell **56:** 731-740.

16. HAVELL, E. A. 1989. Evidence that tumor necrosis factor has an important role in antibacterial resistance. J. Immunol. **143:** 2894-2899.

17. GRAY, P. W., B. B. AGGARWAL, C. V. BENTON, T. S. BRINGMAN, W. J. HENZEL, J. A. JARRETT, D. W. LEUNG, B. MOFFAT, P. NG, L. P. SVEDERSKY, M. A. PALLADINO & G. E. NEDWIN. 1984. Cloning and expression of cDNA for human lymphotoxin, a lymphokine with tumor necrosis activity. Nature **312:** 721-724.

18. ARMITAGE, R. J., W. C. FANSLOW, L. STROCKBINE, T. A. SATO, K. N. CLIFFORD, B. M. MACDUFF, D. M. ANDERSON, S. D. GIMPEL, T. DAVIS-SMITH, C. R. MALISZEWSKI, E. A. CLARK, C. A. SMITH, K. H. GRABSTEIN, D. COSMAN & M. K. SPRIGGS. 1992. Molecular and biological characterization of a murine ligand for CD40. Nature **357:** 80-82.

19. GOODWIN, R. G., M. R. ALDERSON, C. A. SMITH, R. J. ARMITAGE, T. VANDENBOS, R. JERZY, T. W. TOUGH, M. A. SCHOENBORN, T. DAVIS-SMITH, K. HENNEN, B. FALK, D. COSMAN, E. BAKER, G. R. SUTHERLAND, K. H. GRABSTEIN, T. FARRAH, J. G. GIRI & M. P. BECKMANN. 1993. Molecular and biological characterization of a ligand for CD27 defines a new family of cytokines with homology to tumor necrosis factor. Cell **73:** 447-456.

20. GOODWIN, R. G., W. S. DIN, T. DAVIS-SMITH, D. M. ANDERSON, S. D. GIMPEL, T. A. SATO, C. R. MALISZEWSKI, C. I. BRANNAN, N. G. COPELAND, N. A. JENKINS, T. FARRAH, R. J. ARMITAGE, W. C. FANSLOW & C. A. SMITH. 1993. Molecular cloning of a ligand for the inducible T cell gene 4-1BB: A member of an emerging family of cytokines with homology to tumor necrosis factor. Eur. J. Immunol. **23:** 2631-2641.

21. BROWNING, J. L., A. NGAM-EK, P. LAWTON, J. DEMARINIS, R. TIZARD, E. P. CHOW, C. HESSLON, B. O'BRINE-GRECO, S. F. FOLEY & C. F. WARE. 1993. Lymphotoxin β, a novel member of the TNF family that forms a heteromeric complex with lymphotoxin on the cell surface. Cell **72:** 847-856.

22. ECK, M. J., B. BEUTLER, G. KUO, J. P. MERRYWEATHER & S. R. SPRANG. 1988. Crystallization of trimeric recombinant human tumor necrosis factor (cachectin). J. Biol. Chem. **263:** 12816- 12819.

23. ECK, M. J. & S. R. SPRANG. 1989. The structure of tumor necrosis factor-alpha at 2.6A resolution: Implications for receptor binding. J. Biol. Chem. **264:** 17595-17605.

24. ECK, M. J., M. ULTSCH, E. RINDERKNECHT, A. M. DE VOS & S. R. SPRANG. 1992. The structure of human lymphotoxin (TNF-Beta) at 1.9A resolution. J. Biol. Chem. **267:** 2119-2122.

25. SPRANG, S. R. & M. J. ECK. 1992. The 3-D structure of TNF. In Tumor Necrosis Factors: The Molecules and Their Emerging Role in Medicine. B. Beutler, ed.: 11-32. Raven Press. New York.

26. ENGELMANN, H., H. HOLTMANN, C. BRAKEBUSCH, Y. S. AVNI, I. SAROV, Y. NOPHAR, E. HADAS, O. LEITNER & D. WALLACH. 1990. Antibodies to a soluble form of a tumor necrosis factor (TNF) receptor have TNF-like activity. J. Biol. Chem. **265:** 14497-14504.

27. DESCH, C. E., A. DOBRINA, B. B. AGGARWAL & J. M. HARLAN. 1990. Tumor necrosis factor-alpha exhibits greater proinflammatory activity than lymphotoxin *in vitro.* Blood **75:** 2030- 2034.

28. BROUDY, V. C., J. M. HARLAN & J. W. ADAMSON. 1987. Disparate effects of tumor necrosis factor-α/cachectin and tumor necrosis factor-β/lymphotoxin on hematopoietic growth factor production and neutrophil adhesion molecule expression by cultured human endothelial cells. J. Immunol. **138:** 4298-4302.

29. NEDWIN, G. E., L. P. SVEDERSKY, T. S. BRINGMAN, M. A. PALLADINO & D. V. GOEDDEL. 1985. Effect of interleukin 2, interferon-gamma, and mitogens on the production of tumor necrosis factors α and β. J. Immunol. **135:** 2492-2497.

30. BAENS, M., M. CHAFFANET, J. J. CASSIMAN, H. VAN DEN BERGHE & P. MARYNEN. 1993. Construction and evaluation of a hncDNA library of human 12p transcribed sequences derived from a somatic cell hybrid. Genomics **16:** 214-218.

31. HOWARD, S. T., Y. S. CHAN & G. L. SMITH. 1991. Vaccinia virus homologues of the Shope fibroma virus inverted terminal repeat proteins and a discontinuous ORF related to the tumor necrosis factor receptor family. Virology **180:** 633-647.

32. SMITH, C. A., T. DAVIS, J. M. WIGNALL, W. S. DIN, T. FARRAH, C. UPTON, G. MCFADDEN & R. G. GOODWIN. 1991. T2 open reading frame from the Shope fibroma virus encodes a soluble form of the TNF receptor. Biochem. Biophys. Res. Commun. **176:** 335-342.

33. PICKUP, D. J., D. BASTIA, H. O. STONE & W. K. JOKLIK. 1982. Sequence of terminal regions of cowpox virus DNA: Arrangement of repeated and unique sequence elements. Proc. Natl. Acad. Sci. USA **79:** 7112-7116.

34. UPTON, C., J. L. MACEN, M. G. SCHREIBER & G. MCFADDEN. 1991. Myxoma virus expresses a secreted protein with homology to the tumor necrosis factor receptor gene family that contributes to viral virulence. Virology **184:** 370-382.

35. VAN DEN ACKERVEKEN, G. F., J. A. VAN KAN, M. H. JOOSTEN, J. M. MUISERS, H. M. VERBAKEL & D. B. DONNER. 1993. Characterization of two putative pathogenicity genes

of the fungal tomato pathogen *Cladosporium fulvum.* Mol. Plant-Microbiol. Interact. **6:** 210-215.

36. SUGITA, K., T. HIROSE, D. M. ROTHSTEIN, C. DONAHUE, S. F. SCHLOSSMAN & C. MORIMOTO. 1992. CD27, a member of the nerve growth factor receptor family, is preferentially expressed on CD45RA+ CD4 T cell clones and involved in distinct immunoregulatory functions. J. Immunol. **149:** 3208-3216.

37. TARTAGLIA, L. A., M. ROTHE, Y.-F. HU & D. V. GOEDDEL. 1993. Tumor necrosis factor's cytotoxic activity is signaled by the p55 TNF receptor. Cell **73:** 213-216.

38. HELLER, R. A., K. SONG, N. FAN & D. J. CHANG. 1992. The p70 tumor necrosis factor receptor mediates cytotoxicity. Cell **70:** 47-56.

39. HELLER, R. A., K. SONG & N. FAN. 1993. Cytotoxicity by tumor necrosis factor is mediated by both p55 and p70 receptors. Cell **73:** 216.

40. OEHM, A., I. BEHRMANN, W. FALK, M. PAWLITA, G. MAIER, C. KLAS, M. LI-WEBER, S. RICHARDS, J. DHEIN, B. C. TRAUTH, H. PONSTINGL & P. H. KRAMMER. 1992. Purification and molecular cloning of the APO-1 cell surface antigen, a member of the tumor necrosis factor/nerve growth factor receptor superfamily. J. Biol. Chem. **267:** 10709-10715.

41. TRAUTH, B. C., C. KLAS, A. M. J. PETERS, S. MATZKU, P. MOLLER, W. FALK, K.-M. DEBATIN & P. H. KRAMMER. 1989. Monoclonal antibody-mediated tumor regression by induction of apoptosis. Science **245:** 301-305.

42. ITOH, N., S. YONEHARA, A. ISHII, M. YONEHARA, S.-I. MIZUSHIMA, M. SAMESHIMA, A. HASE, Y. SETO & S. NAGATA. 1991. The polypeptide encoded by the cDNA for human cell surface antigen Fas can mediate apoptosis. Cell **66:** 233-243.

43. WATANABE-FUKUNAGA, R., C. I. BRANNAN, N. ITOH, S. YONEHARA, N. G. COPELAND, N. A. JENKINS & S. NAGATA. 1992. The cDNA structure, expression, and chromosomal assignment of the mouse Fas antigen. J. Immunol. **148:** 1274-1279.

44. HOLDER, M. J., H. WANG, A. E. MILNER, M. CASAMAYOR, R. ARMITAGE, M. K. SPRIGGS, W. C. FANSLOW, I. C. M. MACLENNAN, C. D. GREGORY & J. GORDON. 1993. Suppression of apoptosis in normal and neoplastic human B lymphocytes by CD40 ligand is independent of Bc1-2 induction. Eur. J. Immunol. **23:** 2368-2371.

45. TSUBATA, T., J. WU & T. HONJO. 1993. B-cell apoptosis induced by antigen receptor crosslinking is blocked by a T-cell signal through CD40. Nature **364:** 645-648.

46. RABIZADEH, S., J. OH, L. ZHONG, J. YANG, C. M. BITLER, L. L. BUTCHER & D. E. BREDESEN. 1993. Induction of apoptosis by the low-affinity NGF receptor. Science **261:** 345-348.

47. TARTAGLIA, L. A., D. V. GOEDDEL, C. REYNOLDS, I. S. FIGARI, R. F. WEBER, B. M. FENDLY & M. A. PALLADINO, JR. 1993. Stimulation of human T-cell proliferation by specific activation of the 75-kDa tumor necrosis factor receptor. J. Immunol. **151:** 4637-4641.

48. TARTAGLIA, L. A., T. M. AYRES, G. H. W. WONG & D. V. GOEDDEL. 1993. A novel domain within the 55 kd TNF receptor signals cell death. Cell **74:** 845-853.

49. OHNO, S. 1970. Evolution by Gene Duplication. Springer-Verlag. Berlin, Heidelberg, New York.

50. HAVELL, E. A. 1993. *Listeria monocytogenes* induced interferon-gamma primes the host for production of tumor necrosis factor and interferon-α/β. J. Infect. Dis. **167:** 1364-1371.

51. ANDERSON, K. P., Y. S. LIE, M.-A. L. LOW & E. H. FENNIE. 1993. Effects of tumor necrosis factor-α treatment on mortality in murine cytomegalovirus-infected mice. Antiviral Res. **21:** 343-355.

52. SMITH, C. A., T. DAVIS & J. M. WIGNALL. 1991. T2 open reading frame from the shope fibroma virus encodes a soluble form of the TNF receptor. Biochem. Biophy. Res. Commun. **176:** 335-342.

53. GOODING, L. R., L. W. ELMORE, A. E. TOLLEFSON, H. A. BRADY & W. S. M. WOLD. 1988. A 14,700 MW protein from the E3 region of adenovirus inhibits cytolysis by tumor necrosis factor. Cell **53:** 341–346.

54. WOLD, W. S. M. & L. R. GOODING. 1989. Adenovirus region E3 proteins that prevent cytolysis by cytotoxic T cells and tumor necrosis factor. Mol. Biol. Med. **6:** 433–452.

55. CHU, J.-L., J. DRAPPA, A. PARNASSA & K. B. ELKON. 1993. The defect in *Fas* mRNA expression in MRL/*lpr* mice is associated with insertion of the retrotransposon, *ETn.* J. Exp. Med. **178:** 723–730.

56. MATSUZAWA, A., T. MORIYAMA, T. KANEKO, M. TANAKA, M. KIMURA, H. IKEDA & T. KATAGIRI. 1990. A new allele of the lpr locus, lprcg, that complements the gld gene in induction of lymphadenopathy in the mouse. J. Exp. Med. **171:** 519–531.

57. MARSHALL, L. S., A. ARUFFO, J. A. LEDBETTER & R. J. NOELLE. 1993. The molecular basis for T cell help in humoral immunity: CD40 and its ligand, gp39. J. Clin. Immunol. **13:** 165– 174.

58. DURANDY, A., C. SCHIFF, J. Y. BONNEFOY, M. FORVEILLE, F. ROUSSET, G. MAZZEI, M. MILILI & A. FISCHER. 1993. Induction by anti-CD40 antibody or soluble CD40 ligand and cytokines of IgG, IgA and IgE production by B cells from patients with X-linked hyper IgM syndrome. Eur. J. Immunol. **23:** 2294–2299.

59. DISANTO, J. P., J. Y. BONNEFOY, J. F. GAUCHAT, A. FISCHER & G. DE SAINT BASILE. 1993. CD40 ligand mutations in x-linked immunodeficiency with hyper-IgM. Nature **361:** 541– 543.

60. FULEIHAN, R., N. RAMESH, R. LOH, H. JABARA, F. S. ROSEN, T. CHATILA, S. M. FU, I. STAMENKOVIC & R. S. GEHA. 1993. Defective expression of the CD40 ligand in X chromosome-linked imunoglobulin deficiency with normal or elevated IgM. Proc. Natl. Acad. Sci. USA **90:** 2170–2173.

61. JACOB, C. O., S. AISO, S. A. MICHIE, H. O. MCDEVITT & H. ACHA-ORBEA. 1990. Prevention of diabetic in nonobese diabetes mice by tumor necrosis factor (TNF): Similarities between TNF-α and interleukin 1. Proc. Natl. Acad. Sci. USA **87:** 968–972.

62. SATOH, J., H. SEINO, T. ABO, S. TANAKA, S. SHINTANI, S. OHTA, K. TAMURA, T. SAWAI, T. NOBUNAGA, T. OTEKI, K. KUMAGAI & T. TOYOTA. 1989. Recombinant human tumor necrosis factor α suppresses autoimmune diabetes in nonobese diabetic mice. J. Clin. Invest. **84:** 1345–1348.

63. SATOH, J., H. SEINO, S. SHINTANI, S.-I. TANAKA, T. OHTEKI, T. MASUDA, T. NOBUNAGA & T. TOYOTA. 1990. Inhibition of type I diabetes in BB rats with recombinant human tumor necrosis factor-α J. Immunol. **145:** 1395–1399.

64. TAKAHASHI, K., J. SATOH, H. SEINO, X. P. ZHU, M. SAGARA, T. MASUDA & T. TOYOTA. 1993. Prevention of type I diabetes with lymphotoxin in BB rats. Clin. Immunol. Immunopathol. **69:** 318–323.

65. JACOB, C. O. & H. O. MCDEVITT. 1988. Tumour necrosis factor-α in murine autoimmune ''lupus'' nephritis. Nature **331:** 356–358.

66. BAZZONI, F. & B. BEUTLER. 1994. Comparative expression of TNF-α alleles from normal and autoimmune-prone MHC haplotypes. Submitted.

67. BEUTLER, B. & T. BROWN. 1993. Polymorphism of the mouse *TNF*-α locus: Sequence studies of the 3′-untranslated region and first intron. Gene **129:** 279–283.

68. PEPPEL, K. & B. BEUTLER. 1993. Biological properties of a recombinant TNF inhibitor. *In* Bacterial Endotoxin: Recognition and Effector Mechanisms. J. Levin, C. R. Alving, R. S. Munford & P. L. Stütz, eds.: 447–454. Elsevier Science Publishers B. V. Vienna, Austria.

69. PEPPEL, K., A. POLTORAK, I. MELHADO, F. JIRIK & B. BEUTLER. 1993. Expression of a TNF inhibitor in transgenic mice. J. Immunol. **151:** 5699–5703.

70. PEPPEL, K., D. CRAWFORD & B. BEUTLER. 1991. A tumor necrosis factor (TNF) receptor-IgG heavy chain chimeric protein as a bivalent antagonist of TNF activity. J. Exp. Med. **174:** 1483–1489.

71. KOLLS, J., K. PEPPEL, M. SILVA & B. BEUTLER. 1994. Prolonged and effective blockade of tumor necrosis factor activity through adenovirus-mediated gene transfer. Proc. Natl. Acad. Sci. USA **91:** 215–219.

72. FELSENSTEIN, J. 1989. PHYLIP-Phylogeny Inference Package (Version 3.2). Cladistics **5:** 164– 166.

73. HIGGINS, D. G., A. J. BLEASBY & P. M. FUCHS. 1992. Clustal-V-improved software for multiple alignment. Cabio. **8:** 189–191.

74. SANDERS, C., D. I. H. STEWART & L. B. SMILLIE. 1987. Troponin-T and glyceraldehyde-3-phosphate dehydrogenase share a common antigenic determinant. J. Mus. Res. Cell Motil. **8:** 118–124.

75. SAITOU, N. & M. NEI. 1987. The neighbor-joining method: a new method for reconstructing phylogenetic trees. Mol. Biol. Evol. **4:** 406–425.

The Role of Interleukin-8 in the Infectious Process[a]

STEVEN L. KUNKEL,[b,c] NICKOLAS W. LUKACS,[b] AND
ROBERT M. STRIETER[d,e]

Departments of Pathology[b] and Internal Medicine[d]
Division of Pulmonary and Critical Care Medicine[e]
The University of Michigan Medical School
Ann Arbor, Michigan 48109-0602

The recruitment of blood-born leukocytes to a specific site of infection is one of the most fundamental of all inflammatory processes. To successfully elicit the appropriate leukocyte populations, a number of dynamic alterations must first occur in a tightly coordinated manner. The first changes that are evident involve alterations in the endothelium as this structure is converted from a passive to an active role in inflammation.[1,2] The changes that occur in the endothelium are important in localizing the circulating leukocytes to a restricted area of injury where the infectious process is originating. The actual mechanism(s) that leads to the generation of an "inflamed" or activated endothelium is likely multifactoral. Bacteria-derived products, such as lipopolysaccharide (LPS), can serve as powerful agents for stimulating endothelial cells.[2] In addition, early response cytokines, including interleukin-1 alpha (IL-1α), interleukin-1 beta (IL-1β), and tumor necrosis factor alpha (TNFα), are also classic mediators that can activate the endothelium.[1] Interestingly, LPS can either directly stimulate or indirectly activate endothelial cells by induction of resident, tissue macrophage-derived IL-1 or TNF.[3,4] Expression of these cell-derived mediators can establish a cytokine network necessary to fully drive the inflammatory response.[5,6] Independent of an exogenous (LPS) or endogenous (IL-1 or TNF) signal, activation of the endothelium results in the expression of adhesion molecules on the surface of endothelial cells and leukocytes. The net result of this interaction is the localization of specific leukocyte populations to an area of tissue injury. Elegant studies have demonstrated that the endothelial cell–leukocyte adhesion process is comprised of discrete steps, which include an initial "rolling" event followed by tenacious binding by strong leukocyte-to-endothelial cell interactions. Once tethered to endothelial cells in a local area of tissue injury, the leukocyte must next traffic out of the vessel lumen, move through the basement membrane, and successfully arrive at the inflammatory site. Thus, binding of leukocytes to the endothelium is a transient event.

[a] This research was supported in part by National Institutes of Health grants P50HL46487, HL02401, HL31693, and HL35276 and a grant from the Tobacco Research Council.

[c] Address for correspondence: Steven L. Kunkel, Ph.D., Department of Pathology, 1301 Catherine Road/Box 0602, The University of Michigan Medical School, Ann Arbor, Michigan 48109-0602.

CHEMOTACTIC FACTORS

Whereas events involved in the initial binding of leukocytes to an activated endothelium are becoming increasingly clear, the actual movement of certain leukocyte populations from the vasculature to an exact site of tissue injury is not well understood. However, recent information suggests that specific targeting and movement of leukocytes involve the further participation of adhesion molecules and chemotactic factors often expressed by stromal and other resident tissue cells. The idea that leukocytes follow chemical signals is not new, as historic studies have identified chemotactic factors that can induce the directed migration of leukocytes. For example, bacterial peptides (fmetleuphe), polypeptides (C5a), and lipids (LTB and PAF) have all demonstrated the ability to elicit various leukocyte populations.[7–9] There is little doubt that these chemotactic factors play an important role in the initiation of leukocyte recruitment; however, their transient expression, instability, and lack of cell specificity have always left a void in the total explanation of the chemotactic response. The finding that many chemotactic factors possess little specificity for eliciting specific leukocyte populations has been inconsistent with the histopathology of a number of diseases. For example, acute inflammatory reactions are often characterized by the presence of polymorphonuclear leukocytes, whereas other chronic inflammatory diseases are characterized by mononuclear cell infiltration. Further understanding of the mechanism of this biologic response has been attained by studies assessing the role of chemotactic cytokines or chemokines in mediating leukocyte elicitation.[10–12]

The first chemotactic cytokine to be discovered was originally termed monocyte-derived neutrophil chemotactic factor (MDNCF) and later classified as interleukin-8 (IL-8).[13] Subsequent studies proved that most nucleated cells, when appropriately stimulated, have the capacity to generate IL-8.[14–17] As research in the chemotactic cytokine arena progressed, it became increasingly apparent that IL-8 was only one member of a supergene family that possesses chemotactic activity for polymorphonuclear (PMN) leukocytes.[10] Presently, chemokines that possess chemotactic activity for PMNs include epithelial cell-derived neutrophil activating peptide (ENA-78), neutrophil-activating peptide-2 (NAP-2), growth-related oncogene (GRO-alpha, beta, and gamma), and macrophage inflammatory protein-2 alpha and beta (MIP-2 α and β). This supergene family of chemotactic cytokines is structurally characterized by the conserved location of two of four cysteine residues. The first two cysteines are separated by one additional amino acid; therefore, this family is often referred to as the C-X-C chemokine family. The aforementioned chemotactic factors also share a common amino acid motif, ELR (glutamic acid, leucine, and arginine), which is present in juxtaposition to the first NH_2-terminal cysteine amino of the C-X-C.[10] The importance of the ELR is that this sequence is responsible for neutrophil activation via receptor ligand interactions. Interestingly, other C-X-C supergene family members that do not possess the ELR motif are not chemotactic for neutrophils. These polypeptides include platelet factor-4 (PF-4) and an interferon-inducible protein (IP-10). Recent investigations demonstrated that generation of recombinant PF-4, which has been mutated to include the ELR, is indeed chemotactic for neutrophils. On the contrary, ELR-containing chemokines that have been truncated to remove the ELR element dramatically change their binding affinity for the appropriate receptor, subsequently reducing their chemotactic activity. However, the synthesis of short peptides that include the ELR motif is not active, suggesting that interaction of other domains of the chemokine molecule is necessary for biologic activity. The receptor system for the C-X-C chemokines is comprised of two high affinity receptors. One is promiscuous and able to interact with other family members, whereas the other receptor possesses specificity for an individual chemokine. The chemokine receptors are seven transmembrane-spanning proteins that signal via GTP-binding proteins.

Whereas the IL-8 or C-X-C supergene family possesses chemotactic activity mainly for neutrophils, a related polypepide family has been discovered with activity predominantly for mononuclear cells. This class of chemokines is also structurally identified by the location of two of four cysteines. However, the first two cysteines are in juxtaposition and this family is designated as the C-C chemokine family.[11] Monocyte chemoattractant protein-1, 2, and 3 (MCP-1, MCP-2, and MCP-3), macrophage inflammatory protein-1 (MIP-1) alpha and beta, and RANTES are members of this family of chemotactic cytokines. Recent data suggest that the ligand:receptor system for the C-C family is similar to the C-X-C system. Structure/function analysis of these chemokines and the quest for receptor antagonists have greatly accelerated interest in this area of inflammation.

EXPRESSION AND REGULATION OF CHEMOTACTIC CYTOKINES

A striking novel aspect of both the C-C and C-X-C chemokine families is the expression pattern that results in the generation of these mediators. Both inflammatory and noninflammatory cells have been identified as cell sources of these chemotactic factors. Thus, neutrophils, monocytes, smooth muscle cells, fibroblasts, epithelial cells, and endothelial cells have all been identified as rich sources of chemokines, especially IL-8.[14–17] Although these cells do not usually generate high levels of IL-8 during resting conditions, they can produce elevated concentrations when stimulated with an appropriate agonist. One exception is the expression of IL-8 by certain tumor cell lines which possess the ability to constitutively generate significant levels of IL-8. Two of the most potent agents for the induction of IL-8 are IL-1 and TNF. These early response cytokines induce the production of IL-8 by most nucleated cells at picomolar to nanomolar concentrations. Although IL-1 and TNF are potent early response cytokines that are able to induce IL-8 expression, other cytokines such as interleukin-6 (IL-6) do not serve as effective signals for the production of IL-8. Thus, expression of IL-8 depends on both cell and stimulus specificity.[5,6] LPS and other bacteria-derived products can also serve as important activating agents for the production of IL-8; however, LPS-dependent IL-8 production is not routinely observed from all cells. Although both mononuclear phagocytes and polymorphonuclear leukocytes can generate IL-8 in response to LPS, most noninflammatory cells do not generate IL-8 in response to bacteria-derived products.

The inability of LPS to activate specific cells to produce IL-8 does not imply that Gram-negative bacteria are not involved in the process of generating chemotactic cytokines. Evolving scientific information suggests that generation of cytokine networks via LPS-dependent mechanisms is a major pathway for the production of chemokines.[5,6] During the pathogenesis of an infectious process, it is likely that bacterial products activate sentinel, resident macrophages which are ubiquitously dispersed throughout tissue. This activation event results in the production of early response cytokines (IL-1 and TNF), which can "network" with surrounding resident tissue cells and orchestrate the production of more distal cytokines, including IL-8. Therefore, the overall effect of the inciting agent is to activate the inflammatory cascade and cause the up-regulation of appropriate chemotactic factors to insure the successful elicitation of leukocytes to the area of inflammation. Interestingly, noninflammatory cells such as stromal and epithelial cells can no longer be only designated as targets of the inflammatory response, but are more likely to be considered as effector cells via the expression of important cytokines. This scenario was previously shown to be active in the generation of lung and hepatic chemotactic cytokines using _in vitro_ models. For example, the conditioned media from LPS-challenged alveolar macrophages, recovered from nonsmoking, disease-free volunteers, possessed significant activity in stimulating the expression of IL-8 from pulmonary fibroblasts.[5] These same lung fibroblasts were not susceptible to LPS stimulation, suggesting that factors(s) in the alveolar macrophage-conditioned media were providing the signal for noninflammatory cell activation. Similar results were observed using type II-like pneumocyte cell lines challenged with conditioned media from LPS-treated alveolar macrophages.[6] Further studies identified that both IL-1 and TNF are involved in the expression of IL-8 from these noninflammatory cells. In these studies, conditioned media from alveolar macrophages treated with neutralizing antibodies to IL-1 or TNF significantly reduced the production of fibroblast-derived IL-8. This networking phenomenon is not restricted only to the lungs, as previous studies demonstrated that cytokine networking can also occur in the liver. These investigations showed that LPS-activated Kupffer cells can secrete both IL-1 and TNF which can interact with hepatocytes and induce the production of IL-8 from these noninflammatory cells. It is becoming increasingly clear that this pathway of cell activation leading to the production of a potent chemotactic factor for neutrophils is likely a mechanism for leukocyte elicitation common to all tissues. Stimulated resident macrophages signal the surrounding normal resident cells to produce a chemoattractant that elicits a specific population of leukocytes to a local area of inflammation. This scenario is a key component of leukocyte elicitation, as it insures that the recruitment response is timely, specific, and localized only to the area of tissue injury. This latter phenomenon is one of the most fundamental aspects of normal inflammation.

NEUTROPHIL-DEPENDENT CHEMOKINE EXPRESSION

In acute inflammation, the first blood-born leukocyte to arrive at a site of tissue injury or infection is the neutrophil. Historically, these elicited cells have been important in clearing infectious agents by the release of proteolytic enzymes and reactive oxygen metabolites. In addition, these terminally differentiated leukocytes have classically been viewed as possessing limited protein-synthesizing activity. Recent studies showed that neutrophils can produce polypeptides, including heat shock proteins, elastase, plasminogen activator, cytoskeletal proteins, and cell surface receptors.[18–20] Also, stimulated neutrophils have the ability to generate cytokines, that

                     ANNALS NEW YORK ACADEMY OF SCIENCES

are important in maintaining the inflammatory response, such as colony-stimulating factors (G-CSF and GM-CSF), interferon-alpha, interleukin-6, interleukin-1, tumor necrosis factor, and interleukin-8.[21-26] The production of these polypeptide mediators at a site of injury is likely to play a significant role in the subsequent evolution of inflammation by both paracrine and autocrine interactions, involving other leukocytes and/or noninflammatory cells.

Investigations have demonstrated that neutrophils are capable of generating IL-8 in response to both endogenous and exogenous signals. For example, the phagocytic response to zymosan or other particulate material, as well as LPS, may serve as an exogenous agent for neutrophil-derived IL-8. In addition, the adherence response is a significant signal which may lead to the production of IL-8. The mechanism(s) involved in adherence-dependent IL-8 expression may be an adhesion molecule-mediated event, as freshly isolated neutrophils in suspension did not express steady-state levels of IL-8 mRNA or release antigenic IL-8. The concomitant treatment of neutrophils with actinomycin D also blocked any adherence-induced IL-8 mRNA and protein. Subsequent investigations showed that adherence-induced, neutrophil-derived IL-8 is under the regulation of repressor proteins. This was ascertained by the concomitant addition of cycloheximide to neutrophils undergoing adherence, resulting in the superinduction of IL-8 mRNA.

Whereas exogenous stimuli can cause neutrophils to generate IL-8, other endogenous mediators are highly effective in generating neutrophil-derived IL-8. In particular, IL-1 and TNF were effective stimulating agents for neutrophils in both a time- and dose-dependent manner. The findings that IL-1 can stimulate neutrophil-derived IL-8 is intriguing in light of reports demonstrating that IL-1 is not a potent neutrophil-activating compound for direct chemotaxis, exocytosis, or enzyme release. However, IL-1 can induce neutrophils to generate a potent neutrophil chemoattractant, which is likely to perpetuate the recruitment process. Other factors have also been identified as important neutrophil-activating agents and play both direct and indirect roles in leukocyte recruitment. C5a, fMLP, and LTB$_4$ are all known mediators of neutrophil recruitment that also synergize in the presence of LPS to induce neutrophil-derived IL-8. The synergistic activity of bacteria-derived products plus traditional neutrophil-activating agents such as C5a, fMLP, and LTB$_4$ could aid in explaining the rapid elicitation of neutrophils to a site of bacterial infection. At the inflammatory lesion, neutrophils can encounter host-derived cytokines (IL-1 and TNF), endogenous chemotactic and activating agents (C5a, fMLP, and LTB$_4$), as well as bacteria and their products, which can stimulate neutrophils in a synergistic manner for the production of neutrophil-derived IL-8. Although the aforementioned classic neutrophil chemotactic factors (C5a, fMLP, and LTB$_4$) are indeed chemotactic agents, these agonsts have relatively short half-lives. Thus, local generation of IL-8 by mononuclear phagocytes, noninflammatory cells, and neutrophils may sustain the inflammatory response through continued neutrophil recruitment and activation. The importance of the neutrophil as an effector cell via *de novo* cytokine production places this inflammatory cell in a pivotal position to aid in the orchestration of conventional immune responses.

Although increasing evidence supports the role of the neutrophil as an important cytokine-producing leukocyte, less is known about the mechanism(s) that regulates the expression of these neutrophil-derived polypeptides. Interestingly, specific compounds that control the production of monocyte-derived cytokines also appear to have a regulating influence on neutrophil-derived cytokines.

Dexamethasone, interleukin-4 (IL-4), and interleukin-10 (IL-10) have been demonstrated in a time- and dose-dependent manner and in a delayed addition manner to regulate the production of neutrophil-derived IL-8. Neutrophils treated with LPS and dexamethasone at 100, 10, and 1 nM demonstrated a 73%, 47%, and 45% reduction, respectively, in IL-8 levels. Concentrations of dexamethasone less than 1 nM failed to cause any further suppression of neutrophil IL-8 in response to LPS. In similar studies, IL-4 and IL-10 exerted a suppressive effect on neutrophil IL-8 production over a concentration range of 100 pg/ml to 100 ng/ml. Further studies demonstrated that the delayed addition of dexamethasone, IL-4, or IL-10 could still dramatically influence the production of neutrophil-derived IL-8. The production of IL-8 from neutrophils stimulated with LPS at time 0 and given either of the three suppressing agents 2 hours later was still significantly inhibited at the final 18-hour time-point. Additional studies demonstrated that the suppressive effects of IL-4, IL-10, and dexamethasone were at the transcriptional level. Northern blot analyses of neutrophils challenged with LPS plus one of the three immunomodulating agents showed that steady-state levels of IL-8 were significantly reduced as compared to LPS alone. These studies are significant in that they demonstrate the regulation of neutrophil-derived IL-8 at the transcriptional level.

The foregoing investigations are of interest, because IL-4 and IL-10 are phenotypically expressed by TH2 lymphocytes and have been shown to possess pleiotropic activities in a number of cell systems. Although IL-4 was originally described as a B- and T-cell maturation and growth factor, it has also been reported to have the dual role of either enhancing or suppressing monocyte functions. Interleukin-4 can also enhance monocyte major histocompatibility complex expression and augment tumoricidal activity. In contrast, IL-4 has been shown to block the generation of monocyte-derived cytokines, including IL-6, IL-8, TNF, and IL-1, as well as to reduce the generation of reactive oxygen metabolites. Whereas IL-4 can inhibit important phagocyte functions, it appears to be a general activating agent for endothelial cells. This cytokine can stimulate endothelial cells to induce the expression of specific adhesion molecules for lymphocytes and monocytes but not neutrophils, suggesting that IL-4 is important in driving the switch from an acute to a chronic inflammatory response. These studies demonstrating a reduction of IL-8 by IL-4-treated neutrophils support this hypothesis, as the continued generation of IL-8 would propagate the acute inflammatory response by continued neutrophil recruitment.

Interleukin-10 may mechanistically play a key role in the leukocyte switch in a manner similar to that of IL-4. Originally, IL-10 was found to be able to inhibit the production of gamma interferon from CD4$^+$ T cells; however, this cytokine can also suppress a number of cytokines necessary to maintain an inflammatory response. Monocytes treated with LPS in the presence of graded doses of IL-10 produced significantly less IL-1, TNF, IL-6, IL-8, and G-CSF. In addition, IL-10 can suppress macrophage cytotoxic activity, parasite killing, and macrophage-derived nitric oxide production. Thus, the cytokine networks that function in both a positive and negative manner for the production and regulation of IL-8 are an important yet complex system.

BACTERIAL INFECTIONS AND IL-8 EXPRESSION

Cytokines unquestionably represent an important communication link necessary to combat infectious processes. Previous studies identified cytokines, such as TNF, IL-1, and IL-6, as being elevated in infectious disease states and suggested that they are indicators of clinical severity. Although these cytokines undoubtedly play a role in disease progression, other chemotactic cytokines appear to be involved in the initiation and maintenance of bacterial infection. Elevated concentrations of IL-8 were identified after injection of intravenous *Escherichia coli* in primates and after an injection of LPS into human volunteers.[27,28] The kinetics of the *in vivo* expression pattern for IL-8 was similar to that for IL-6 in that the detection of IL-8 was delayed about 3 hours postchallenge. These data suggest that *in vivo* cytokine networking could account for the mechanism of IL-8 production, because IL-8 production was distal to the acute production of TNF in these experiments.

Recently, IL-8 levels were identified in human patients with either severe bacterial infections, septicemia, or adult respiratory distress syndrome. A detailed longitudinal study assessing the plasma concentrations of TNF, IL-6, and IL-8 was reported for patients with melioidosis.[29] This infection is caused by *Pseudomonas pseudomallei* and is endemic throughout Southeast Asia. Clinically, melioidosis caused a serious septicemic illness with a 40% death rate. In this study, 18 patients were monitored for circulating levels of plasma IL-8, IL-6, and TNF. Elevated concentrations of plasma IL-8 were found in 8 of 18 subjects, including four who subsequently died. Three of the four who died had the highest levels of IL-8, 161–362 pg/ml; therefore, IL-8 levels may have value as a predictor of mortality. Qualitative plasma IL-6 levels followed a pattern similar to those of IL-8 in that the highest levels of IL-6 were found in three of the four patients who died of this disease. On the contrary, no correlation was noted between plasma TNF levels and concentrations of IL-8 or IL-6. Additional clinical studies demonstrated a close correlation between plasma levels of TNF, IL-6, and IL-8 and the pathophysiology of the Jarisch-Herxheimer reaction (J-HR) associated with the treatment protocol for certain infectious diseases.[30] In this clinical study, 14 of 17 patients (82%) diagnosed with relapsing fever due to *Borrelia recurrentis* and treated with penicillin subsequently experienced J-HR. This acute reaction is characterized by rigors, fever, leukopenia, and a decrease in mean arterial blood pressure. Although no fatalities occurred, plasma TNF, IL-6, and IL-8 levels rose seven, six, and fourfold, respectively, over admission levels. Interestingly, a pulsatile release of the three different cytokines was associated with J-HR which occurred between 2 and 4 hours after antibiotic treatment. The peak values for TNF, IL-6, and IL-8 were 126 ± 38, 9,578 ± 1,808, and 8,102 ± 4,491 pg/ml, respectively.

In further studies, 105 of 151 patients undergoing mechanical ventilation in an intensive care unit had detectable IL-8 levels in bronchial secretions.[31] However, IL-8 levels could not be detected in arterial blood, mixed venous blood, or urine samples. The occurrence of IL-8 in bronchial secretions of the pulmonary air space was significantly associated with patients with multiple injuries and nosocomial pneumonia. Interestingly, 66% of the patients who had positive IL-8 levels were diagnosed as having nosocomial pneumonia. Most of the patients tested positive for IL-8 within the first 36 hours of admission, suggesting that the production of IL-8 was a relatively rapid event. In addition, detectable IL-8 levels were associated with significant pulmonary dysfunction, as evidenced by static lung compliance and a low PaO_2/FIO_2 ratio.

Finally, recent investigation of 29 patients with adult respiratory distress syndrome (ARDS) demonstrated a significant correlation between the early appearance of IL-8 in the bronchoalveolar lavage (BAL) fluid and the development of clinical ARDS.[32] The 29 patients were grouped into three at-risk categories: multiple trauma, perforated bowel, and pancreatitis. Both BAL and plasma from each patient were assessed for antigenic IL-8 within a mean of 2 hours of trauma, 34 hours of diagnosed pancreatitis, and 33 hours of diagnosed perforated bowel. Although no significant difference was noted between the groups in plasma IL-8 levels, a significant difference was found in the BAL fluid IL-8 levels in the group that progressed to ARDS as compared to the non-ARDS group (p value = 0.0006). Patients with clinical ARDS had IL-8 levels of 3.06 ng/ml *versus* 0.53 ng/ml in the non-ARDS group.

Immunocytochemical analyses for antigenic IL-8 demonstrated more intense staining of alveolar macrophages from patients who subsequently progressed to ARDS than of alveolar macrophages from non-ARDS patients. The latter findings support the concept that activated alveolar macrophages are a potent source of cytokines, such as IL-8, during the initiation of ARDS. These findings suggest that measurement of IL-8 levels in the BAL fluid of at-risk patients could aid in early identification of those likely to progress to ARDS.

REFERENCES

1. POBER, J. S., P. BEVILACQUA, D. L. MENDRICK, L. A. LAPIERRE, W. FIERS & M. A. GIMBRONE. 1986. Two distinct monokines, interleukin-1 and tumor necrosis factor, each independently induce biosynthesis and transient expression of the same antigen on the surface of cultured human vascular endothelial cells. J. Immunol. **137:** 1680–1693.
2. CYBULSKY, M. I., M. K. W. CHAN & H. Z. MOVAT. 1988. Acute inflammation and microthrombosis induced by endotoxin, interleukin-1, and tumor necrosis factor, and their implication in gram negative infection. Lab. Invest. **58:** 365–378.
3. CHENSUE, W., P. D. TEREBUH, D. G. REMICK, W. E. SCALES & S. L. KUNKEL. 1991. *In vivo* biologic and immunohistochemical analysis of interleukin-1 alpha, beta, and tumor necrosis factor during experimental enotoxemia: Kinetics, Kupffer cell expression and glucocorticoid effects. Am. J. Pathol. **138:** 395–402.
4. STRIETER, R. M., D. G. REMICK, J. P. LYNCH & S. L. KUNKEL. 1989. Differential regulation of tumor necrosis factor-alpha in human alveolar macrophages and peripheral blood monocytes: A cellular and molecular analysis. Am. J. Respir. Cell Mol. Biol. **1:** 57–63.
5. ROLFE, M. W., S. L. KUNKEL, T. J. STANDIFORD & R. M. STRIETER. 1992. Pulmonary fibroblasts expression of interleukin-8: A model for alveolar macrophage derived cytokine networking. Am. J. Respir. Cell Mol. Biol. **5:** 579–585.
6. STANDIFORD, T. J., S. L. KUNKEL, M. A. BASHA & R. M. STRIETER. 1990. Interleukin-8 expression by pulmonary epithelial cells: A model for cytokine networks in the lung. J. Clin. Invest. **86:** 1945–1953.
7. FERNANDEZ, H. N., P. M. HENSON, A. OTANI & T. E. HUGLI. 1978. Chemotactic response to human C3a and C5a anaphylatoxins. 1. Evaluation of C3a and C5a leukotaxis *in vitro* and under stimulated *in vivo* conditions. J. Immunol. **120:** 109–115.

8. FORD-HUTCHINSON, A. W., M. A. BRAY, M. V. DOIG & M. J. SMITH. 1980. Leukotriene B4 a potent chemokinetic and aggregating substance released from polymorphonuclear leukocytes. Nature **286:** 262-265.

9. SHIFFMAN, E., B. A. CORCORAN, S. M. WAHL, H. J. SHOWELL & E. BECKER. 1975. N-formylmethionyl peptides as chemoattractants for leukocytes. Proc. Natl. Acad. Sci. USA **72:** 1059- 1062.

10. MATSUSHIMA K. & J. J. OPPENHEIM. 1990. Interleukin-8 and MCAF: Novel inflammatory cytokines inducible by IL-1 and TNF. Cytokine **1:** 2-13.

11. LEONARD, E. J. & T. YOSHIMURA. 1990. Human monocyte chemoattractant protein-1 (MCP-1). Immunol. Today **11:** 97-100.

12. STRIETER, R. M., S. L. KUNKEL, H. J. SHOWELL, D. G. REMICK, S. H. PHAN, P. A. WARD & R. M. MARKS. 1989. Endothelial cell gene expression of a neutrophil chemotactic factor by TNF-alpha, LPS, and IL-1 beta. Science **243:** 1467-1469.

13. MATSUSHIMA, K., K. MOISHITA, T. YOSHIMURA, S. LAVU, Y. OBAYASHI, W. LEW, E. APPELLA, E. J. LEONARD & J. J. OPPENHEIM. 1988. Molecular cloning of human monocyte-derived neutrophil chemotactic factor (MDNCF) and induction of MDNCF by interleukin-1 and tumor necrosis factor. J. Exp. Med. **167:** 1883-1893.

14. THORNTON, A. J., J. HAM & S. L. KUNKEL. 1991. Kupffer cell-derived cytokines induce the synthesis of a leukocyte chemotactic peptide, interleukin-8, in human hepatoma and primary heptocyte cultures. Hepatology **14:** 1112-1122.

15. SCHMOUDER, R. L., R. M. STRIETER, R. C. WIGGINS & S. L. KUNKEL. 1992. *In vitro* and *in vivo* interleukin-8 production in human renal cortical epithelia. Kidney Int. **41:** 191-198.

16. STRIETER, R. M., S. H. PHAN, H. J. SHOWELL, D. G. REMICK, J. P. LYNCH, R. M. MARKS & S. L. KUNKEL. 1989. Monokine-induced neutrophil chemotactic factor gene expression in human fibroblasts. J. Biol. Chem. **264:** 10621-10626.

17. DIBB, C. R., R. M. STRIETER, M. BURDICK & S. L. KUNKEL. 1992. Expression of interleukin-8 by LPS-stimulated bone marrow derived mononuclear cells. Infect. Immunol. **60:** 3052- 3058.

18. GRANELLI-PIPERNO, A., J. D. VASSALLI & E. REICH. 1979. RNA and protein synthesis in human polymorphonuclear leukocytes. J. Exp. Med. **149:** 284-289.

19. JACK, R. M. & D. T. FEARON. 1988. Selective synthesis of mRNA and proteins by human peripheral blood neutrophils. J. Immunol. **140:** 4286-4293.

20. EID, N. S., R. E. KRAVATH & K. W. LANKS. 1987. Heat-shock protein synthesis by human polymorphonuclear cells. J. Exp. Med. **165:** 1148-1153.

21. DUBRAVEC, D. B., D. R. SPRIGGS, J. A. MANNICK & M. L. RODRICK. 1990. Circulating human peripheral blood granulocytes synthesize and secrete tumor necrosis factor-alpha. Proc. Natl. Acad. Sci. USA **87:** 6758-6761.

22. TIKU, K., M. L. TIKU & J. L. SKOSEY. 1986. Interleukin-1 production by human polymorphonuclear neutrophils. J. Immunol. **136:** 3677-3685.

23. LINDEMANN A., D. RIEDEL, W. OSTER, S. C. MEUER, D. BLOHM, R. H. MERTELSMANN & F. HERRMANN. 1988. Granulocyte/macrophage colony-stimulating factor induces interleukin-1 production by human polymorphonuclear neutrophils. J. Immunol. **140:** 837-839.

24. CICCO, N. A., A. LINDEMANN, J. CONTENT, P. VANDENBUSSCHE, M. LUBBERT, J. GAUSS, R. H. MERTELSMANN & F. HERRMANN. 1990. Inducible production of interleukin-6 by human polymorphonuclear neutrophils. Blood **75:** 2049-2052.

25. STRIETER, R. M., K. KASAHARA, R. ALLEN, H. J. SHOWELL, T. J. STANDFORD & S. L. KUNKEL. 1990. Human neutrophils exhibit disparate chemotactic factor gene expression. Biochem. Biophys. Res. Comm. **173:** 725-730.

26. STRIETER, R. M., K. KASAHARA, R. A. ALLEN, T. J. STANDIFORD, M. W. ROLFE, F. S. BECKER, S. W. CHENSUE & S. L. KUNKEL. 1992. Cytokine-induced neutrophil-derived interleukin-8. Am. J. Pathol. **141:** 397–407.

27. MARTICH, G., R. L. DANNER, M. CESKA & A. F. SUFFREDINI. 1991. Detection of interleukin-8 and tumor necrosis factor in normal humans after intravenous endotoxin: The effect of antiinflammatory agents. J. Exp. Med. **173:** 1021–1024.

28. VAN ZEE, K. J., L. E. DEFORGE, E. FISCHER, M. A. MARANO, J. S. KENNEY, D. G. REMICK, S. F. LOWRY & L. L. MOLDAWER. 1991. IL-8 in septic shock, endotoxemia, and after IL-1 administration. J. Immunol. **146:** 3478–3482.

29. FRIEDLAND, J. S., Y. SUPUTTAMONGKOL, D. G. REMICK, W. CHAOWAGUL, R. M. STRIETER, S. L. KUNKEL, N. J. WHITE & G. E. GRIFFIN. 1992. Prolonged elevation of interleukin-8 and interleukin-6 concentrations in plasma and of leukocyte interleukin-8 mRNA levels during septicemic and localized *Pseudomonas pseudomallei* infection. Infect. Immunol. **60:** 2402–2408.

30. NEGUSSIE, Y., D. G. REMICK, L. E. DEFORGE, A. EYNON, S. L. KUNKEL & G. E. GRIFFIN. 1992. Detection of plasma tumor necrosis factor, interleukin-6, and interleukin-8 during the Jarisch-Herxheimer reaction of relapsing fever. J. Exp. Med. **127:** 1207–1212.

31. RODRIGUEZ, J. L., C. G. MILLER, L. E. DEFORGE, L. KELTY, S. J. SHANLEY, R. H. BARLETT & D. G. REMICK. 1992. Local production of interleukin-8 is associated with nosocomial pneumonia. J. Trauma **33:** 74–82.

32. DONNELLY, S. C., R. M. STRIETER, S. L. KUNKEL, A. WALZ, C. R. ROBERTSON, D. C. CARTER, I. S. GRANT, A. J. POLLOK & C. HASLETT. 1993. Interleukin-8 and development of adult respiratory distress syndrome in at-risk patient groups. Lancet **341:** 643–647.

The Development of Effective Vaccine Adjuvants Employing Natural Regulators of T-Cell Lymphokine Production *in Vivo*[a]

RAYMOND A. DAYNES [b,c] AND
BARBARA A. ARANEO [b]

[b]*Division of Cell Biology and Immunology*
Department of Pathology
University of Utah
Salt Lake City, Utah 84132

[c]*Geriatric Research, Education and Clinical Center*
Veterans Affairs Medical Center
Salt Lake City, Utah 84148

The adaptive immune system of mammals has evolved to possess a great degree of cellular, biochemical, and molecular complexity. In fully immunocompetent animals, optimal protection provided by this essential system generally requires the simultaneous or sequential mobilization of both cell-mediated and antibody-mediated effector mechanisms.

The vast majority of microorganisms capable of causing disease initially interact, colonize, and infect mammalian host tissues at some mucosal surface. The mucosal interface has direct contact with the external environment and covers a tremendously large surface area. The lungs and gastrointestinal tract of humans alone, for example, possess a membrane surface area of approximately 400 m^2. Specialized immunologic mechanisms have evolved to provide the mucosal surfaces of appropriately immunized animals with the ability to produce secretory antibodies having specificity for a variety of microbial antigens.[1-4] This "common mucosal immune system" is considered by most investigators in the field to represent a "first line of adaptive immunologic defense."

Secretory antibodies within mucosal secretions having specificity for bacterial, fungal, or viral antigens function by reducing the likelihood of infection of host tissues following an encounter with these potentially infectious agents. This generally is accomplished by diminishing the potential for successful bacterial or viral colonization with antibodies capable of binding those molecules that allow microbial adhesion to epithelial surfaces. If these mucosal tissue barriers are breached, the microorganisms can gain direct access to the internal organ systems of the host. Systemically acting

[a]This work was supported in part by US Public Health Service grants R37-CA25917 and R01-AG11475, awarded by the National Institutes of Health, and by a research grant from the Department of Veterans Affairs Medical Research Funds.

cellular and antibody-mediated immune effector mechanisms need to then become actively mobilized to eliminate, neutralize, or sequester the offending agent or any of its toxic products. Systemic immunity, and the large number of effector mechanisms that are available to an immunocompetent host, may actually represent the backup adaptive system of immune protection.

The vast diversity in immune effector mechanisms available to a normal mammalian host, coupled with the specialization that often occurs when establishing effective protective immunity to a particular pathogen, indicates that elaborate mechanisms must exist to control the unique developmental processes necessary for the induction of any specific type of immune response. Present evidence suggests that lymphokines, molecules produced by helper T cells in response to antigen stimulation, play essential roles in controlling these developmental processes. Lymphokines function *in vivo* via their capacities to influence a vast array of cellular, biosynthetic, and differentiation processes.[5,6] It is now appreciated that qualitative fluctuations in the patterns of lymphokines produced by T cells in response to an antigenic insult lead to variations in the dominant effector mechanisms that ultimately develop.[5] Understanding the natural processes that operate to regulate the pattern of individual lymphokine species could therefore lead to methods of control over the various types of immune effector mechanisms.

In recent reports we argued that variations in the patterns of lymphokines produced by activated T cells isolated from distinct (mucosal *versus* nonmucosal) lymphoid organs of normal animals are not due to a mechanism that allows only selective activation of a particular preexisting T-cell subset.[7,8] Rather, we advocate that the potential of most T cells *in vivo* to produce lymphokines following activation represents a flexible and dynamic phenotype, with lymphokine output being dependent on microenvironmental factors provided uniquely within distinct secondary lymphoid organs.[7-11] According to this working hypothesis, T cells within the recirculating lymphocyte pool become programmed upon their migration from the bloodstream into a particular lymphoid organ microenvironment. These cells are rapidly deprogrammed when they leave that microenvironment without being activated and are reprogrammed with new information, that is lymphoid organ specific, after their extravasation into a new secondary lymphoid compartment. We therefore believe that ''resting T cells'' are constantly receiving and losing information able to control the species of lymphokines that they would produce, qualitatively and quantitatively, should they become activated by antigen while residing within a particular lymphoid compartment.[7,8]

We previously determined that dehydroepiandrosterone (DHEA) augments T-cell production of lymphokine interleukin-2 (IL-2) following cellular activation.[12] High levels of IL-2 can be produced by T cells residing in peripheral lymph nodes and the spleen, and the steroid sulfatase activity (DHEAS→DHEA) within these same lymphoid tissues is greater than the sulfatase activity found in mucosal lymph nodes that contain T cells having minimal potential for IL-2 production. This finding led to the hypothesis that tissue-compartmentalized end-organ metabolism of DHEAS to DHEA may help to control the unique responsiveness of T cells during their residence in nonmucosal lymphoid organs.[7]

By testing the concept that some end-organ metabolized steroid hormones may play essential roles in programming T-cell functions *in vivo*, we recently established a linkage between the well-known age-associated losses in immunocompetence, with the equally well-established age-related declines in the endogenous production of DHEA and its sulfated derivative (DHEAS).[9,10] Replacement therapy of old animals with DHEAS was found to quickly restore a normal mature adult phenotype of T-cell lymphokine production by T cells, from all lymphoid compartments tested. We, and others, have now extended these observations to further establish that aged animals can be effectively vaccinated to either protein or polysaccharide antigens, so long as the immunomodulatory or reconstituting activities of this steroid hormone are present.[9,10,13,14]

Aging of the immune system, therefore, especially some of its more pronounced immunologic consequences, may actually be due, at least in part, to a loss in production of the molecules that convey appropriate information to peripheral lymph node and splenic T cells during their transient residence periods within these lymphoid organs. Such a defect would result in a depression in lymphocyte responsiveness to stimulation by neoantigens, a condition well documented to exist in aged animals and elderly humans. Normalization of lymphocyte responsiveness would be expected under those conditions in which the precursor steroid hormone deficiency (DHEAS) is corrected therapeutically. In preclinical animal systems, this appears to be the case.[9–11,13,14]

The primary objective of the present investigation was to experimentally evaluate whether our working hypothesis concerning the mechanisms associated with regulation of T-cell function by particular steroid hormones could be used therapeutically not only to reconstitute normal immune function when appropriate (e.g., aged animals), but also to manipulate the immunologic outcome following selected types of vaccinations of normal animals. We reasoned that it might be possible to therapeutically alter the patterns of lymphokines produced by T cells within any selected lymphoid compartment to patterns and activities normally only found in other lymphoid organs. Such changes should translate into definable alterations in the type of immune effector mechanism ultimately induced following an antigen challenge to the manipulated lymphoid organ. Our experimental findings support the validity of this concept, as the results indicate that common mucosal immune responses can be induced after a standard subcutaneous vaccination. These findings suggest the possibility that it may be unnecessary to use oral, intranasal, or other routes of mucosal immunization to induce secretory immune responses.

RESULTS

Immunomodulation of T-Cell Function with Topically Applied Steroid Hormones

Our laboratory previously reported that the topical application of particular types of naturally occurring steroid hormones can quickly and significantly alter the patterns of lymphokines capable of being produced by T cells residing within the draining, but not the contralateral lymphoid organs.[15] The data presented in TABLE 1 represent the results of a typical experiment of this type in which 1.0 μg of 1,25 dihydroxyvitamin D_3 $(1,25(OH)_2D_3)$ was topically applied to one forepaw of normal mice 3 hours before sacrifice and collection of the draining (popliteal and brachial) and contralateral lymph nodes. The lymphocytes were cultured for 24 hours in serum-free tissue culture

TABLE 1. *In Vivo* Modulation of Cytokine-Producing Potential by Topical Application of 1,25(OH)$_2$D$_3$

Assessment of Lymph Node Cells[a]	Amount of Immunoactive Cytokine in Supernatants of Activated Cells[b]				
	IL-2 (SD; pg/ml)	IL-4 (SD; pg/ml)	IL-5 (SD; pg/ml)	IFNγ (SD; pg/ml)	IL-10 (SD; U/ml)
Vehicle-treated side	1180 (160)	1050 (215)	678 (121)	3680 (350)	24 (2)
1,25(OH)$_2$D$_3$-treated side	575 (25)	2650 (175)	1580 (120)	1470 (57)	68 (9)

[a]One microgram of 1,25(OH)$_2$D$_3$ was topically applied in an ethanol vehicle to a single front paw of a group of age- and sex-matched mice. The ethanol carrier was applied to the opposite paw in the same group of treated mice. After 3 hours mice were sacrificed and pools of lymph node cells representing the steroid and control treatments were cultured with 1 μg anti-CD3 to elicit cytokine production. Culture supernatants were collected after a 24-hour culture period to quantify the amounts of cytokine.

[b]Cytokines were detected by quantitative capture ELISA using reagents and standards as previously described in detail.[9,11]

medium and stimulated by the addition of anti-CD3$_\epsilon$. The supernatants were then quantitatively analyzed for lymphokine content. The results of this particular study demonstrate that 1,25(OH)$_2$D$_3$ treatment has modulatory influences on many different lymphokines analyzed. 1,25(OH)$_2$D$_3$ treatment, as previously documented by others,[16,17] was able to reduce T-cell production of IL-2 and gamma interferon (IFN-γ) (greater than 50%). In addition, we found that this treatment enhanced the production of IL-4 (250%), IL-5 (230%), and IL-10 (280%). In essence, 1,25(OH)$_2$D$_3$ could alter a normal Th-1 type pattern of lymphokine production into one that was more Th-2-like.[5] 1,25(OH)$_2$D$_3$ was also reported to stimulate some cell types to produce the active form of transforming growth factor β.[18] This fact, coupled with our present results, indicated that exposure of peripheral lymph node T cells to the action of 1,25(OH)$_2$D$_3$ was able to closely mimic the types of T-cell responses normally produced by Peyer's patch T cells.[9] This pattern of responsiveness is presently believed to be essential for promoting the development of a common mucosal immune response to an immunizing antigen.[2,4,19,20]

Hormonal Immunomodulation with Subcutaneous Vaccination Allows Successful Induction of Common Mucosal Immunity

The microenvironment of lymphoid organ inductive sites for mucosal immunity (e.g., Peyer's patches) must have evolved to selectively promote the induction of secretory immune responses. It is possible that unique microenvironmental factors being provided by these gut-associated secondary lymphoid organs actually promote

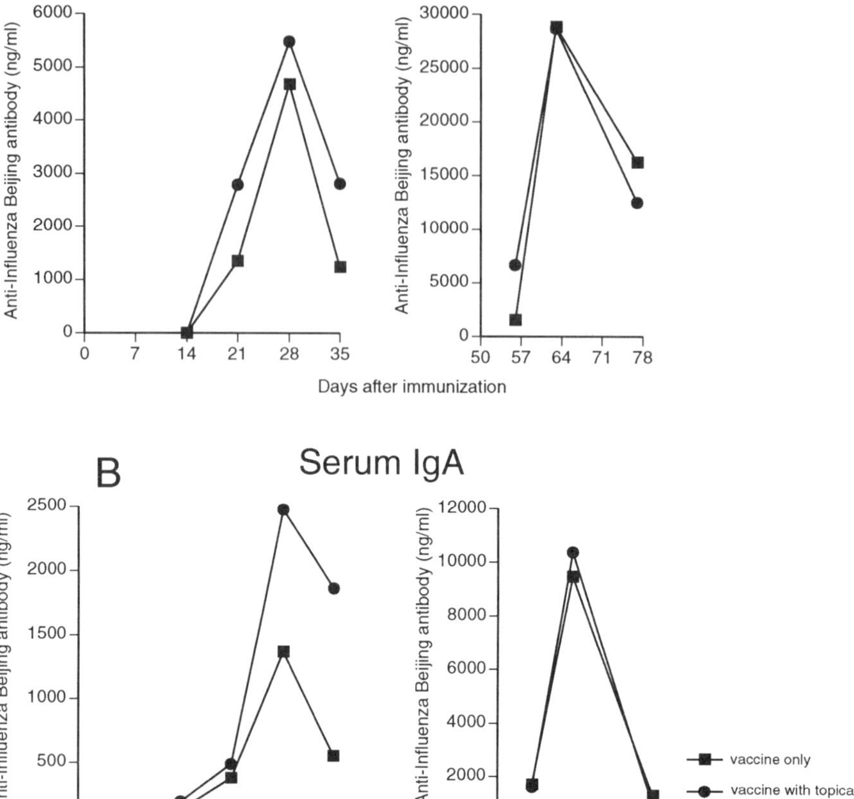

FIGURE 1. Antibody responses in the serum (**A,B**) and mucosal secretions (**C,D**, *facing page*) of animals vaccinated subcutaneously with inactivated influenza virus. Groups of mature adult (12–15-week-old) C3H/HEN strain mice received either vaccine alone (■) or vaccine plus a topical application of $1,25(OH)_2D_3$ to the inoculation site (●).

the induction of common mucosal immune responses by controlling the specific patterns of lymphokines produced following T-cell activation. If this is indeed the case, we reasoned that the anatomic site of antigen presentation may be less important for induction of particular types of immune effector responses than the appropriate epigenetic programming that regulates the specific patterns of specific lymphokine production. Inasmuch as it appeared possible to modify, in lymphoid organs, the types of lymphokines produced by their resident activated T cells, the possibility of

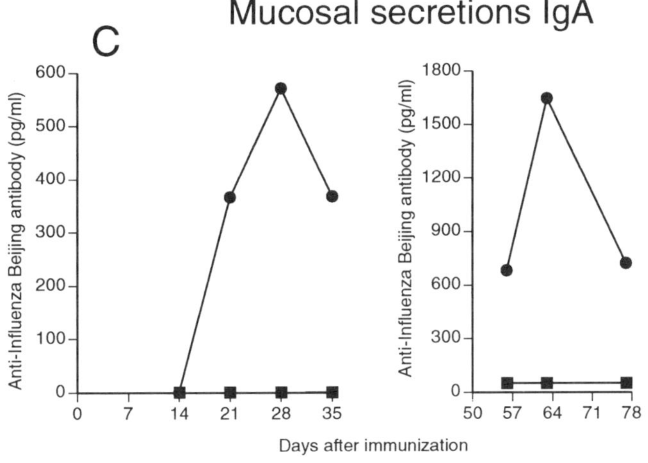

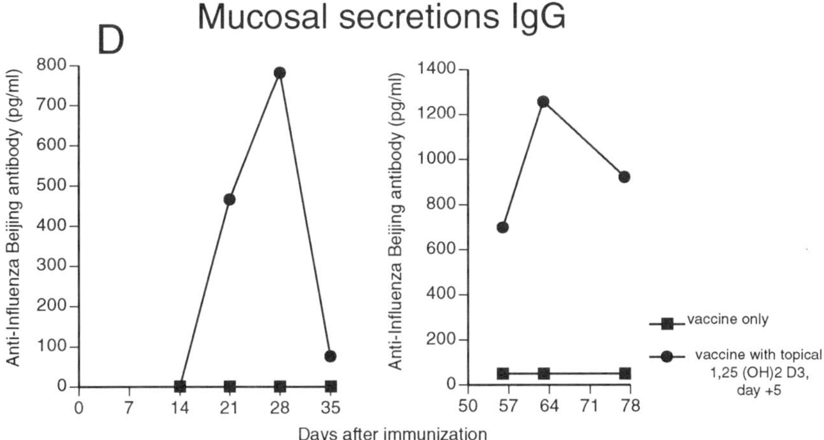

FIGURE 1. C and D.

being able to similarly modify the type of effector responses elicited following vaccination was explored.

Normal mature adult mice were immunized with 0.1 μg of inactivated influenza virus vaccine subcutaneously in the hind footpad. Five days later, an optimum time determined by preliminary experimentation, a 1-μg dose of 1,25(OH)$_2$D$_3$ was topically applied to the site of vaccination in one half the vaccinated animals. Serum and vaginal lavage samples were collected at various times postimmunization for analysis of systemic and mucosal immunity. All animals were given a second immunization with antigen alone 50 days after the primary inoculation. Serum plus mucosal secretion samples were collected and analyzed at the times specified in FIGURE 1. The results indicate that serum IgG and serum IgA responses were similar in both experimental groups, with very good antibody titers being observed after both primary and secondary exposures to antigen (FIG. 1A and B). A very different result was observed when the mucosal secretions were analyzed for antibody content (FIG. 1C and D). Mucosal IgA and IgG antibody was consistently present in the mucosal lavage fluids, but it was only found in the group of mice given $1,25(OH)_2D_3$ during the primary immunization process. This particular type of experiment has now been repeated many times, employing eight different microbial protein (native or recombinant) or bacterial polysaccharide antigens with equivalent results. These data include an ability to induce mucosal antibodies to hepatitis B surface antigen, gp120 of HIV, peptides derived from the outer membranes of *Chlamydia trachomatis* and pilin proteins isolated from *Neisseria gonorrhoeae* (data not shown). Each of these antigen preparations was capable of inducing specific common mucosal immunity after a simple subcutaneous injection of antigen when coupled with appropriate immunomodulation.

To verify that a common mucosal immune response to influenza virus antigen had been successfully induced, a micro dot blot analysis of lacrimal, vaginal, oral, and colorectal secretions was performed on groups of hormonally modulated and conventionally immunized animals. Mucosal samples from the specified sites were collected 14 days after secondary immunization and blotted onto a moistened nitrocellulose membrane previously derivatized with influenza virus antigen. The results presented in TABLE 2 demonstrate that secretory antibody was present in all of the mucosal samples analyzed from the group of mice that were hormonally manipulated during the course of the primary immunization.

An ELISPOT analysis on dissociated spleen cells and collagenase-digested lung cells of influenza-immunized mice further supported the existence of common mucosal immunity (TABLE 3). Both IgG and IgA antibody-producing cells were uniquely detected in the lungs of the animals vaccinated in conjunction with hormonal manipulation, but their spleens were found to contain significant numbers of B cells producing specific antibody. Further analysis of the lamina propria of the small intestine confirmed by ELISPOT the presence of influenza virus-specific antibody producing cells in the gut of appropriately immunized, but not conventionally immunized animals (data not shown).

The data presented in FIGURE 2 support the concept that common mucosal immune responses can also be induced employing protein vaccine preparations containing directly incorporated $1,25(OH)_2D_3$. Parallel groups of mature adult mice were immunized with $0.1\mu g$ of influenza virus vaccine alone or mixed in combination with $0.1\mu g$ of $1,25(OH)_2D_3$. Elicited serum antibody responses were comparable in the two test groups after primary and secondary immunization (data not shown). Evaluation of the antibody responses in the mucosal secretions, however (FIG. 2), established that only animals immunized with $1,25(OH)_2D_3$ incorporated into the vaccine were capable of responding with secretory antibody. The direct incorporation of the selective immunomodulator $1,25(OH)_2D_3$ into a vaccine preparation, or its topical application to vaccination sites, appears to represent a safe, efficient, and cost-effective way to promote the successful induction of common mucosal immunity to many types of antigens.

TABLE 2. Micro Dot-Blot Analysis of Influenza-Specific Secretory Immunoglobulins

Mucosal Epithelium[a]	IgG[b] Vaccine[c] Only	Vaccine with D₃	IgA[b] Vaccine Only	Vaccine with D₃
Lacrimal	−[d]	+++	−	+++
Oral	−	+++	−	+++
Vaginal	−	+++	−	+++
Colorectal	−	+	−	+

[a]Specimen collections consisted of swabbing each of the indicated mucosas with a pre-wet cotton sponge (1–2 mm in diameter). The swab is then rinsed in a small volume (50 μl) of buffer which releases the absorbed immunoglobulins. Samples are frozen at −20°C until assessment.

[b]Influenza-specific immunoglobulins were detected using goat anti-mouse heavy chain-specific antibodies.

[c]Each mouse was immunized with 0.1 μg monovalent, inactivated influenza virus (Beijing strain) in the hind footpad in a 25-μl volume of aluminum hydroxide (273 μg/ml). When indicated, mice were subsequently treated with 1 μg 1,25(OH)$_2$D$_3$ by topical application at the site of immunization, 5 days after immunization.

[d]The reactivity of each sample for nitrocellulose-bound antigen (influenza) was equated with the detection of murine IgG and IgA standards.[26] Negative reactions gave undetectable binding (a predicted value of >10 pg/ml). Positive detection ranged from + to +++, where + had an approximate value of 50–100 pg/ml, ++ had an approximate value of 200 mg/ml, and +++ had an approximate value of 500–1000 pg/ml.

Stimulation of Common Mucosal Immunity in Aged Animals Using Selective Hormone Immunomodulation Requires Their Simultaneous Supplementation with DHEAS

Aging is often associated with depression in a host's capacity to mount protective immune responses to vaccination with neoantigens. Whereas most research information in this area has focused attention on age-related alterations in systemic humoral and cellular responses, some strongly suggestive experimental data that mucosal immune responses are also negatively affected by aging also exist.[21–23]

We recently reported that one reason the mammalian immune system becomes less efficient with advancing age is linked to the age-associated decline in endogenous DHEAS production.[9,10] In essence, old animals having a markedly reduced capacity to mount humoral antibody responses to protein and polysaccharide antigens respond very efficiently to similar immunizations when provided with supplemental DHEAS.

Influenza represents an important respiratory disease, especially in the susceptible elderly. Although yearly vaccination can reduce disease severity, presently employed immunization strategy does not successfully eliminate infection of lung tissue. It is possible, therefore, that better protection against disease could be achieved if a common mucosal immune response specific for influenza antigens could also be induced.

TABLE 3. Analysis of Influenza-Specific Antibody-Secreting Cells by ELISPOT

	IgG[b]		IgA[b]	
Tissue Assayed[a]	Vaccine[c] Only	Vaccine with Topical 1,25(OH)$_2$D$_3$	Vaccine Only	Vaccine with Topical 1,25(OH)$_2$D$_3$
Spleen	4,800[d]	6,700	670	4,400
	(410)	(730)	(56)	(460)
Lung	20	650	20	320
	(3)	(55)	(2)	(37)

[a]Spleens and lungs of two individual mice were dissociated in balanced salt solution. Lung tissue was further dissociated in collagenase using a modification of the method of Sedgwick and Holt.[27]

[b]Detection of antibody-secreting cells was performed on antigen-coated, nitrocellulose-backed 96-well microtiter plates, with biotinylated goat–anti-mouse heavy chain-specific antibodies, avidin-alkaline phosphatase, and BCIP and NBT substrates.

[c]Each mouse was immunized with 0.1 μg monovalent, inactivated influenza A virus (Beijing strain) in the hind footpad in a 25-μl volume of aluminum hydroxide (273 μg/ml). Half of the immunized mice were administered 1 μg 1,25(OH)$_2$D$_3$ by topical application at the site of immunization, 5 days after immunization. C3H mature adult (≈6 months at time of evaluation, 4 days after second immunization.

[d]Mean (± SEM) number of spot-forming cells/10^6 cells.

We recently attempted to expand on our approaches to promote the development of mucosal immunity by addressing whether the elderly might have special immunobiologic problems which differentiate them from mature adults. Two parallel groups, consisting of mature adult (12–16 weeks), aged (>30 months), and aged mice provided with supplemental DHEAS (≈100 μg/day in their drinking water), were vaccinated subcutaneously with inactivated influenza virus (0.1 μg). One of the groups received topical treatment with 1,25(OH)$_2$D$_3$ 5 days later at the vaccination site. At various times after immunization as well as after a booster immunization on day 50 with vaccine alone, blood and vaginal lavage samples were collected for antibody quantitation.

The results of this experiment (FIGS. 3 and 4A-D) provided us with a great deal of new information. Quantitative analysis of serum IgG (FIG. 3A and B) and serum IgA (FIG. 3C and D) responses established that the mature adult and DHEAS-supplemented aged animals, regardless of whether 1,25(OH)$_2$D$_3$ was given, were able to mount very significant antibody responses to the initial vaccine exposure and recall challenge. As expected, the untreated aged animals responded poorly to immunization with influenza virus antigens.

Evaluation of the titers of antibody specific for influenza virus antigens in the mucosal secretions, however, provided some interesting findings (FIG. 4A-D). No antibody could be detected in the mucosal secretions of conventionally immunized animals (FIG. 4A and C). In animals immunized with viral antigen followed by topical 1,25(OH)$_2$D$_3$ treatment, significant levels of both IgA (FIG. 4B) and IgG (FIG. 4D)

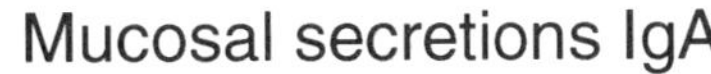

Mucosal secretions IgA

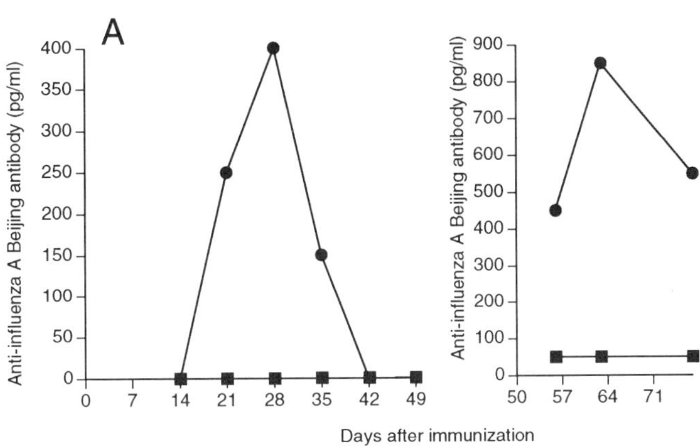

Mucosal secretions IgG

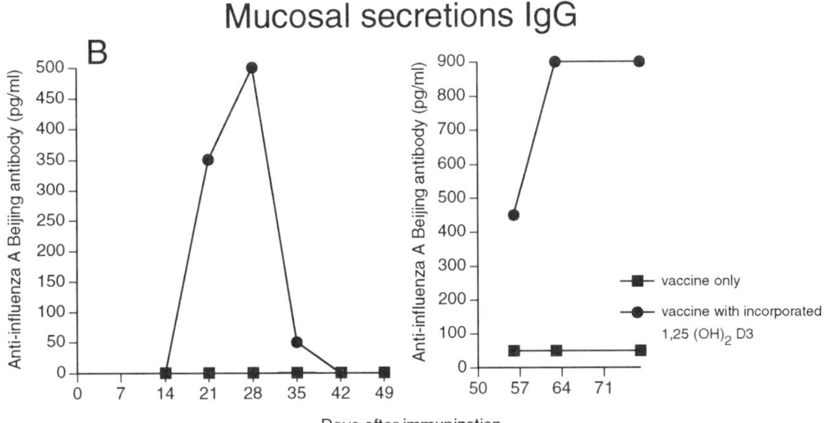

FIGURE 2. Antibody responses in the mucosal secretions of mature adult mice vaccinated with inactivated influenza virus alone (■) or influenza virus vaccine containing 0.1 μg of 1,25(OH)$_2$D$_3$ (●).

were found, but only in the secretions from mature adult and DHEAS-supplemented aged animals. Minimal to no antibody was detectable in the mucosal secretions of immunized aged animals. Therefore, the capacity of aged animals to elicit a common mucosal immune response to vaccine antigens apparently depends on whether the host has retained/regained the ability to mount other types of systemic immune responses after antigen exposure, a situation that has now had an established link to whether endogenous DHEAS levels are adequate.

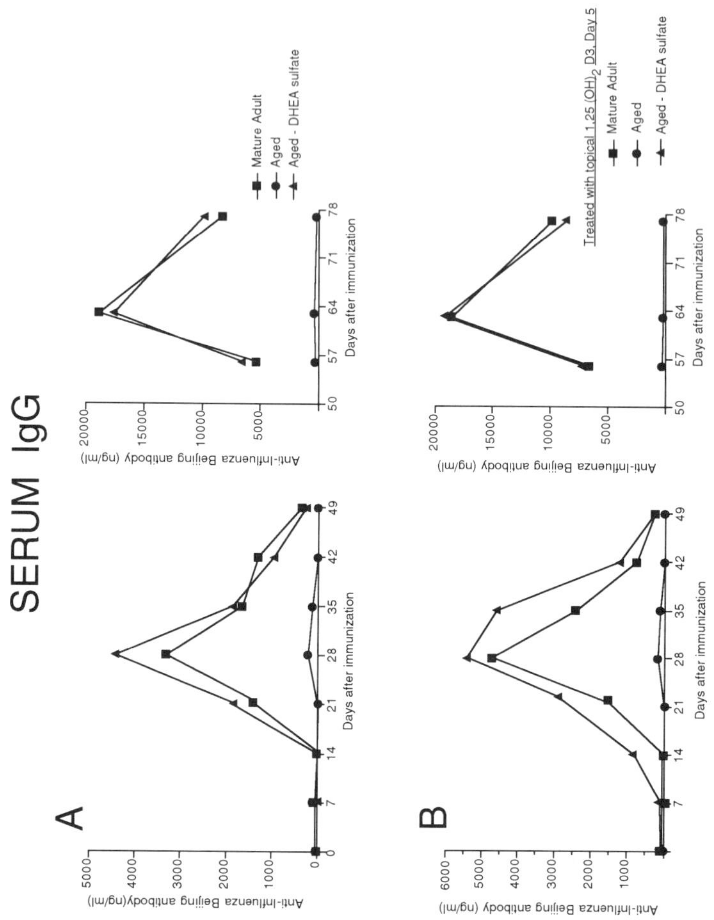

SERUM IgG
A
B
Mature Adult
Aged
Aged - DHEA sulfate
Treated with topical 1,25 (OH)_2 D3, Day 5
Mature Adult
Aged
Aged - DHEA sulfate
Anti-Influenza Beijing antibody (ng/ml)
Days after immunization

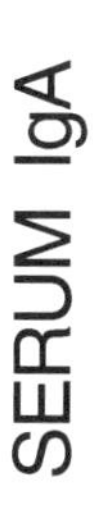

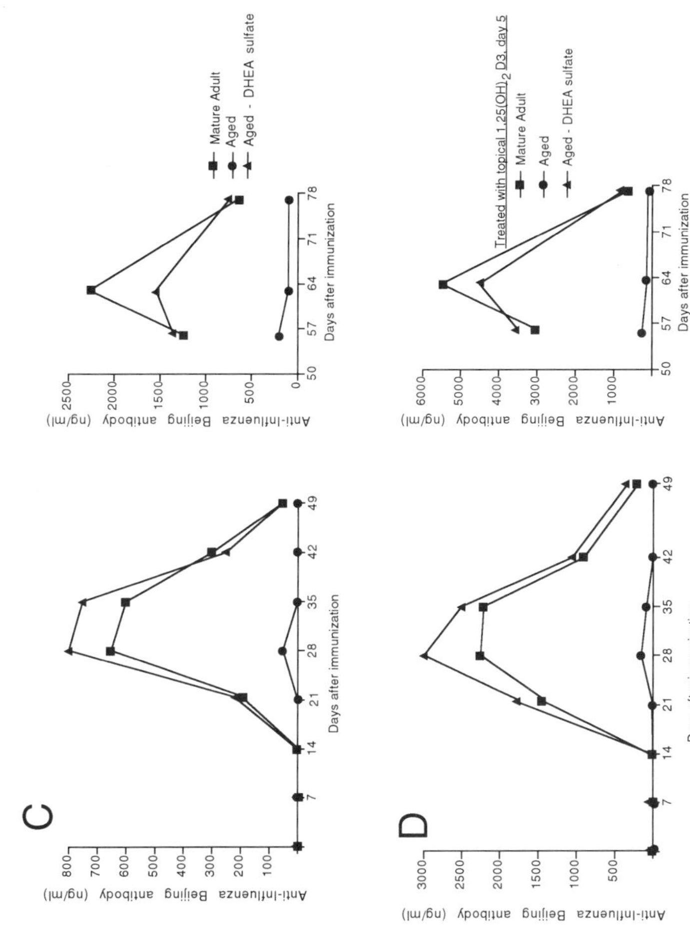

FIGURE 3. Serum antibody responses to influenza virus by mature adult (12–15-week-old), aged (>100 weeks old), or aged mice provided with supplemental DHEA sulfate in their drinking water. (**A,C**) Animals vaccinated with influenza virus antigen alone; (**B,D**) animals vaccinated with influenza virus antigen followed 5 days later by topical application of 1,25(OH)$_2$D$_3$ to the site of inoculation.

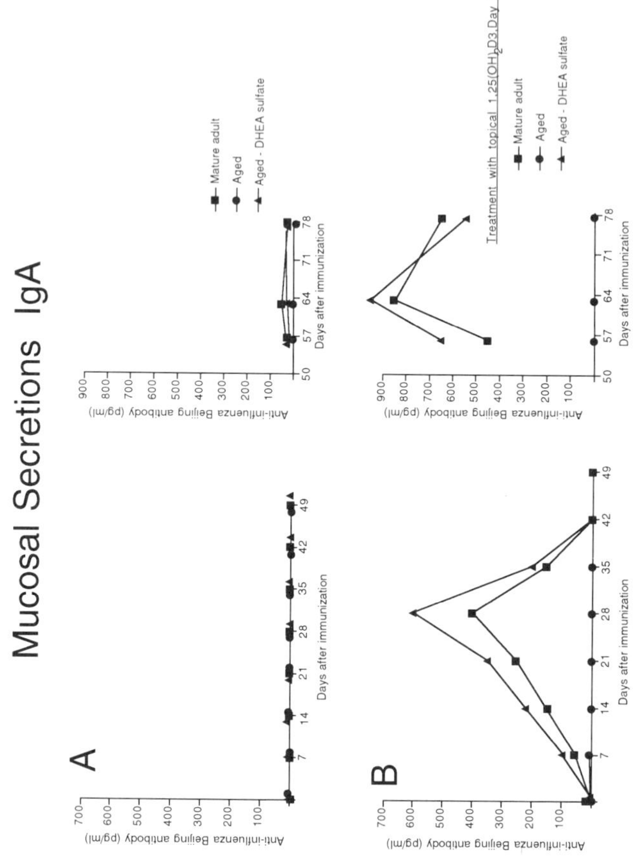
Mucosal Secretions IgA
A
B
Anti-influenza Beijing antibody (pg/ml)
Days after immunization
Mature adult
Aged
Aged - DHEA sulfate
Treatment with topical 1,25(OH)₂D3 Day 5

Mucosal Secretions IgG

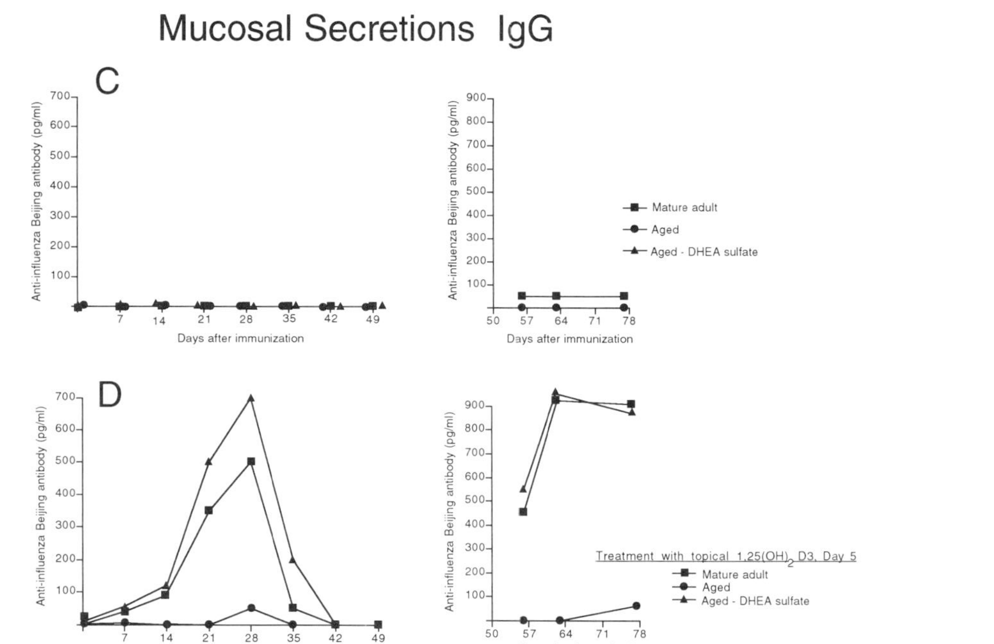

FIGURE 4. Mucosal antibody responses to influenza virus by mature adult, aged, and aged mice provided with supplemental DHEA sulfate. (**A,C**) Animals vaccinated with influeza virus antigen alone; (**B,D**) animals immunized with influenza virus antigen followed 5 days later by topical application of 1,25(OH)$_2$D$_3$ to the site of inoculation.

DISCUSSION

Vaccination represents the most effective and economical means to control infectious disease. The new molecular approaches that were recently developed provide researchers the means to easily define relevant antigen epitopes and produce recombinant subunit antigens for many disease-causing microorganisms. Many of these engineered or recombinant substances are able to elicit protective states of immunity under those conditions where appropriate types of effector responses can be stimulated.

Despite our tremendous knowledge about the molecular and cellular workings of the mammalian immune system, little attention is presently being given to better defining the many host factors that can affect outcomes of immune responses. It is well known, for example, that factors such as age, stress, secondary infection, and many other environmental influences are able to significantly modify the types and intensities of immune responses to vaccination. A working understanding of how these types of host factors function to influence the effectiveness of vaccination is presently an unresolved problem. As future research gains answers to the many questions that remain concerning the molecular aspects of immunoregulation, new and novel approaches to successfully promote the development of long-lasting protective immune responses should emerge.

Many naturally produced molecules such as steroid hormones, prostaglandins, certain cellular growth factors, and even lymphokines themselves serve to naturally control the types and patterns of lymphokines produced by T cells in response to cellular activation after antigen challenge. A comprehensive T-cell regulatory system that is guided by molecules that can be produced by many tissues and organ systems offers many distinct advantages for controlling the various types of immune responses available to a host *in vivo* because it provides a working system whereby the induction and release of bioactive lymphokines can be anatomically restricted.

We attempted to employ recent mechanistic information about how the production of lymphokines might be microenvironmentally controlled *in vivo,* to design novel therapeutic strategies capable of promoting more effective immune responses to vaccination. The problem of immunosenescence, for example, can be linked to the age-related loss in the production of DHEA, an adrenal steroid hormone whose levels drop with advancing age.[24] Successful vaccination can be accomplished by simultaneously providing elderly animals with the missing hormone at the time of immunization or by simply supplementing aged animals with precursor hormone (DHEAS) at the time of vaccination. In essence, natural regulators of T-cell lymphokine production can be effectively used as vaccine adjuvants to promote the successful induction of immunity.

We next challenged the paradigm held by most investigators in the field that induction of common mucosal immunity (secretory antibodies) requires antigen presentation across a mucosal surface.[25] These experiments provided an additional test for our working hypothesis that flexibility in responses is available to individual T cells. It was rewarding to find that the types of immune responses elicited from hormone-manipulated lymph nodes were consistent with the types of responses that would be predicted from the patterns of lymphokines capable of being made by the steroid hormone-influenced T cells.

We are led by our studies to believe that hormone manipulation coupled with a standard peripheral vaccination offers an easy means to guide the immune system down a desirable differentiation pathway. The protocol described in this report represents a means to promote the successful induction of a common mucosal immune response to a number of test antigens. There is little doubt that other types of control over immune effector responses are possible, because a variety of steroid and polypeptide hormones exist that can influence T-cell lymphokine production in their own unique and definable ways. Hormonal manipulation of T-cell responsiveness, when coupled with vaccination, offers a variety of unique therapeutic possibilities for the future.

SUMMARY

Steroid hormones are important regulators of gene function *in vivo*. A number of naturally occurring species of steroid hormones are able to qualitatively and quantitatively influence the production of lymphokines by activated T cells *in vitro*. Similar mechanisms are probably also occurring naturally *in vivo* and could explain why mucosal and nonmucosal lymphoid organs harbor T cells having unique potentials for lymphokine production. It was established that the topical application of 1,25 dihydroxyvitamin D_3 (1,25(OH)$_2$D$_3$) to normal mice changed the pattern of lymphokines produced by activated T cells isolated from the draining peripheral lymph nodes. The hormone-treated T cells produced a pattern of lymphokines similar to that normally found in Peyer's patches. Subcutaneous vaccination with a protein antigen, in a site afferent to 1,25(OH)$_2$D$_3$-manipulated lymph nodes, resulted in an enhanced serum antibody response and was uniquely capable of also stimulating a common mucosal immune response to the antigen as well. Common mucosal immunity was confirmed by demonstrating the presence of antigen-specific IgA and IgG responses in a number of mucosal secretions and by further establishing that antibody-secreting plasma cells had migrated to the lungs and small intestines of the hormone-treated and vaccinated animals. Additional experiments established that common mucosal immunity could also be induced in aged animals as long as the immune system of the vaccinated animals was functioning normally. This was accomplished by providing the aged animals with a dietary supplement of dehydroepiandrosterone sulfate (DHEAS). Previous studies by us have documented that aged animals provided with replacement levels of DHEAS, a natural steroid hormone whose endogenous production declines with advancing age, are able to mount normal systemic humoral and cellular immune response following subcutaneous vaccination with a variety of protein and polysaccharide antigens. The combination of supplemental DHEAS therapy with topical 1,25(OH)$_2$D$_3$ treatment at the time of vaccination provided the conditions needed to generate mucosal and systemic immune responses to inactivated influenza virus antigen by old animals.

REFERENCES

1. BEAGLEY, K. & C. ELSON. 1992. Cells and cytokines in mucosal immunity and inflammation. Gastroenterol. Clin. North Am. **21:** 347–366.

2. KIYONO, H., J. BIENENSTOCK, J. McGHEE & P. ERNST. 1992. The mucosal immune system: Features of inductive and effector sites to consider in mucosal immunization and vaccine development. Regul. Immunol. **4:** 54–62.

3. MESTECKY, J. 1987. The common mucosal immune system and current strategies for induction of immune responses in external secretions. J. Clin. Immunol. **7:** 265–276.

4. McGEE, J., J. MESTECKY, M. DERTZBAUGH, J. ELDRIDGE, M. HIRASAWA & H. KIYONO. 1992. The mucosal immune system: From fundamental concepts to vaccine development. Vaccine **10:** 75–89.

5. MOSMANN, R. & R. COFFMAN. 1989. TH1 and TH2 cells: Different patterns of lymphokine secretion lead to different functional properties. Ann. Rev. Immunol. **7:** 145–173.

6. FINKELMAN, F., J. HOLMES, I. KATONA, J. URBAN, JR., M. BECKMANN, L. PARK, K. SCHOOLEY, R. KOFFMAN, T. MOSMANN & W. PAUL. 1990. Lymphokine control of *in vivo* immunoglobulin isotype selection. Ann. Rev. Immunol. **8:** 303–333.

7. DAYNES, R. A., B. A. ARANEO, T. D. DOWELL, K. HUANG & D. DUDLEY. 1990. Regulation of murine lymphokine production *in vivo*. III. The lymphoid tissue microenvironment exerts regulatory influences over T helper cell function. J. Exp. Med. **171:** 979–996.

8. DAYNES, R. A. & B. A. ARANEO. 1992. Programming of lymphocyte responses to activation: Extrinsic factors, provided microenvironmentally, confer flexibility and compartmentalization to T-cell function. Chem. Immunol. **54:** 1–20.

9. ARANEO, B. A., M. L. WOODS, II & R. A. DAYNES. 1993. Reversal of the immunosenescent phenotype by dehydroepiandrosterone: Hormone treatment provides an adjuvant effect on the immunization of aged mice with recombinant hepatitis B surface antigen. J. Infect. Dis. **167:** 830–840.

10. DAYNES, R. A. & B. A. ARANEO. 1992. Prevention and reversal of age-associated changes in immunologic responses by supplemental dehydroepiandrosterone sulfate therapy. Aging: Immunol. Infect. Dis. **3:** 135–154.

11. DAYNES, R. A., T. DOWELL & B. A. ARANEO. 1991. Platelet derived growth factor is a potent biologic response modifier of T cells. J. Exp. Med. **174:** 1323–1334.

12. DAYNES, R. A., D. J. DUDLEY & B. A. ARANEO. 1990. Regulation of murine lymphokine production *in vivo*. II. Dehydroepiandrosterone is a natural enhancer of IL-2 synthesis by helper T cells. Eur. J. Immunol. **20:** 793–802.

13. GARG, M. & S. BONDADA. 1993. Reversal of age associated decline in immune response to Pnu-immune vaccine by supplementation with the steroid hormone dehydroepiandrosterone. Infect. Immun. **61:** 2238–2241.

14. RASMUSSEN, K. & M. HEALEY. 1992. Dehydroepiandrosterone-induced reduction of *Cryptosporidium parvum* infections in aged syrian golden hamsters. J. Parasitol. **78:** 554–557.

15. ARANEO, B. A., T. DOWELL, T. TERUI, M. DIEGEL & R. A. DAYNES. 1991. Dihydrotestosterone exerts a depressive influence on the production of IL-4, IL-5, and γIFN, but not IL-2 by activated murine cells. Blood **78:** 688–699.

16. BHALLA, A., E. AMENTO & S. KRANE. 1986. Differential effects of 1,25-dihydroxyvitamin D_3 on human lymphocytes and monocyte/macrophages. Inhibition of interleukin-2 and augmentation of interleukin-1 production. Cell. Immunol. **98:** 311–317.

17. REICHEL, H., H. KOEFFLER, A. TOBLER & A. NORMAN. 1987. 1α,25-Dihydroxyvitamin D_3 inhibits γ-interferon synthesis by normal human peripheral blood lymphocytes. Proc. Natl. Acad. Sci. USA **84:** 3385–3389.

18. PETKOVICH, P., J. WRANA, A. GRIGORIODIS, J. HEERSCHE & J. SODEK. 1987. 1,25-dihydroxyvitamin D_3 increases epidermal growth factor receptors and transforming growth factor β-like activity in a bone-derived cell line. J. Biol. Chem. **262:** 13424–13428.

19. XU-AMANO, J., K. BEAGLEY, J. MEGA, K. FUJIHASHI, H. KIYANO & J. McGHEE. 1992. Induction of helper T cells and cytokines for mucosal IgA responses. Adv. Exp. Med. Biol. **327:** 107–117.

20. WILSON, A., M. BAILEY, N. WILLIAMS & C. STOKES. 1991. The *in vitro* production of cytokines by mucosal lymphocytes immunized by oral administration of keyhole limpet hemocyanin using cholera toxin as an adjuvant. Eur. J. Immunol. **21:** 2333–2339.

21. EBERSOLE, J. & M. STEFFEN. 1989. Aging effects on secretory IgA immune responses. Immunol. Invest. **18:** 59–68.

22. SENDA, S., E. CHENG & H. KAWANISHI. 1989. IgG in murine intestinal secretions: Aging effect and possible physiological role. Scand. J. Immunol. **29:** 41–47.

23. SENDA, S., E. CHENG & H. KAWANISHI. 1988. Aging-associated changes in murine intestinal immunoglobulin A and M secretions. Scand. J. Immunol. **27:** 157–164.

24. ORENTREICH, N., J. BRIND, R. RIZER & J. VOGELMAN. 1984. Age changes and sex differences in serum dehydroepiandrosterone sulfate concentrations throughout adulthood. J. Clin. Endocrinol. Metab. **59:** 551–555.

25. HUSBAND, A. 1993. Novel vaccination strategies for the control of mucosal infection. Vaccine **11:** 107–112.

26. OBATA, T. & S. CHENG. 1991. Development of a simplified method for subclass isotyping and screening monoclonal antibodies. Biotechniques **10:** 574–576.

27. SEDGWICK, J. & P. HOLT. 1986. The ELISA-plaque assay for the detection and enumeration of antibody-secreting cells. J. Immunol. Methods **87:** 37–44.

Bacterial Adherence and Mucosal Cytokine Production

C. SVANBORG, W. AGACE, S. HEDGES,
R. LINDSTEDT, AND M. L. SVENSSON

Department of Medical Microbiology
Section of Clinical Immunology
Lund University
Lund, Sweden

This review focuses on the interaction of uropathogenic *Escherichia coli* with mucosal surfaces, a model that has proven useful in addressing questions on mechanisms of mucosal infection. The pathogenesis of urinary tract infections, like other mucosal infections, involves: (1) The localization of bacteria to the site of infection and the establishment of a population at this site. This may be guided by the specific attachment of bacteria to receptors at the mucosal surface. (2) Induction of localized inflammation which may occur through the secretion of bacterial exotoxins, through inflammatogenic cell wall or outer membrane components, or through localized invasion into or through the epithelial cells. (3) Systemic responses possibly caused by the release of mediators from the local site or by microbial invasion to distant tissues.

Uropathogenic *E. coli* colonize the human large intestine, spread to the urinary tract, and establish bacteriuria. The infection may remain asymptomatic, may cause localized inflammation in the lower urinary tract, or may reach the kidneys and blood stream and activate a systemic response. The site of infection and magnitude of the host response is influenced by the properties of the infecting strain. Severe infections (acute pyelonephritis and urosepsis) are often caused by a genetically restricted subset of *E. coli* clones that may be identified by their OKH serotype, their electromorph type, and the ability to express several virulence factors (adherence factors, hemolysin, iron binding proteins, etc). (For a review see refs. 1 and 2.)

BACTERIAL LECTINS

Bacterial adhesins are lectins, that is, proteins with carbohydrate specifity. They recognize as receptors, cell surface carbohydrates linked to lipids or proteins.[3]

Pioneering studies on bacterial adhesion to host tissues were performed by Duguid *et al.*[4] and Brinton *et al.*[5] in the 1950s. *E. coli* strains were shown to bind to intestinal epithelial cells and to agglutinate erythrocytes. Duguid and coworkers[4] found that only mannose, among other monosaccharides and low molecular weight substances tested, could inhibit hemagglutination, suggesting that binding to cells was carbohydrate specific. They also showed that long hair-like structures on the bacteria were responsible for the mannose-sensitive hemagglutination and named these structures fimbriae.

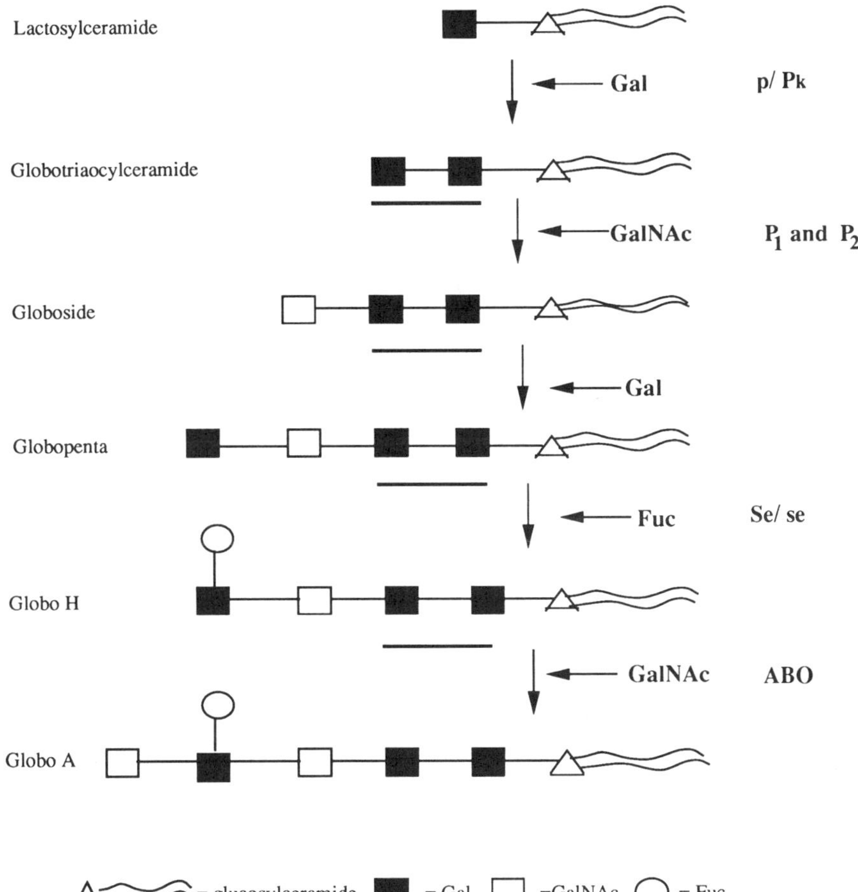

FIGURE 1. Biosythetic pathway of the globoseries of glycolipids. The first two steps, the addition of Gal and GalNAc, depend on the P blood group system. Both P_1 and P_2 individuals synthesize the P antigen globoside, but in addition, P_1 individuals sythesize the P_1 antigen. Addition of Fuc at mucosal surfaces depends on the secretor state of the individual, and the last step depends on the ABO blood group. The $Gal\alpha_1$-4Galβ disaccharide is underlined.

Uropathogenic *E. coli* clones may express a variety of fimbrial adhesins including P fimbriae, type 1 fimbriae, and S fimbriae.[2] The association with virulence is stronger for P fimbriae than for the other adherence factors.[6,7] P fimbriae mediate the attachment of *E. coli* to intestinal[8] and uroepithelial cells[9] and were recently shown to enhance activation of the inflammatory host response.[10] The symbol P was chosen because of the association with pyelonephritis and the specificity for receptors that are antigens

TABLE 1. GALα_1–4Galβ-Containing Glycolipids

Glycolipid Structures	Blood Group Antigens and/or Names of Glycolipids
Gal$\alpha_1\rightarrow$Gal$\beta_1\rightarrow$1Cer	Galabiosylceramide
Gal$\alpha_1\rightarrow$Gal$\beta_1\rightarrow$4Glc$\beta_1\rightarrow$1Cer	P_k, globotriaosylceramide
GalNAc$\beta_1\rightarrow$3Gal$\alpha_1\rightarrow$4Gal$\beta_1\rightarrow$4Glc1$\rightarrow$1Cer	P globotetraosylceramide
Gal$\alpha_1\rightarrow$4Gal$\beta_1\rightarrow$4GlcNAc$\beta_1\rightarrow$3Gal$\beta_1\rightarrow$4Glc$\beta_1\rightarrow$1Cer	P_1
Gal$\beta_1\rightarrow$3GalNAc$\beta_1\rightarrow$3Gal$\alpha_1\rightarrow$4Gal$\beta_1\rightarrow$4Glc$\beta_1\rightarrow$1Cer	SSEA-3, globopenta
Fuc$\alpha_1\rightarrow$2Gal$\beta_1\rightarrow$3GalNAc$\beta_1\rightarrow$3Gal$\alpha_1\rightarrow$4Gal$\beta_1\rightarrow$4Glc$_1\rightarrow$1Cer	Globo H
GalNAc$\alpha_1\rightarrow$3(Fuc$\alpha_1\rightarrow$2)Gal$\beta_1\rightarrow$3GalNAc$\beta_1\rightarrow$3Gal$\alpha_1\rightarrow$4Gal$\beta_1\rightarrow$4Glc1$\rightarrow$1Cer	Globo A
Gal$\alpha_1\rightarrow$3(Fuc$\alpha_1\rightarrow$2)Gal$\beta_1\rightarrow$3GalNAc$\beta_1\rightarrow$3Gal$\alpha_1\rightarrow$4Gal$\beta_1\rightarrow$4Glc1$\rightarrow$1Cer	Globo B
NeuAc$\alpha_2\rightarrow$3Gal$\beta_1\rightarrow$3GalNAc$\beta_1\rightarrow$3Gal$\alpha_1\rightarrow$4Gal$\beta_1\rightarrow$4Glc1$\rightarrow$1Cer	LKE, SSEA-4
GalNAc$\alpha_1\rightarrow$3GalNAc$\beta_1\rightarrow$3Gal$\alpha_1\rightarrow$4Gal$\beta_1\rightarrow$4Glc1$\rightarrow$1Cer	Forssman
GalNAc$\beta_1\rightarrow$3GalNAc$\beta_1\rightarrow$3Gal$\alpha_1\rightarrow$4Gal$\beta_1\rightarrow$4Glc1$\rightarrow$1Cer	para-Forssman

in the P blood system.[11] The P fimbriae are encoded by the *pap* family of chromosomal gene clusters[12] consisting of 11 genes (*pap*A-*pap*K).[13,14] The *pap*A sequences encode the major subunit which polymerizes into the fimbrial filamentous structure. The proteins encoded by *pap*E, *pap*F, and *pap*G are expressed at the tip of the fimbriae.[15] The protein encoded by the *pap*G sequences is the actual adhesin that is responsible for receptor binding. *Pap* gene clusters from different *E. coli* strains show extensive sequence homology except for *pap*A and *pap*G. Nucleotide sequence alignment of *pap*G genes from different *E. coli* isolates distinguished three classes of adhesins with approximately 70% sequence homology. Sequences within each class were highly conserved (>97%). These three types of adhesin genes were named *pap*G$_{J96}$, *pap*G$_{IA2}$, and *prs*G$_{J96}$.[16] These differ in disease association; the *pap*G$_{IA2}$ type of P fimbriae dominate in patients with severe infection.[17]

RECEPTOR IDENTIFICATION

Identification of the receptors for P fimbriae was based on the observation that adherence varied between cells from different species, tissues, and individuals.[6,18] Glycolipid extracts of uroepithelial cells from individuals of blood group P_1 or P_2 inhibited bacterial adhesion to these cells. Glycolipid extracts of uroepithelial cells from blood group p individuals lacked inhibitory activity. The glycolipids acting as receptors were identified as members of the globoseries of glycolipids. It was concluded that the bacteria recognize Galα1-4Galβ-containing oligosaccharide epitopes on the globoseries of glycolipids.

The globoseries of glycolipids are abundant in kidney and ureteral epithelial cells.[19] At least 11 Galα1-4Galβ-containing glycolipids have been found (TABLE 1). The glycolipid core structure of epithelial cells can be further elongated with carbohydrates such as the ABH antigens[18] (FIG. 1). The ABH determinants are created by glycosyltransferases acting on a terminal galactose. The H determinant is formed by the transferases encoded by the H or the secretor gene. Which of the two transferases act on the precursors depends on the tissue and glycolipid chain. The H gene-encoded transferase is active on the neolacto-series of glycolipids, which are found in cells such as erythrocytes. The secretor gene (Se) product elongates glycolipids with the H determinant but acts preferentially on core structures other than the H gene product. Expression of the H and Se gene products is also tissue specific. The glycosyltransferases act in a sequential manner; the H or Se glycosyltransferases have to act on the glycolipid precursors before the A or B glycosyltransferases. Individuals with positive secretor (Se) status express ABH determinants on their glycolipids in the epithelium, whereas individuals with negative secretor (se) status do not (FIG. 1). Consequently the type of glycolipid expressed by the individual will be determined by a combination of factors including blood group and secretor status.

FUNCTIONS OF *E. coli* P FIMBRIAE

The fecal flora is the reservoir for uropathogenic *E. coli*. We have proposed that P fimbriae increase the ability of *E. coli* to colonize the intestine as well as to infect the urinary tract.[20] Receptors for P fimbriae are expressed on human colonic epithelial cells,[8] and P-fimbriated *E. coli* have been shown to attach to these cells *in vitro*. P-fimbriated *E. coli* persist longer in the large intestine of children prone to urinary tract infections than do other *E. coli* strains.[21] They spread to the urinary tract more effectively than do P fimbriae negative strains. Indeed, P fimbriae negative strains were only recovered from the urinary tract of children in whom no P-fimbriated fecal strain was detected.[22]

The role of P fimbriae in the persistence of *E. coli* in the urinary tract remains unclear. Studies in animal models show that P-fimbriated *E. coli* persist longer in kidneys and bladders than do isogenic strains lacking *pap* DNA sequences.[23,24] Observations in patients with urinary tract infection provide conflicting evidence. Persisting bacteriuria is found mainly in patients with asymptomatic bacteriuria (ABU). If left untreated, these patients may carry the same *E. coli* strain for several years. ABU strains rarely express P fimbriae.[6,25,26] This suggests that P fimbriae are not required for persistence of bacteria in the urinary tract.

Colonization studies in humans confirmed this hypothesis. After deliberate colonization with isogenic strains expressing P fimbriae (J96) or type 1 fimbriae, the P fimbriated and type 1 fimbriated isogens were eliminated more rapidly than was the nonfimbriated clinical isolate. We therefore proposed that the persistence of *E. coli* in the human urinary tract is determined by factors other than or in addition to adherence.[27] The P fimbriae play an important role in virulence by enhancing the inflammatory response to infection.

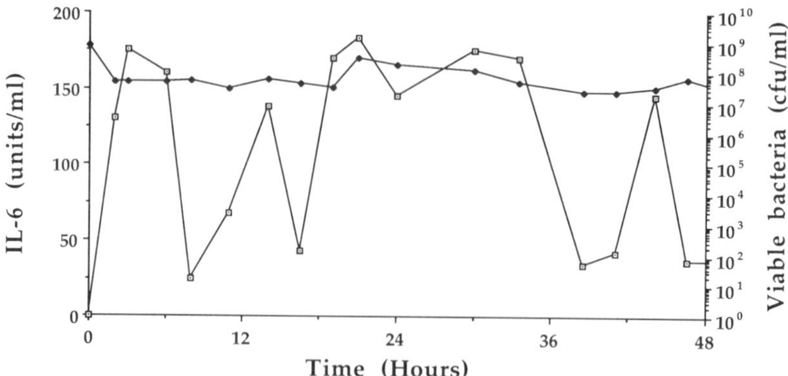

FIGURE 2. Urinary IL-6 response to deliberate colonization of the human urinary tract with *E. coli.* Deliberate colonization of the human urinary tract with nonvirulent bacteria was used in patients with recurrent urinary tract infections that are refractory to other therapy.[27] During such a study, urine and serum samples were collected and the levels of IL-6 and IL-8 were measured. The aim was to analyze whether mucosal challenge with *E. coli* induced a local and/or systemic cytokine response. IL-6 was not detected in urine or serum samples obtained prior to bacterial instillation, and catheterization without infection did not induce a response. Urinary IL-6 levels increased in all patients after bacterial instillation. IL-6 was secreted intermittently. A threshold concentration of bacteria was required to induce an IL-6 response ($>10^5$/ml). As a point of interest, this bacterial concentration agrees with levels used to define significant bacteriuria.[34]

E. coli ACTIVATE A MUCOSAL CYTOKINE RESPONSE IN HUMANS

Uropathogenic *E. coli* cause disease by activating a local and a systemic inflammatory response.[28] Local responses include the influx of granulocytes into the urine[29] and the production of cytokines.[30] Systemic responses include fever and elevated levels of acute phase reactants such as CRP and erythrocyte sedimentation rate. These responses may be explained in part by the ability of *E. coli* to induce the local production of cytokines leading to activation of the host response.

The existence of a mucosal cytokine response in the urinary tract was first recognized in mice.[30] We found interleukin-6 (IL-6) in the urine of mice within minutes after intravesical instillation of *E. coli* bacteria or isolated P fimbriae. Subsequently, deliberate colonization of the human urinary tract with nonvirulent bacteria was shown to cause a local production of IL-6 and IL-8 (FIGS. 2 and 3).[31,32] The IL-6 production was further examined in patients with different forms of urinary tract infection.[33] Most patients (86%) had elevated urinary IL-6 levels at the time of diagnosis. In contrast, serum IL-6 was only detected in patients with acute pyelonephritis (50%).

The profile of cytokines produced in response to human urinary tract infection was different from that observed during gram-negative systemic infection. During gram-negative systemic infections, tumor necrosis factor α (TNFα), IL-1, and IL-6

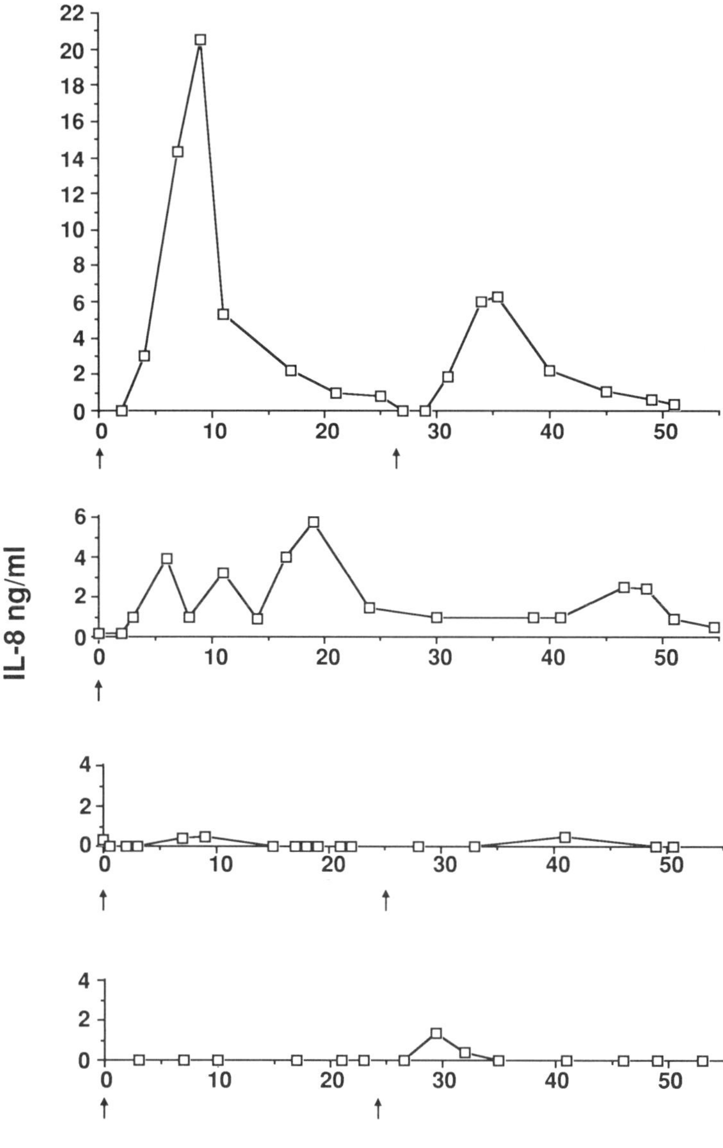

FIGURE 3. Urinary IL-8 response to deliberate colonization of the human urinary tract with *E. coli* in four patients. ↑ indicates the atime of bacterial instillation into the bladder of the patients. IL-8 was not detected in urine or serum prior to bacterial instillation. Urinary IL-8 levels increased in all colonized patients, but the levels varied. IL-8 was not detected in serum samples from colonized patients. We concluded that bacteria induce a local IL-8 response in the human urinary tract. (See reference 32.)

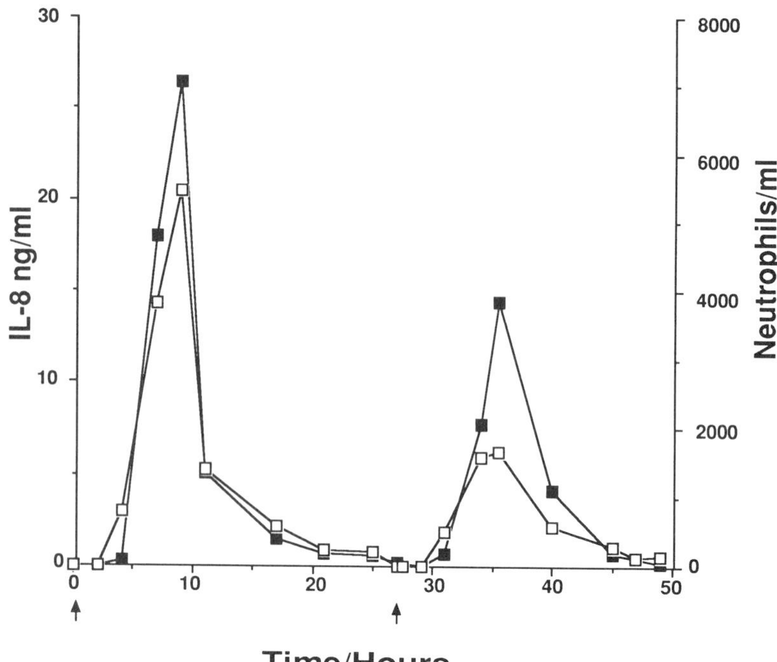

FIGURE 4. Urinary IL-8 and the neutrophil response of one deliberately colonized patient. —□— = levels of IL-8; —■— = number of neutrophils; ↑ = time of bacterial instillation into the bladder of the patients. (See reference 32.)

are detected. TNFα is found prior to IL-1 or IL-6. It is believed that lipopolysaccharide stimulates TNF production, leading to a cytokine cascade and the production of IL-1 and IL-6.[35-37] This is based on evidence that (1) TNFα stimulated IL-1 and IL-6 secretion *in vivo* and (2) anti-TNF antibodies given after endotoxin administration lowered the serum levels of TNF, IL-1, and IL-6.[38] Thus TNFα is though to act as an obligate precursor of further cytokine responses during systemic infections.[39,40] During urinary tract infection, no significant amounts of IL-1α, IL-β, or TNFα are detected. At the onset of urinary tract infection, IL-6 was detected in urine within 30 minutes of bacterial instillation. The rapid kinetics of the IL-6 responses to bacteria *in vivo* argued against a sequential activation of IL-6 production by cytokines and suggested that bacteria can directly stimulate a mucosal IL-6 and IL-8 response. Such TNF independent IL-6 secretion has also been demonstrated in other models.[41,42]

UROEPITHELIAL CELLS ARE A SOURCE OF MUCOSAL CYTOKINES

Epithelial cells are the first mucosal cells to make contact with bacteria. We therefore tested urinary tract epithelial cell lines and normal bladder epithelial cells for their ability to secrete cytokines in response to *E. coli* (FIG. 4). Cell lines from the human kidney (A-498) and bladder (J82) were exposed to bacteria or bacterial components. The cytokine response was analyzed as secreted and intracellular cytokine protein and as cytokine mRNA. *E. coli* Hu734 caused IL-6 and IL-8 secretion by urinary tract cell lines. Secreted IL-1α, and IL-1β, and TNFα were not detected. IL-1α, IL-1β, IL-6, and IL-8 mRNA were detected in both uroepithelial cell lines at different times. TNFα mRNA was not detected. These results were partly confirmed using nontransformed urinary tract epithelial cells. Human bladder epithelial cells isolated from patients undergoing cystoscopy for bladder neck obstruction were exposed to *E. coli*. The epithelial cells secreted IL-6 and IL-8 and contained intracellular IL-8; however, intracellular IL-6 was not detected.[32]

Before these studies it was not known that bacteria induced epithelial cell cytokine production. Subsequently, these results were confirmed in other epithelial cells and with other techniques.[43–45] The similarity between the cytokine response to urinary tract infection and the cytokines secreted by the epithelial cell lines supports the hypothesis that epithelial cells can be a major source of the cytokines detected during urinary tract infection.

BACTERIAL ADHERENCE CAN INFLUENCE UROEPITHELIAL CELL IL-6 AND IL-8 SECRETION

P-fimbriated *E. coli* induce higher levels of fever, CRP, and IgA than do other *E. coli* strains.[7] Children with urinary tract infection who were infected with P-fimbriated *E. coli* had higher IL-6 responses than did children infected with other *E. coli* strains.[46] This suggested that bacterial adherence may modify the mucosal cytokine response. This hypothesis was examined *in vitro* by comparing the levels of IL-6 and IL-8 secreted by the epithelial cell lines in response to adhering and non-adhering *E. coli* strains. Adhering bacteria induced higher IL-6 and IL-8 levels than did nonadhering bacteria. This effect was seen for both type 1 fimbriated and P fimbriated strains.[10,32]

Fimbrial activation of the epithelial cell IL-6 response was examined using P and S fimbrial preparations with or without the receptor binding domain. All fimbrial preparations induced IL-6 secretion above the constitutive levels. In addition, P fimbriae induced adhesin and cell receptor dependent enhancement of the IL-6 response. These results paralleled the IL-6 responses to isolated P fimbriae *in vivo*.[47] The P fimbrial preparations contained low levels of lipopolysaccharide; however, these concentrations of LPS on their own were not stimulatory for kidney epithelial cells.

E. coli STIMULATE URINARY TRACT EPITHELIAL CELLS TO INDUCE NEUTROPHIL INFLUX

The mucosal inflammatory response to urinary tract infection includes a rapid influx of neutrophils into the urine. This occurs both in patients with natural urinary tract infection and in individuals deliberately colonized with *E. coli*.[27,31,32] Two prerequisites for neutrophil influx to sites of mucosal infection are: (1) the local release of

TABLE 2. Migration of Neutrophils through *E. coli*-Stimulated A-498 Kidney Epithelial Cells

	Percent of Neutrophils Added	
	24 Hours	48 Hours
Control	2	13
E. coli *stimulation*	34	88
+ anti-CD18	3	6
+ anti-ICAM-1	7	24
+ anti-VCAM-1	34	83
IL-1 stimulation	43	94
+ anti-CD18	2	8
+ anti-ICAM-1	25	26
+ anti-VCAM-1	34	91

chemoattractants from the infected site, and (2) the interaction of neutrophils with cells of the mucosa via specific adhesion molecules.

Production of Chemoattractants. IL-8 is a powerful neutrophil chemoattractant/ activator. Deliberate colonization of the human urinary tract with nonvirulent bacteria leads to local secretion of IL-8 within hours of infection.[32] The IL-8 levels varied greatly from patient to patient (FIG. 3). A strong correlation between IL-8 levels and neutrophil numbers was observed (FIG. 4). We concluded that bacteria induce a mucosal IL-8 response in the human urinary tract and proposed IL-8 to be an important mediator of neutrophil influx during urinary tract infection. The cellular origin of the mucosal IL-8 was analyzed *in vitro*. *E. coli* stimulated the production of IL-8 in normal bladder epithelial cells as well as urinary tract epithelial cell lines. *E. coli* also stimulated IL-8 production in neutrophils. The level of IL-8 secretion in both cell types was influenced by the ability of the bacteria to adhere to the cells.

Expression of Adhesion Molecules. During neutrophil influx to mucosal sites, cells must traverse both the endothelial cells lining the blood vessel and the mucosal epithelium (lung, intestine, and urinary tract). The first site of neutrophil contact occurs at the blood vessel wall. Endothelial leukocyte adhesion molecule-1 (ELAM-1) and intercellular adhesion molecules (ICAM-1, ICAM-2) expressed on the surface of the endothelium, and L-selectin and B_2 integrins expressed on the neutrophils, all appear to be involved in transendothelial neutrophil migration.[48]

We examined the expression of adhesion molecules by uroepithelial cell lines. The kidney epithelial cell line expressed ICAM-1 constitutively (FIG. 5). The bladder epithelial cell line and epithelial cells isolated from bladder irrigation fluid expressed ICAM-1. Expression of adhesion molecules was augmented after stimulation with either *E. coli* bacteria or IL-1α (FIG. 6a and b). In contrast to endothelial cells, neither epithelial cell line expressed ELAM-1.

Transepithelial Neutrophil Migration. E. coli stimulated transepithelial neutrophil migration. Epithelial cells were grown to confluency on the underside of transwell polycarbonate units.[49] Neutrophils were placed in the upper well, bacteria in the

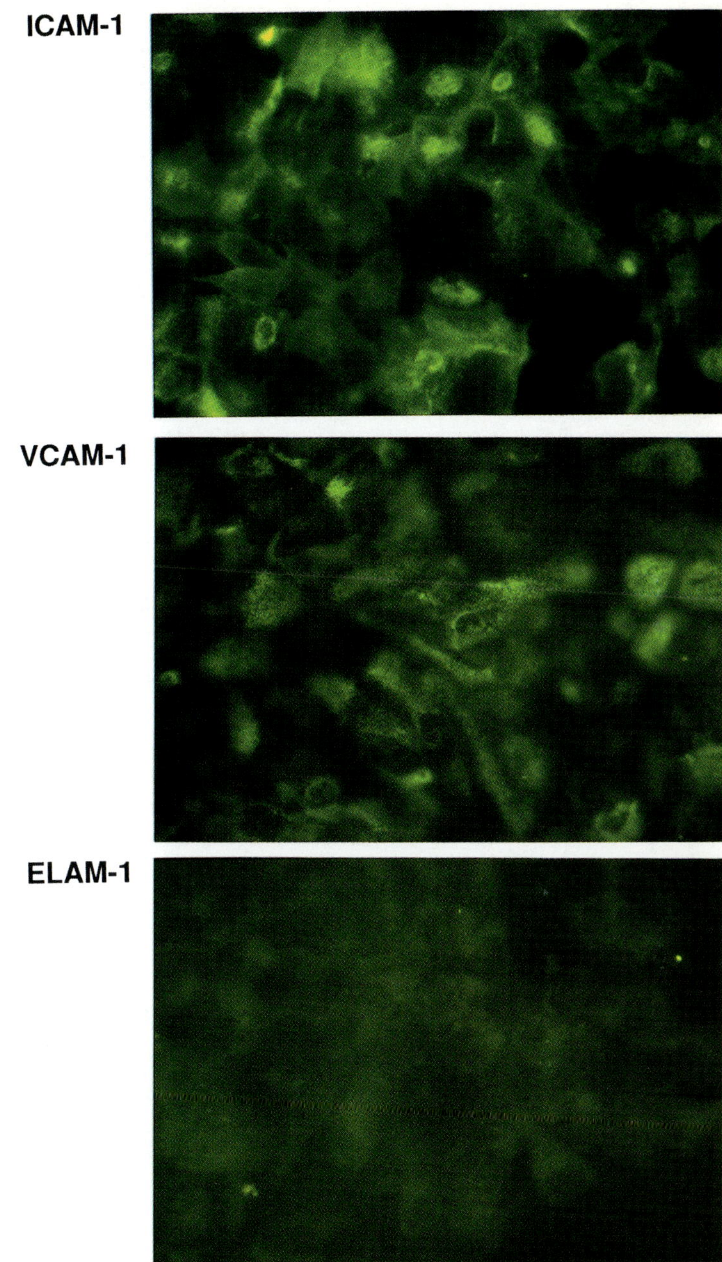

FIGURE 5. Adhesion molecule expression by the A-498 kidney epithelial cell line, as determined by indirect immunofluorescence, 4 hours after stimulation with *E. coli.*

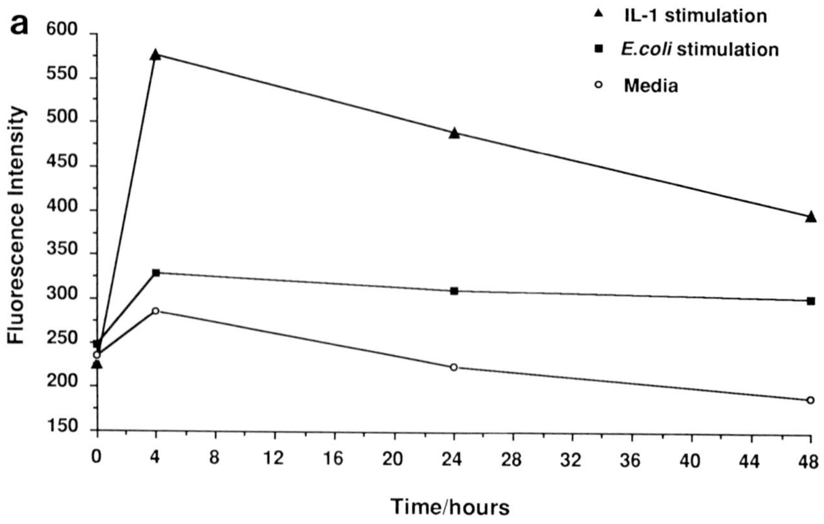

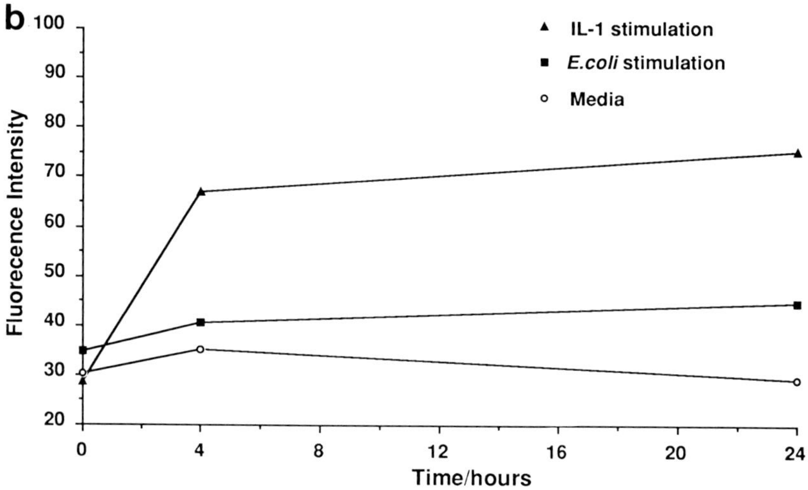

% positive cells

	0h	4h	24h
IL-1	52	83	92
E.coli	65	77	81
Control	56	67	58

FIGURE 6. Kinetics of ICAM expression by the A-498 epithelial cell line after stimulation with IL-1, *E. coli,* or media. (**a**) ICAM-1 expression; positive cells >95% at all time points.

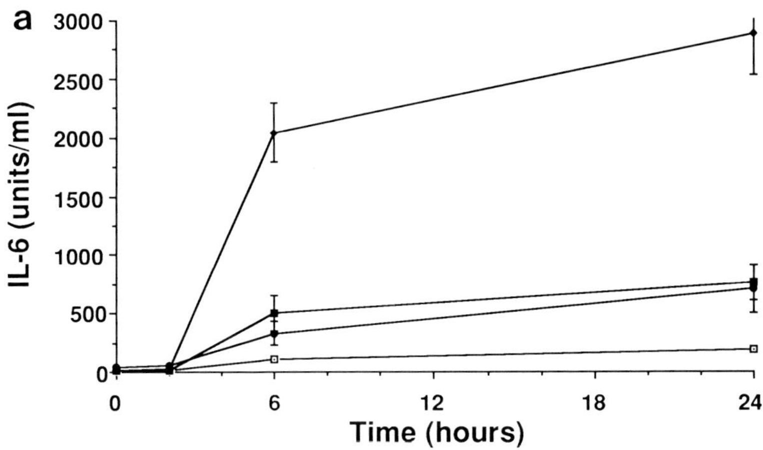

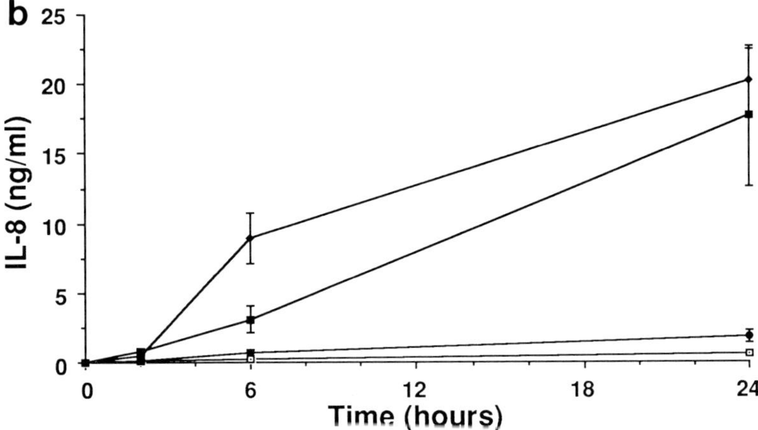

FIGURE 7. Cytokine secretion by epithelial cell lines exposed to TNFα, IL-1α, *E. coli,* or media. (**a**) IL-6 secretion by the A-498 cell line; (**b**) IL-8 secretion by the A-498 cell line.

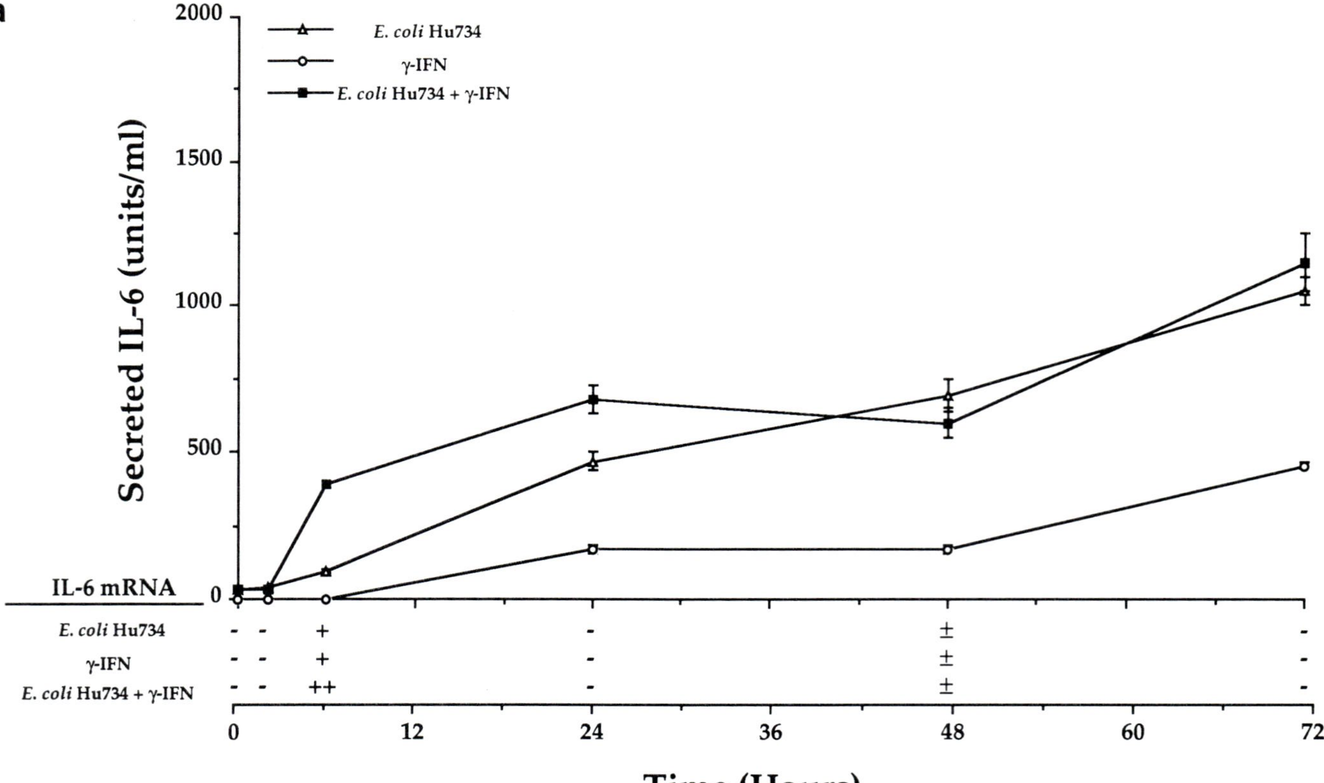
a
E. coli Hu734
γ-IFN
E. coli Hu734 + γ-IFN
Secreted IL-6 (units/ml)
2000
1500
1000
500
0
IL-6 mRNA
E. coli Hu734
γ-IFN
E. coli Hu734 + γ-IFN
0
12
24
36
48
60
72
Time (Hours)

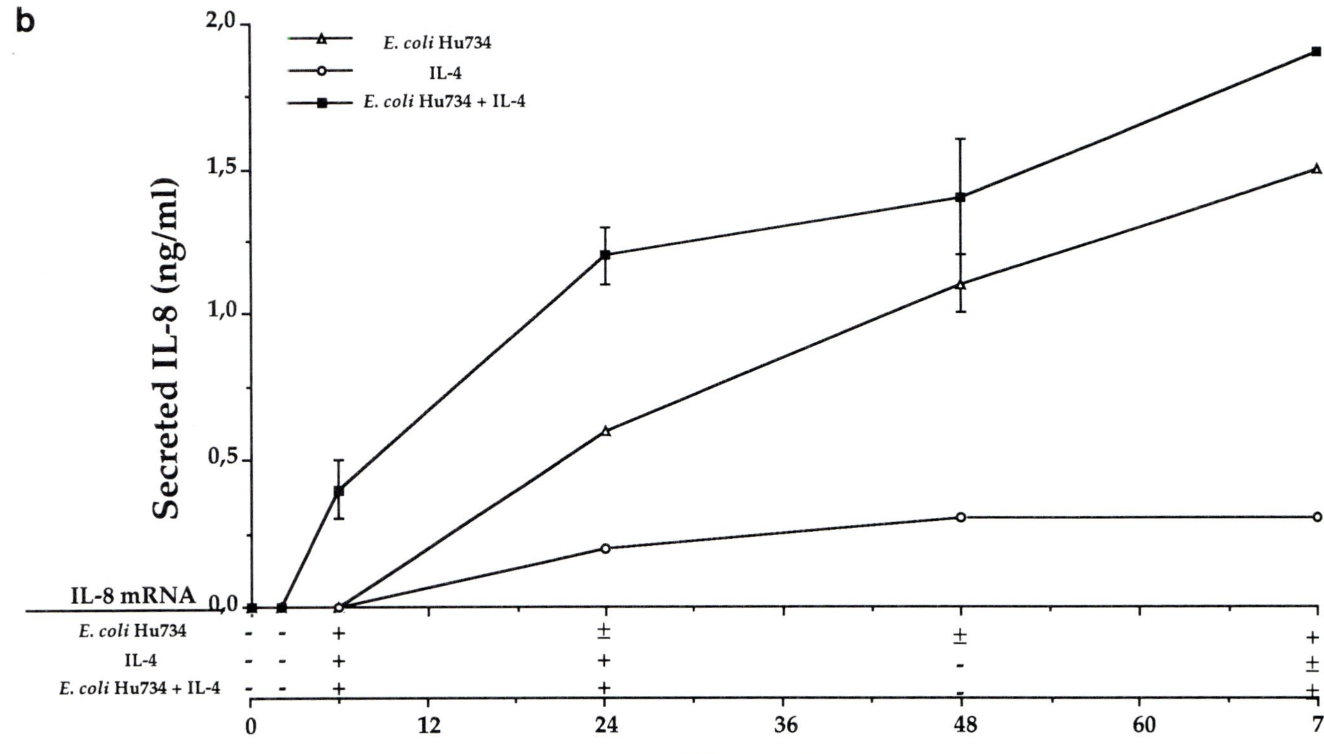

FIGURE 8. Influence of T-cell cytokines on the epithelial cytokine response to *E. coli.* (a) IL-6 secretion by the A-498 cell line; (b) IL-8 secretion by the A-498 cell line.

lower. *E. coli* stimulated the migration of neutrophils among epithelial cell layers (TABLE 2). Anti-CD18 antibodies completely blocked this migration. Anti-ICAM-1 antibodies blocked up to 70% of the neutrophil transepithelial migration. Anti-VCAM-1 antibodies did not influence neutrophil migration.

Together, these results show that *E. coli* can stimulate epithelial cells to initiate the two prerequisites necessary for neutrophil migration; (1) release of neutrophil chemoattractants, and (2) induction of adhesion molecules necessary for transepithelial neutrophil migration. Urinary tract epithelial cells appear to play an important role in directing neutrophil migration into the urine during urinary tract infection.

PROINFLAMMATORY CYTOKINES INDUCE UROEPITHELIAL CELL CYTOKINE PRODUCTION

The mucosal compartment contains cells that migrate to the mucosal site in response to chemotactic signals and resident nonepithelial cells such as macrophages and intraepithelial lymphocytes. These cells can be stimulated to secrete cytokines by bacterial components as well as by cytokines released from the epithelial cells. In this way, complicated networks of interactions can be formed that depend on the type of responding cell and the type of cytokines present in the local environment. We tested whether IL-1α or TNFα could stimulate epithelial cell lines to produce IL-6 (FIG. 7a). IL-1α and TNFα induced a rapid IL-6 response. IL-1α or TNFα also stimulated IL-8 production (FIG. 7b).

IL-1α and IL-β as well as IL-6 and IL-8 mRNAs were detected by RT-PCR in both kidney and bladder cell lines after IL-α and TNFα stimulation. In addition, TNFα mRNA was upregulated in the bladder cell line in response to TNFα stimulation. These results demonstrate that uroepithelial cells produce cytokines in response to IL-1α or TNFα stimulation. Epithelial cells from other mucosal sites produced IL-6 and IL-8 after IL-1α or TNFα stimulation.[50,51] The results emphasize the potential role of epithelial cells in mucosal cytokine networks.

T-CELL CYTOKINES STIMULATE AND MODIFY CYTOKINE PRODUCTION BY UROEPITHELIAL CELL LINES

Interactions between epithelial cells and intraepithelial lymphocytes or other lymphocytes may be a common event in the mucosal compartment. Intraepithelial lymphocytes modulate Ia expression on intestinal epithelial cells.[52] It has also been suggested that intestinal epithelial cells may be competent antigen presenting cells.[53–56] T-cell cytokines affect epithelial cell functions. IFN-γ up-regulated the expression of ICAM and class II antigens and enhanced the secretion of secretory component by epithelial cells.[57–59]

We examined the effects of T-cell cytokines on epithelial cell cytokine responses to *E. coli.* IL-6 secretion was rapidly induced by the combination of IL-4 and bacteria. This result was confirmed by the IL-6 mRNA detected in stimulated cells; IL-6 mRNA was detected earlier and more often than after bacterial stimulation alone. IFN-γ transiently enhanced *E. coli*-induced IL-6 secretion and IL-6 mRNA production, but no difference was noted in total levels of IL-6 detected after 24 hours (FIG. 8a).

IL-4 increased the bacterially induced IL-8 response as determined by both secretion and mRNA. In contrast, the IL-8 response to *E. coli* Hu734 was significantly lowered by the addition of IFN-γ (Fig. 8b).

IFN-γ and IL-4 were previously shown to have opposing effects on activated monocytes. IFN-γ enhanced and IL-4 inhibited cytokine production in lipopolysaccharide-stimulated monocytes.[60-63] In comparison, the epithelial cell IL-6 response to *E. coli* was enhanced by IL-4, whereas IL-4 stimulated and IFN-γ inhibited IL-8 secretion. Similarly, the production of IL-8 in polymorphonuclear cells was recently shown to be inhibited by IFN-γ.[64]

The results of these experiments provide a mechanism whereby T cells may regulate the epithelial cell response to bacteria.

SUMMARY

1. Uropathogenic *E. coli* adhere to mucosal sites.

2. In the urinary tract, adherence is followed by inflammation, including a mucosal cytokine response.

3. Bacteria activate epithelial cells to secrete IL-6 and IL-8. IL-6 may cause the fever and acute phase response that accompany systemic urinary tract infections. IL-8 may function as a neutrophil chemoattractant.

4. *E. coli* up-regulate adhesion molecule expression on epithelial cell lines and neutrophil migration through epithelial cell monolayers. This process is inhibited by antibodies to CD18 and ICAM-1.

5. Cytokines released by nonepithelial cells (T cells and monocytes) modify the epithelial cell cytokine response to bacteria.

REFERENCES

1. SVANBORG-EDÉN, C., S. HANSSON, U. JODAL, G. LIDIN-JANSON, K. LINCOLN, H. LINDER, H. LOMBERG, P. DE MAN, S. MÅRILD, J. MARTINELL, K. PLOS, T. SANDBERG & K. STENQVIST. 1988. Host parasite interaction in the urinary tract. J. Infect Dis. **157:** 421–148.

2. JOHNSON, J. R. 1991. Virulence factors in *Escherichia coli* urinary tract infection. Clin. Microbiol. Rev. **4:** 80–128.

3. MIRELMAN, D., ED. 1986. Microbial Agglutinins and Lectins: Properties and Biological Activity. John Wiley & Sons. New York.

4. DUGUID, J. P., G. DEMPSTER & P. N. EDMUND. 1955. Non-flagellar filamentous appendages ("fimbriae") and hemagglutinating activity in Bacterium coli. J. Path. Bact. **70:** 335–348.

5. BRINTON, C. C. 1959. Non-flagellar appendages of bacteria. Nature **183:** 782–786.

6. LEFFLER, H. & C. SVANBORG-EDÉN. 1981. Glycolipid receptors for uropathogenic *Escherichia coli* on human erythrocytes and uroepithelial cells. Infect. Immun. **34:** 920–929.

7. DE MAN, P., U. JODAL, K. LINCOLN & C. SVANBORG-EDÉN. 1988. Bacterial attachment and inflammation in the urinary tract. J. Infect. Dis. **158:** 29–35.

8. WOLD, A. E., M. THORSSEN, S. HULL & C. SVANBORG-EDÉN. 1988. Attachment of *Escherichia coli* via mannose- or Galα1-4Galβ-containing receptors to human colonic epithelial cells. Infect. Immun. **56:** 2531–2537.

9. LEFFLER, H. & C. SVANBORG-EDÉN. 1980. Chemical identification of a glycosphingo-lipid receptor for *Escherichia coli* attaching to human urinary tract epithelial cells and agglutinating human erythrocytes. FEMS Microbiol. Lett. **8:** 127–134.

10. HEDGES S., M. SVENSSON & C. SVANBORG. 1992. Interleukin-6 response of epithelial cell lines to bacterial stimulation *in vitro.* Infect. Immun. **60:** 1295–1301.

11. KÄLLENIUS, G., R. MÖLLBY, S. B. SVENSSON, J. WINBERG, A. LUNDBLAD, S. SVENSSON & B. CEDERGREN. 1980. The P antigen as receptor for the hemagglutination of pyelonephritic *Escherichia coli.* FEMS Microbiol. Lett. **7:** 297–302.

12. HULL, R. A., R. E. GILL, P. HSU, B. H. MINSHEW & S. FALKOV. 1989. Construction and expression of recombinant plasmids encoding type 1 or D-mannose-resistant pili from a urinary tract infection *Escherichia coli* isolate. Infect. Immun. **51:** 693–695.

13. HULTGREN, S. J., S. ABRAHAM, M. CAPARON, P. FALK, J. W. S. (III) GEME & S. NORMARK. 1993. Pilus and nonpilus bacterial adhesins: Assembly and function in cell recognition. Cell **73:** 887–901.

14. LINDBERG, F. P., B. LUND & S. NORMARK. 1984. Genes of pyelonephritogenic *E. coli* required for digalactoside specific agglutination of human cells. EMBO J. **3:** 1167–1173.

15. LUND, B., F. B. LINDBERG, B.-I. MARKLUND & S. NORMARK. 1987. The Pap G protein is the α-D-galactopyranosyl-(1-4)-β-D-galactopyranose-binding adhesin of uropathogenic *Escherichia coli.* Proc. Natl. Acad. Sci. USA **84:** 5898–5902.

16. MARKLUND, B.-I., J. M. TENNENT & E. GARCIA. 1992. Horizontal gene transfer of the *E. coli pap* and *prs* operons as mechanism for the development of tissue specific adhesive properties. Molec. Microbiol. **6:** 2225–2242.

17. JOHANSSON, I. M., K. PLOS, B.-I. MARKLUND & C. SVANBORG. 1993. Pap, pap G, and prs G DNA sequences in *Escherichia coli* from the fecal flora and the urinary tract. Microbial. Pathog.

18. CLAUSEN, H. & S.-I. HAKOMORI. 1989. ABH and related histo-blood group antigens: Immunochemical differences and carrier isotypes and their distribution. Vox. Sang. **56:** 1–20.

19. HOLGERSSON, J., M. E. BREIMER & B. E. SAMULESSON. 1992. Basic biochemistry of cell surface carbohydrates and aspects of the tissue distribution of histo-blood group ABH and related glycosphingolipids. APMIS **100:** 18–27.

20. SVANBORG-EDÉN C. S., S. HULL, H. LEFFLER, S. NORGREN, K. PLOS & A. WOLD. 1989. The large intestine as a reservoir for *Escherichia coli* causing extraintestinal infections. Wenner-Gren International Symposium Series **52:** 47–58.

21. WOLD, A., D. A. CAUGANT, G. LINDEN-JANSSON, P. DE MAN & C. SVANBORG. 1992. Resident colonic *Escherichia coli* strains frequently display uropathogenic characteristics. J. Infect. Dis. **165:** 46–52.

22. PLOS, K., H. CONNELL, U. JODAL, B.-I. MARKLUND, S. MÅRILD, B. WETTERGREN & C. SVANBORG. Intestinal carriage of P fimbriated *Escherichia coli* and the susceptibility to urinary tract infection in young children. In manuscript.

23. HAGBERG, L., R. HULL, S. HULL, S. FALKOV, R. FRETER & C. SVANBORG-EDÉN. 1983. Contribution of adhesion to bacterial persistence in the mouse urinary tract. Infect. Immun. **40:** 265.

24. O'HANLEY, P., D. LARK, S. FALKOW & G. SCHOOLNIK. 1985. Molecular basis of *Escherichia coli* colonisation of the upper urinary tract in BALB/c mice. Gal-Gal pili immunization prevents *Escherichia coli* pyelonephritis in the BALB/c mouse model of human pyelone-phritis. J. Clin. Invest. **75:** 347–360.

25. SVANBORG-EDÉN, C., L. HANSON, U. JODAL, U. LINDBERG & A. ÅKERLUND. 1976. Variable adherence to normal human urinary tract epithelial cells of *Escherichia coli* strains associated with various forms of urinary tract infection. Lancet 490–492.

26. PLOS, K., T. CARTER, S. HULL & R. HULL. 1990. Frequency and organization of *pap* homologous DNA in relation to clinical origin of uropathogenic *E. coli*. J. Infect. Dis. **161:** 518.

27. ANDERSON, P., I. ENGBERG, G. LIDIN-JANSON, K. LINCOLN, R. HULL, S. HULL & C. SVANBORG. 1991. Persistence of *E. coli* bacteriuria not determined by bacterial adherence. Infect. Immun. **59:** 2915-2921.

28. DE MAN, P., U. JODAL & C. SVANBORG. 1991. Dependence among host response parameters used to diagnose urinary tract infection. J. Infect. Dis. **163:** 331-335.

29. SHAHIN, R. D., I. ENGBERG, L. HAGBERG & C. SVANBORG-EDÉN. 1987. Neutrophil recruitment and bacterial clearance correlated with LPS responsiveness in local gram-negative infection. J. Immunol. **138:** 3475.

30. DE MAN, P., L. AARDEN, I. ENGBERG, H. LINDER, C. SVANBORG-EDÉN & C. VAN KOOTEN. 1989. Interleukin-6 induced at mucosal surfaces by Gram-negative bacterial infection. Infect. Immun. **57:** 3383.

31. HEDGES, S., P. ANDERSON, G. LIDIN-JANSON, P. DE MAN & C. SVANBORG. 1991. Interleukin-6 response to deliberate colonization of the human urinary tract with Gram-negative bacteria. Infect. Immun. **59:** 421.

32. AGACE, W., S. HEDGES, M. CESKA & C. SVANBORG. 1993. Interleukin-8 and the neutrophil response to mucosal Gram-negative infection. J. Clin. Invest. **92:** 780-785.

33. HEDGES, S., G. LIDIN-JANSON, J. MARTINELL, T. SANDBERG, K. STENQVIST & C. SVANBORG. 1992. Comparison of urine and serum concentrations of interleukin-6 in women with acute pyelonephritis or asymptomatic bacteriuria. J. Infect. Dis. **166:** 653.

34. KASS, E. H. 1956. Asymptomatic infection of the urinary tract. Trans. Assoc. Am. Physicians **69:** 56-63.

35. WAAGE, A. 1987. Production and clearance of tumor necrosis factor in rats exposed to endotoxin and dexamethasone. Clin. Immunol. Immunopathol. **45:** 348-355.

36. MATHISON, J. C., E. WOLFSON & R. J. ULEVITCH. 1988. Participation of tumour necrosis factor in the mediation of bacterial lipopolysaccharide-induced injury in rabbits. J. Clin. Invest. **81:** 1925.

37. WAAGE, A., P. BRANDTZEG, A. HALSTENSEN, P. KIERULF & T. ESPEVIK. 1989. The complex pattern of cytokines in serum from patients with meningococcal septic shock. Association between interleukin 6, interleukin 1, and fatal outcome. J. Exp. Med. **169:** 333.

38. FOND, Y., K. J. TRACEY, L. L. MOLDAWER, D. G. HESSE, K. MANOGUE, J. S. KENNEY, A. T. LEE, G. C. KUO, A. C. ALLISON, S. F. LOWRY & A. CERAMI. 1989. Antibodies to cachectin/ tumour necrosis factor reduce interleukin 1β and interleukin 6 appearance during lethal bacteremia. J. Exp. Med. **170:** 1627-1633.

39. DINARELLO, C. A., J. G. CANON, S. M. WOLFF, H. A. BERNHEIM, B. BEUTLER, A. CERAMI, I. S. FIGARI, M. A. PALLADINO & J. V. O'CONNOR. 1986. Tumor necrosis factor (cachectin) is an endogenous pyrogen and induces production of interleukin-1. J. Exp. Med. **163:** 1433- 1450.

40. VAN DAMME, J., G. OPDENAKKER, R. J. SIMPSON, M. R. RUBIRA, S. CAYPHAS, A. VINK, A. BILLIAU & J. VAN SNICK. 1987. Identification of the human 26kDa protein, interferon β2 (IFNβ2) as a B cell hybridoma/plasmacytoma growth factor induced by interleukin 1 and tumor necrosis factor. J. Exp. Med. **165:** 914-919.

41. HAVELL, E. A. & P. B. SEHGAL. 1991. Tumour necrosis factor-independent IL-6 production during murine Listeriosis. J. Immunol. **146:** 756-761.

42. ZANETTI, G., D. HEUMANN, J. GÉRAIN, J. KOHLER, P. ABBET, C. BARRAS, R. LUCAS, M. GLAUSER & J. BAUMGARTNER. 1992. Cytokine production after intravenous or peritoneal Gram-negative bacterial challenge in mice. J. Immunol. **148:** 1890-1897.

43. AGACE, W., S. HEDGES, U. ANDERSSON, M. CESKA & C. SVANBORG. 1993. Selective cytokine production by epithelial cells following exposure to *Escherichia coli*. Infect. Immun. **61:** 602-609.

44. KREFT, B., S. BOHNET, O. CARSTENSEN, J. HACKER & R. MARRE. 1993. Differential expression of interleukin-6, intracellular adhesion molecule 1, and major histocompatibility complex class II molecules in renal carcinoma cells stimulated with S fimbriae of uropathogenic *Escherichia coli*. Infect. Immun. **61:** 3060-3063.

45. ARNOLD, R., J. SCHEFFER, B. KÖNIG & W. KÖNIG. 1993. Effects of *Listeria monocytogenes* and *Yersinia enterocolitica* on cytokine gene expression and release from human polymorphonuclear granulocytes and epithelial (HEP-2) cells. Infect. Immun. **61:** 2545-2552.

46. BENSON, M., A. ANDRESSON, U. JODAL, Å. KARLSSON, J. RYDBERG & SVANBORG. Interleukin-6 in childhood urinary tract infection. Pediatr. Infect. Dis.

47. LINDER, H., I. ENGBERG, H. HOSCHÜTZKY, I. MATTSBY-BALTZER & C. SVANBORG-EDÉN. 1991. Adhesion dependent activation of mucosal IL-6 production. Infect. Immun. **59:** 4357-4362.

48. ZIMMERMAN, G. A., S. M. PRESCOTT & T. M. MCINTYRE. 1992. Endothelial cell interactions with granuloyctes: Tethering and signalling molecules. Immunol. Today. **13:** 93-99.

49. PARKOS, C. A., C. DELP, M. A. ARNOULT & J. L. MADARA. 1991. Neutrophil migration across a cultured epithelium: Dependence on a CD11b/CD18 mediated event and enhanced efficiency in the physiological direction. J. Clin. Invest. **88:** 1605-1612.

50. CROMWELL, O., W. HAMID, C. J. CORRIGAN, J. BARKANS, Q. MENG, P. D. COLLINS & A. B. KAY. 1992. Expression and generation of interleukin-8, IL-6 and granulocyte-macrophage colony-stimulating factor by bronchial epithelial cells and enhancement by IL-1β and tumour necrosis factor-α. Immunology **77:** 330-337.

51. STANDIFORD, T. J., S. L. KUNKEL, M. A. BASHA, S. W. CHENSUE, L. E. LYNCH, G. B. TOEWS, J. WESTWICK & R. M. STRIETER. 1990. Interleukin-8 gene expression by a pulmonary epithelial cell line. A model for cytokine networks in the lung. J. Clin. Invest. **86:** 1945-1953.

52. CERF-BENSUSSAN, N., A. QUARONI, J. KURNICK & A. BHAN. 1984. Intraepithelial lymphocytes modulate Ia expression by intestinal epithelial cells. J. Immunol. **132:** 2244-2252.

53. BLAND, P. W. & L. G. WARREN. 1986. Antigen presentation by epithelial cells of the rat small intestine. I. Kinetics, antigen specificity and blocking by anti-Ia antisera. Immunology **58:** 1-7.

54. BLAND, P. W. & L. G. WARREN. 1986. Antigen presentation by epithelial cells of ther at small intestine. II. Selective induction of suppressor T cells. Immunology **58:** 9-14.

55. KAISERLIAN, D., K. VIDAL & J.-P. REVILLARD. 1989. Murine enterocytes can present soluble antigen to specific class II restricted CD4+ T cells. Eur. J. Immunol. **19:** 1513-1516.

56. KALB, T. H., M. T. CHUANG, Z. MAROM & L. MAYER. 1991. Evidence for accessory cell function by class II MHC antigen-expressing airway epithelial cells. Am. J. Respir. Cell. Mol. Biol. **4:** 320-329.

57. KVALE, D., P. BRANDTZAEG & D. LÖVHAUG. 1988. Up-regulation of the expression of secretory component and HLA molecules in a human colonic cell line by tumour necrosis factor-a and gamma interferon. Scand. J. Immunol. **28:** 351-357.

58. KVALE, D., P. KRACJI & P. BRANDTZAEG. 1992. Expression and regulation of adhesion molecules ICAM-1 (CD54) and LFA-3 (CD58) in human intestinal epithelial cell lines. Scand. J. Immunol. **35:** 669-676.

59. SOLLID, L. M., D. KVALE, P. BRANDTZAEG, G. MARKUSEN & E. THORSBY. 1987. Interferon-γ enhances expression of secretory component, the epithelial receptor for polymeric immunoglobulins. J. Immunol. **138:** 4303.

60. GIFFORD, G. E. & M. L. LOHAMANN-MATTHES. 1987. Gamma-interferon priming of mouse and human macrophages for induction of tumour necrosis factor production by bacterial lipopolysaccharide. J. Natl. Cancer Inst. **78:** 121.

61. HART, P. H., G. F. VITTI, D. R. BURGESS, G. A. WHITTY, D. S. PICCOLI & J. A. HAMILTON. 1989. Potential anti-inflammatory effects of interleukin-4: Suppression of human monocyte tumor necrosis factor α, interleukin-1, and prostaglandin E_2. Proc. Natl. Acad. Sci. USA **86:** 3803–3807.

62. ESSNER, R., K. RHOADES, W. H. MCBRIDE, D. MORTON & J. S. ECONOMOU. 1989. IL-4 down regulates IL-1 and TNF gene expression in human monocytes. J. Immunol. **142:** 3857–3861.

63. CHEYNG, D. L., P. H. HART, G. F. VITTI, G. A. WHITTY & J. A. HAMILTON. 1988. Contrasting effects of interferon-gamma and interleukin-4 on the interleukin-6 activity of stimulated human monocytes. Immunology **71:** 70–75.

64. CASSATELLA, M. A., I. GUASPARRI, M. CESKA, F. BAZZONI & F. ROSSI. 1993. Interferon gamma inhibits interleukin-8 production by human polymorphonuclear leukocytes. Immunology **78:** 177–184.

Interaction of Pathogenic *Neisseria* with Host Defenses

What Happens *in Vivo*?[a]

RICHARD F. REST,[b] JUNTAO LIU,
RUDRANATH TALUKDAR, JOSEPH V. FRANGIPANE,
AND DANIEL SIMON

Department of Microbiology and Immunology
Hahnemann University School of Medicine
Philadelphia, Pennsylvania 19102–1192

Gonorrhea is characterized by a cervical or urethral purulent exudate comprising serum, high concentrations of neutrophils, and significant numbers of free and cell-associated *Neisseria gonorrhoeae* (reviewed in ref. 1). Most studies of gonococcal pathogenesis have been performed *in vitro*, using isolated peripheral blood neutrophils, epithelial cell lines, or serum. Some studies, however, including a series of investigations by Smith and Parsons and their colleagues, investigated the interactions of human neutrophils and gonococci by studying urethral exudates from males with gonorrhea.[2-4] Their studies suggest that a percentage of gonococci grown *in vivo* remain viable after prolonged exposure to exudate neutrophils. Such results are in stark contrast to results of other *in vitro* studies in which gonococci are killed quite readily by neutrophils over a relatively short time, generally <3 hours.[5-7] Thus, gonococci grown *in vivo* apparently are quite different from gonococci grown *in vitro* in their interaction with human neutrophils.

Yet another set of experiments by Smith and Parsons and their colleagues and collaborators culminated in an exciting and unique set of observations (reviewed in refs. 8-10), observations that have completely altered our view of gonococcal pathogenesis. Whereas most strains of gonococci taken directly from urethral exudates are resistant to serum killing, the same gonococci passaged one or more times on laboratory medium become serum sensitive.[11] Conversely, serum-sensitive gonococci grown *in vitro* in the presence of human serum, genital secretions, or erythrocytes, or their extracts, become phenotypically serum resistant. This serum resistance is due, at least in part, to the covalent transfer of sialic acid (*N*-acetylneuraminic acid)

[a] This work was supported in part by grant AI20897 from the National Institute of Allergy and Infectious Diseases and from an in-house grant from Hahnemann, Office of the Dean of the Graduate School, and Vice President for Research.

[b] Please address all correspondence to: Richard F. Rest, PhD, Department of Microbiology and Immunology, Mail stop 410, Hahnemann University School of Medicine, Philadelphia, PA 19102–1192.

by a gonococcal sialytransferase (STase) from CMP-NANA (cytidine monophospho-*N*-acetyl neuraminic acid, or CMP-sialic acid) to gonococcal lipooligosaccharide (LOS).[12] Thus, most strains of gonococci grown *in vitro* interact with human serum quite differently than do gonococci grown *in vivo*.

Gonococci interact with human neutrophils by nonopsonic (antibody- and complement-independent) mechanisms if they possess one or more of a family of heat-modifiable outer membrane proteins termed opacity-associated (Opa) proteins (previously called PII proteins).[5,6,13–17] Opa proteins are one of several gonococcal outer membrane components that undergo frequent antigenic and/or phase variation.[18,19] An individual gonococcus possesses about a dozen Opa genes and can express from 0 to 3 or more Opa proteins at a time.[18,20–22] *In vitro*, most Opa$^+$ gonococci are phagocytized and killed by human neutrophils.[5–7] CMP-NANA is present in human tissue, probably including cervical epithelial cells, and is used by cellular STases to donate sialic acid to glycoproteins, carbohydrates, and gangliosides. Apicella *et al.*[23] and Mandrell *et al.*[12] showed that gonococci associated with neutrophils in urethral exudates from males with gonorrhea are sialylated, indicating that sialylation indeed occurs *in vivo*, within phagocytic cells.

Gonococci have been isolated in the presence of obligate anaerobes from the genitourinary tract and from individuals with pelvic inflammatory disease. These primary isolates can survive and grow for long periods without oxygen; however, after passage *in vitro*, gonococci grow anaerobically only if provided with millimolar concentrations of nitrite, which they use as a terminal electron acceptor.[24] Nitrite is readily available in the human host from biologic fluids and as a result of the metabolism of normal anaerobic flora. Anaerobic gonococci express at least three novel outer membrane proteins (PANs 1 to 3) and repress at least five aerobically induced outer membrane proteins (POXs 1 to 5).[25] Such induction and repression of outer membrane components could be crucial to colonization or pathogenesis at anaerobic sites of infection, but the function, if any, of these proteins remains unknown. Sera from patients recovering from gonorrhea contain antibodies that react strongly with PAN 1 on Western immunoblots, whereas sera from healthy individuals do not, indicating that gonococci express PAN 1 at some point during infection, probably as a result of anaerobic growth.[26] In one of the few such studies, Keevil *et al.*[27] showed that gonococci grown under oxygen-limited conditions were more virulent in a mouse model of *in vivo* growth. Thus, anaerobic cultivation of gonococci may more closely resemble *in vivo* conditions than may the routine aerobic incubation performed in most laboratories.

MATERIALS AND METHODS

Neisseria gonorrhoeae *and Plasmids*. Nonpiliated Opa variants of strain F62 were used in these studies and have been used extensively in our laboratory. Strain F62 is a serum-sensitive cervical isolate. Of the two Opa variants, one expressed no Opa protein (Opa$^-$) and one expressed an Opa protein termed Opa4.[28] For daily use, passaged gonococci were either (1) resuspended in warm Dulbecco's phosphate-buffered saline solution with 0.1% (w/v) gelatin (PBSG, pH 7) to 2×10^8 to 4×10^8

gonococci/ml and kept at room temperature or 37°C until used, or (2) resuspended in 5 or 10 ml of warm GC broth plus added supplements and grown for about 3 hours to mid-log phase, washed once in PBSG, and resuspended as just described.[29]

For CMP-NANA experiments, various concentrations of CMP-NANA (indicated in the text) were added to growth medium from a 1,250-μg/ml stock of CMP-NANA in water, as described.[30,31] For experiments comparing anaerobic and aerobic gonococci, GC agar plates streaked confluently with a suspension of gonococci at ~6 × 10^8 cfu/ml were incubated in an anaerobic jar containing a BBL GasPak Plus system, or inside an anaerobic chamber, or aerobically for 15 to 16 hours at 37 °C in 5% CO_2. Anaerobic growth of gonococci was achieved using the nitrite-disk method of Knapp and Clark,[24] as slightly modified by Frangipane and Rest.[32]

Plasmids were extracted from gonococci by classical methods or by using Promega Magic Minipreps according to the manufacturer's directions.

Neutrophils and Granule Extract. For functional studies, neutrophils were isolated from heparinized fresh human blood by a single-step separation through a mixture of Ficoll and Hypaque, were suspended to 1 or 2 × 10^7/ml in PBSG without calcium or magnesium, and kept on ice until use. For granule extract, total neutrophil granules were isolated from approximately 1 × 10^{10} neutrophils obtained by leukapheresis and extracted with 0.2 M sodium acetate buffer, pH 4.0.[29]

Adherence Assay. Neutrophils (1 × 10^6, treated with 3 × 10^{-7} M formylmethionyl-leucylphenylalanine [fmlp] for 5 minutes at 37°C, to upregulate neutrophil Opa receptors) were mixed with 5 × 10^7 gonococci in a total volume of 0.5 ml of PBSG and tumbled in 1.5-ml centrifuge tubes for 20 minutes at 37°C.[33] Aliquots (150 μl) were removed, cytocentrifuged (Shandon Southern), stained with Wright stain, and examined by light microscopy (1,000X magnification).

Phagocytic Killing Assay. Ten million neutrophils and 1 × 10^7 Opa4 gonococci were tumbled end over end (12 rpm) in 1 ml of PBSG in 1.5-ml conical snap-cap tubes at 37°C. At 0, 45, 90, and 135 minutes 10-μl aliquots were removed, appropriately diluted in warm PBSG, and plated on GC agar plates. Viability was quantitated by counting colony-forming units after 20–24 hours of incubation. Results are expressed as % viable gonococci, determined as ([cfu at sampling time]/[input cfu at zero time]) × 100.

Serum Bactericidal Assay. Pooled normal human serum (NHS) was diluted to various concentrations in 450 μl of sterile warm PBSG plus Ca^{2+}/Mg^{2+}. Gonococci (1 × 10^7 in 50 μl of PBSG plus Ca and Mg) were added to the mixture, which was incubated at 37°C without agitation. After 30 minutes, 10-μl samples were appropriately diluted in sterile buffer and plated in duplicate on GC agar for overnight incubation. Following quantitation of colonies, values from duplicate plates were averaged. Results are expressed as % viable gonococci, determined as 100 × (cfu of NHS-treated gonococci at 30 minutes)/ (cfu of untreated gonococci at 0 minute).[30]

Isolation and Purification of LOS from Whole Gonococci. Crude LOS was isolated from whole gonococci by the method of Hitchcock,[34] using proteinase K. Purified LOS was prepared from ethanol plus acetone-dried gonococci of strain F62 according to Darveau and Hancock.[35] Identification of gonococcal LOS was determined by tricine SDS-PAGE of proteinase K-treated whole gonococci, performed according

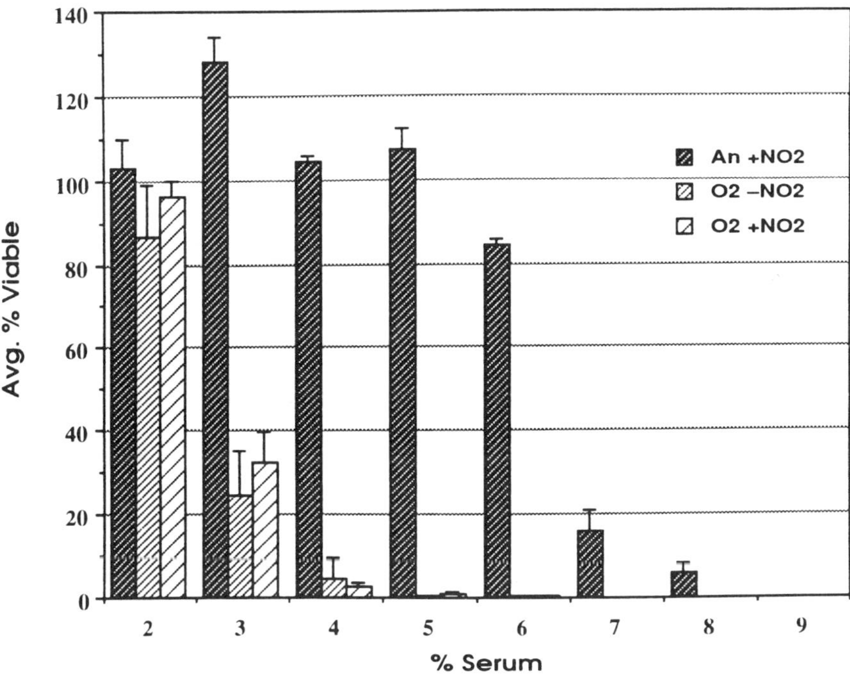

FIGURE 1. Anaerobic gonococci are less sensitive than aerobic gonococci to killing by normal human serum (NHS). Gonococci of strain F62 were grown anaerobically (An) or aerobically (O_2) on plates in the presence (+) or absence (−) of sodium nitrite (NO_2) and mixed with NHS. Serum killing was measured as detailed in *Methods*. Bars = 1 standard deviation (n = 3). Reprinted from Frangipane and Rest,[30] with permission.

to Lesse *et al.*[36] using 14% acrylamide and 2.67 M urea. All electrophoresis reagents were from BioRad Laboratories (Richmond, California).

RESULTS

Effects of Growth in the Absence of Oxygen and the Presence of CMP-NANA on the Susceptibility of Gonococci to Killing by Human Serum

Anaerobic gonococci are less sensitive to serum killing than are aerobic gonococci. Initially, we compared the serum sensitivities of anaerobic and aerobic gonococci grown in the absence of CMP-NANA. Gonococci, grown in the presence or the absence of oxygen, were suspended in sterile PBSG plus Ca^{2+}/Mg^{2+} and mixed with 0 to 9% pooled NHS for 30 minutes at 37°C. Aerobic gonococci were not killed by 2% NHS, but were readily killed by NHS concentrations ≥3% (FIG. 1). Anaerobic gonococci, on the other hand, remained between 128% and 84% viable after treatment with up to 6% NHS and were effectively killed only by ≥7% NHS. Similar results

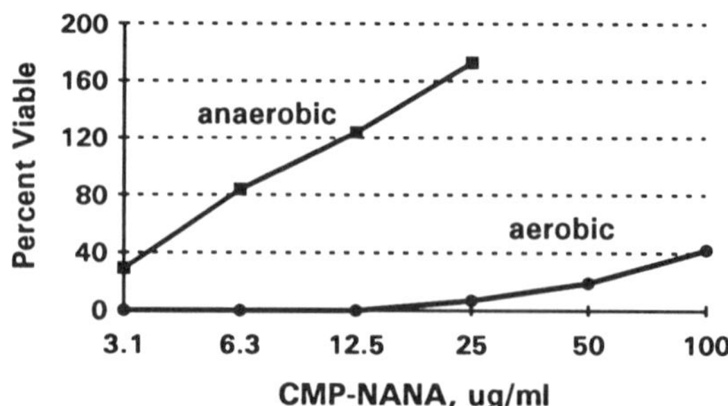

FIGURE 2. Anaerobic growth and CMP-NANA synergistically induce high level serum resistance in gonococci. Gonococci of strain F62 were grown anaerobically or aerobically on plates in the presence of increasing concentrations of CMP-NANA, harvested, washed, and mixed with normal human serum (NHS). Serum killing was measured as detailed in *Methods.* Gonococci incubated without CMP-NANA were 100% killed by NHS (data not shown); $n = 3$.

were obtained whether the experiments were performed in ambient air, as described, or inside an anaerobic chamber (data not shown).[30] The mechanisms responsible for the ability of anaerobically grown gonococci to resist killing by low concentrations of human serum remain to be determined.

Anaerobic growth and CMP-NANA act synergistically to increase gonococcal serum resistance. Next, we determined whether anaerobic and aerobic gonococci differed in their ability to become serum resistant when grown in the presence of CMP-NANA. We grew strain F62 gonococci anaerobically or aerobically on GC agar containing various concentrations of CMP-NANA. After suspension in sterile buffer, gonococci were mixed with 45% or 90% NHS for 30 minutes at 37°C. Gonococci grown in the absence of CMP-NANA were 100% killed regardless of anaerobic or aerobic phenotype. Aerobic gonococci grown on agar containing 25.0, 50.0, or 100.0 μg/ml of CMP-NANA remained only 6%, 18%, or 41% viable, respectively, in assays using 90% NHS (FIG. 2). Similar results were obtained with 45% NHS (data not shown). Growth of aerobic gonococci with CMP-NANA concentrations ≤12.5 μg/ml resulted in no serum resistance. By contrast to the limited ability of CMP-NANA to convert aerobic agar-grown gonococci to serum resistance, anaerobic gonococci grown on agar containing 6.2, 12.5, or 25.0 μg/ml of CMP-NANA remained 83%, 122%, or 175% viable, respectively (FIG. 2). Thus, anaerobic growth of gonococci in the presence of CMP-NANA synergistically enhances their resistance to NHS compared to aerobic growth in the presence of CMP-NANA.

Anaerobic gonococci synthesize different LOS than do aerobic gonococci. Enhanced sialylation of anaerobic gonococcal LOS could be due to a change in LOS phenotype. To explore this possibility, we examined the LOS bands on SDS-PAGE from anaerobic and aerobic gonococci grown without CMP-NANA (FIG. 3). We observed that although anaerobic and aerobic gonococci appear to possess the same two LOS bands, anaerobic gonococci express more of the lower molecular weight band, which now has a terminal *N*-acetylgalactosamine and which does not accept sialic acid, than do anaerobic gonococci. Increased expression of the LOS acceptor molecular for sialic acid could result in uptake of greater amounts of sialic acid by anaerobic gonococci, resulting in enhanced resistance to NHS. Indeed, Frangipane and Rest[30] showed that anaerobic gonococci incorporate more siliac acid from CMP-NANA than do aerobic gonococci.

Anaerobic gonococci possess more sialyltransferase (STase) activity than do aerobic gonococci. It is possible that in addition to the change in LOS expression, anaerobic growth causes the expression of greater gonococcal STase activity. To compare the relative STase activity of anaerobic and aerobic gonococci, we prepared 0.5% triton X-100 extracts of whole gonococci using identical amounts of both gonococcal phenotypes. Extracts were diluted in phosphate-buffered saline solution containing an excess of CMP-NANA (250 μg/ml) and 66 μg/ml LOS purified from aerobic gonococci and were incubated at 37°C. Samples were removed at 10-minute intervals, solubilized in SDS, and treated with proteinase K to degrade all protein, but not LOS. The LOS was then analyzed by 14% acrylamide SDS-PAGE and stained with periodate oxidation and silver. As evidenced by the upward shift in the 4.5-kD LOS band (which now co-migrates with the higher molecular weight LOS molecular form), anaerobic extract caused the complete sialylation of gonococcal LOS after only 40 minutes (FIG. 4, lane G). By contrast, extract of aerobic gonococci required 120 minutes to sialylate only ~90% of the same purified LOS (FIG. 4, lane Y). Such a level of sialylation was achieved by the anaerobic extract after only 30 minutes of incubation with LOS and CMP-NANA (FIG. 4, lane E). These results suggest that anaerobic gonococci possess up to 4 times as much STase activity as do aerobic gonococci. Thus, gonococci apparently have evolved at least two mechanisms for increased serum resistance in the presence of CMP-NANA under anaerobic conditions: they make more LOS that can be sialylated, and they make more STase; together, there is a synergistic increase in serum resistance.

Anaerobic growth increases supercoiling of gonococcal DNA. To investigate how gonococcal LOS and STase could be regulated by anaerobic growth, we determined the degree of supercoiling of a gonococcal 4.1-kbp cryptic plasmid as an indication of chromosomal DNA supercoiling. The 4.1-kbp cryptic plasmid was extracted from gonococcal strains F62 or FA1090 grown anaerobically or aerobically on plates. The plasmid DNA was then electrophoresed through 1% agarose in the presence of 2 or 10 μg/ml of chloroquine to enhance the separation of plasmid subpopulations

FIGURE 3. Anaerobic and aerobic gonococci synthesize different LOS phenotypes. Gonococci of strain F62, grown anaerobically (−) or aerobically (+) on plates (in the absence of CMP-NANA), were solubilized in SDS and treated with proteinase K. The LOS content of these samples was analyzed by 14% acrylamide SDS-PAGE and silver staining, as outlined in *Methods*. The *lower band* has an apparent molecular weight of ~4,500; the *higher band* of ~4,800.

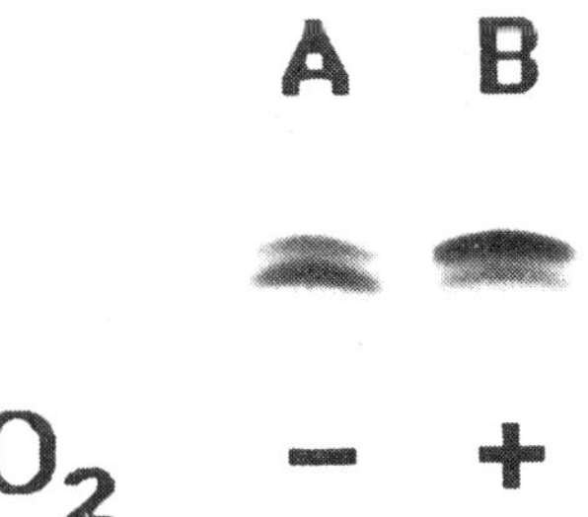

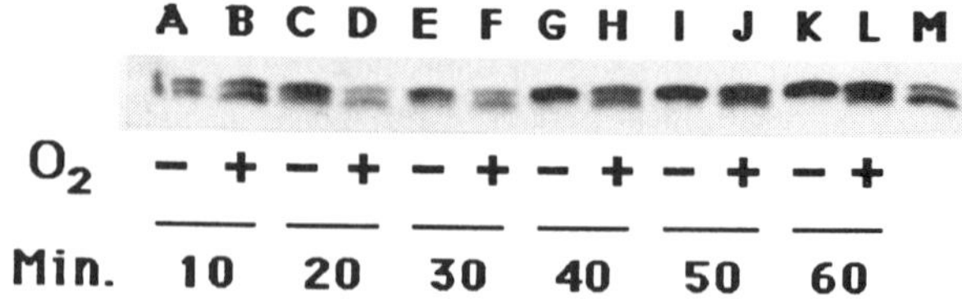

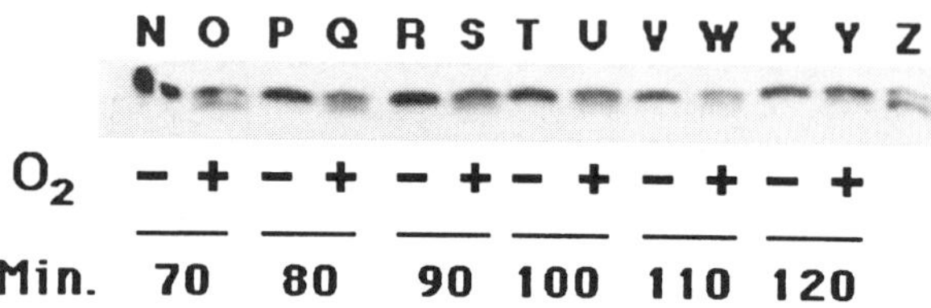

FIGURE 4. Extracts of anaerobic gonococci contain ~fourfold greater sialyltransferase activity than do extracts of aerobic gonococci. Triton X-100 extracts of anaerobic (–) and aerobic (+) plate-grown gonococci were prepared, mixed with CMP-NANA and purified gonococcal LOS, and incubated as described in *Methods.* Samples were removed at 10-minute intervals, and their LOS content was analyzed by 14% acrylamide SDS-PAGE and silver staining. Reprinted from Frangipane and Rest,[30] with permission.

(topoisomers) supercoiled to different degrees. Anaerobic conditions yielded more highly supercoiled DNA than did aerobic conditions, as indicated by the shifting of the band patterns in the different chloroquine concentrations (FIG. 5). These preliminary observations suggest a correlation between DNA supercoiling and induction of increased sialylation, both of which are induced by anaerobic conditions.

Effects of Growth in the Absence of Oxygen and the Presence of CMP-NANA on the Association of Gonococci with Human Neutrophils

Anaerobic and aerobic gonococci interact with human neutrophils in the same manner. Our next attempt at looking at the effects of anaerobiosis on gonococcal pathogenesis was to determine if human neutrophils bind or kill anaerobic gonococci differently than they do aerobic gonococci. Simply stated, aerobic and anaerobic gonococci bound to and were phagocytically killed by human neutrophils to the same extent.[32] What these "negative" results told us, however, was very important. They indicated that anaerobically grown gonococci do not express additional neutrophil adhesins, nor do they express components that inhibit the function of Opa proteins (or other, possibly cryptic adhesins).

Growth of gonococci in the presence of CMP-NANA decreases their ability to adhere to neutrophils. Neisseria gonorrhoeae strain F62 possessing an adherence-promoting Opa protein (Opa4) was grown in the presence of increasing concentrations of CMP-NANA (0 to 50 μg/ml) and mixed with neutrophils for 20 minutes, and

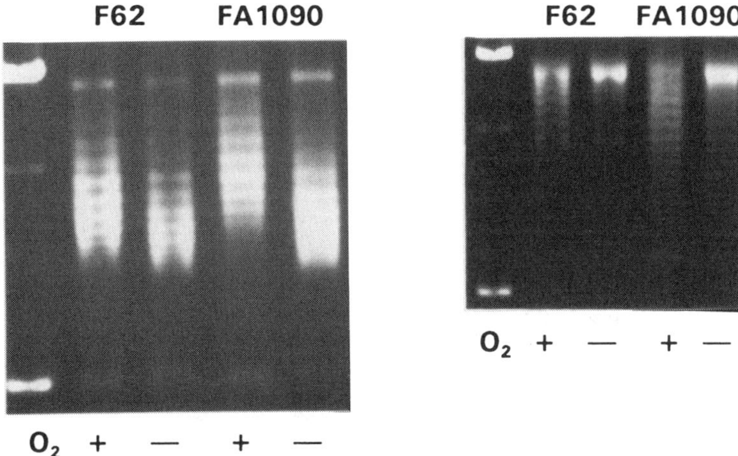

FIGURE 5. Anaerobic growth increases supercoiling of gonococcal DNA. The 4.2-kb cryptic plasmid of *N. gonorrhoeae* strains F62 and FA1090 was extracted from bacteria grown aerobically or anaerobically on plates. Both growth conditions yielded similar growth rates. The plasmid preparations were then electrophoresed through 1% agarose gels containing 2 (*left*) or 10 (*right*) μg/ml chloroquine. (The 1X TAE buffer also contained chloroquine.) After electrophoresis the gels were rinsed, soaked in ethidium bromide, rinsed again, and photographed above a UV light source.

Background. Bacterial DNA is usually negatively supercoiled. Chloroquine, which is uncharged, intercalates into DNA and causes it to positively coil. Thus, as more chloroquine is added to a negatively supercoiled plasmid, it becomes less negatively supercoiled (relaxed), then not supercoiled at all, then positively supercoiled. Regardless of whether it is positively or negatively supercoiled, more highly supercoiled DNA migrates faster than does less highly supercoiled DNA. Finally, plasmids are not as homogeneous as they appear on ethidium bromide-stained agarose gels. They are actually composed of families of distinct topological isomers, each of which has one or more "twists" than the other. In the presence of chloroquine, these topoisomers become visibly distinct.

Interpretation. In the presence of 2 μg/ml chloroquine, the plasmid topoisomers from anaerobic (–O₂) gonococci migrate faster than do the topoisomers from aerobic (+O₂) gonococci; thus, they are more negatively supercoiled. Upon the addition of a bit more chloroquine (10 μg/ml) the anaerobic topoisomers migrate as a thick band near the top of the photograph, having been almost completely relaxed; they have not yet become positively supercoiled by the chloroquine. The aerobic topoisomers, however, have bound enough chloroquine to have become slightly positively supercoiled. Thus, they now migrate faster than do the anaerobic topoisomers. As expected, upon the addition of 20 μg/ml chloroquine, the aerobic topoisomers migrate significantly faster than do the anaerobic topoisomers (data not shown), that is, just the opposite of what is observed in the photograph with 2 μg/ml chloroquine. Representative experiment of four. Both gonococcal strains yield similar results.

gonococcal adherence to neutrophils was quantitated. CMP-NANA caused a dose-dependent inhibition of gonococcal adherence to human neutrophils, up to about 86% of controls (FIG. 6). Sialidase treatment completely restored the ability of Opa⁺ gonococci grown in the presence of CMP-NANA to adhere to neutrophils.[31]

We isolated a naturally occurring stable LOS variant of strain F62, which possessed an LOS phenotype that lacked the faster migrating LOS band and which was

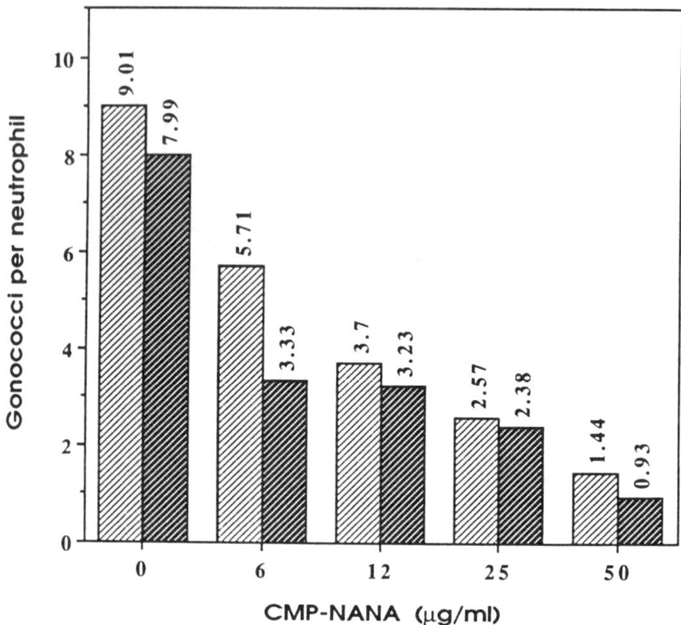

FIGURE 6. Growth of Opa4 gonococci in CMP-NANA inhibits their adherence to human neutrophils. Opa4 (strain F62) gonococci grown in broth with 0 to 50 μg/ml CMP-NANA were tumbled with neutrophils and their adherence was quantitated as described in *Methods*. The two different *bar shadings* represent two independent experiments, each done in duplicate. Reprinted from Rest and Frangipane,[31] with permission.

not sialylated when grown in the presence of up to 50 μg/ml CMP-NANA.[31] An Opa[+] variant of this stable LOS variant, which possessed the same apparent Opa as did the parent F62, adhered to neutrophils to the same degree whether grown in the presence or the absence of 50 μg/ml CMP-NANA (12.3 ± 1.7 and 11.8 ± 1.3 gonococci per neutrophil, respectively; $n = 3$). Thus, if LOS was not sialylated, Opa[+] gonococci remained able to adhere to neutrophils, even after being grown in the presence of CMP-NANA.

Growth of gonococci in CMP-NANA does not affect their phagocytic killing by human neutrophils. Gonococci possessing most Opa proteins not only adhere to human neutrophils, they are also phagocytically killed by them.[6] Thus, we studied whether sialylation of Opa[+] gonococci affected their ability to be phagocytically killed. We observed no differences in the ability of human neutrophils to kill Opa4 gonococci grown in the presence or absence of 50 μg/ml CMP-NANA (data not shown).[31] These results suggested that neutrophil endogenous sialidase or other glycosidases were slowly removing sialic acid from gonococcal LOS, allowing gonococci to adhere and be subsequently killed over the relatively long (135-minute) assay. Alternatively, sialylated LOS was being slowly turned over on the gonococcal surface, allowing nonsialylated LOS to dilute out the sialylated LOS. Thus, whereas growth in 50 µg/ml CMP-NANA is sufficient to sialylate gonococci and prevent their nonopsonic adherence to neutrophils in 20-minute assays, it appears that long-term (2-3 hours) incubation of gonococci with neutrophils *in vitro* results in the loss of sialylation. To address this question, we performed adherence assays for 90 minutes, instead of the standard 20 minutes, to see if sialylated gonococci would regain their ability to adhere to neutrophils over time. Indeed, gonococci grown in 50 µg/ml CMP-NANA gradually regained their ability to adhere to neutrophils over the 90-minute adherence assay (data not shown).[31]

Growth of gonococci in CMP-NANA does not affect their killing by human neutrophil lysosomal enzymes (granule extracts). Apicella and Mandrell and their colleagues[12,23] determined, by immunoelectron microscopic analyses of pus from patients with gonorrhea, that at least some gonococci within neutrophils are sialylated. In addition, Smith and collaborators[9] showed that at least a small percentage of gonococci within urethral pus neutrophils survive and perhaps multiply for extended periods of time. This raises the question if, similar to their resistance to killing by human serum, sialylated gonococci might be resistant to killing by the contents of human neutrophil phagolyosomes. In this vein, gonococci grown under different conditions, such as in broth to log-phase, in broth to stationary-phase, on plates, and in chicken eggs to log- or stationary-phase, are killed to different degrees by human neutrophil lysosomal enzymes, that is, granule extracts.[37] For instance, log-phase gonococci are more sensitive to granule extracts than are stationary-phase gonococci.

To determine if sialylation affected gonococcal sensitivity to granule extract, we exposed gonococci, grown to mid log-phase in broth with or without 50 µg/ml CMP-NANA, to increasing concentrations of granule extract. Assays were performed in Gonococcal Broth (Difco) for 30 minutes. No significant differences were observed in the sensitivity of gonococci to granule extract regardless of the presence or the absence of CMP-NANA in the growth medium (FIG. 7). If anything, gonococci grown in the presence of CMP-NANA are slightly more sensitive to granule extract. These same gonococci, grown in the presence of CMP-NANA, are completely resistant to serum killing. Thus, sialylated gonococci (at least strain F62) are just as sensitive to granule extract killing as are nonsialylated gonococci. We are presently investigating whether sialylated gonococci are more sensitive or less sensitive to oxygen-dependent killing systems.

DISCUSSION

We and others are continuing to study different aspects of gonococcal pathogenesis that may be affected by the *in vivo* microenvironment. To date, several potential virulence factors have been shown to be modulated by anaerobic conditions and by the presence of CMP-NANA in the growth medium. The results suggest that serum-sensitive gonococci can use available CMP-NANA more efficiently in anaerobic sites than in oxygen-replete sites and, in so doing, can significantly increase their resistance to NHS and decrease their association with neutrophils.

Gonococci grown in the presence of increasing concentrations of CMP-NANA (up to 50 µg/ml) adhere to neutrophils, in the absence of serum, significantly less than do Opa4 gonococci grown without CMP-NANA. All of the effects we observed

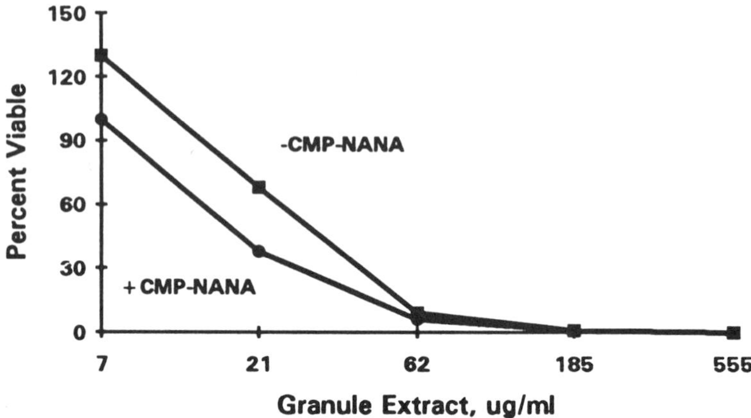

FIGURE 7. Human neutrophil granule extracts kill gonococci regardless of their sialylation. Gonococci of strain F62 were grown aerobically in broth with (+) or without (–) 50 μg/ml CMP-NANA, harvested, washed, and immediately exposed to increasing concentrations of granule extract for 30 minutes, as described in *Methods.* Viability was determined by plate counting. Representative experiment of three.

appear to be due to sialylation of LOS, because (1) SDS-PAGE LOS profiles (i.e., LOS phenotypes) were altered after growth in CMP-NANA, consistent with the addition of sialic acid, (2) sialidase treatment of CMP-NANA-grown gonococci reversed all effects, and (3) a stable LOS variant that was not sialylated when grown in the presence of up to 50 μg/ml of CMP-NANA adhered to the same degree as did gonococci grown without CMP-NANA.

It is interesting that a dichotomy exists in the effects of CMP-NANA on gonococcal interactions with host humoral and cellular defenses. On the one hand, Opa4 gonococci grown in the presence of 50 μg/ml CMP-NANA have a dramatically decreased association with neutrophils and are totally resistant to the bactericidal action of serum. On the other hand, CMP-NANA has minimal effects on the ability of Opa gonococci to be opsonized by the same serum towards which they are resistant.[31] Thus, whereas sialylated gonococci resist the bactericidal activity of normal human serum, they do have the capacity to be coated with opsonic complement.[38] The various mechanisms behind these observations remain to be investigated.

We observed a small decrease in serum sensitivity of anaerobic gonococci compared to aerobic gonococci grown in the absence of CMP-NANA. Whether this slight difference has biologic significance for gonococcal pathogenesis is unknown. Perhaps a slight decrease in serum sensitivity is advantageous to gonococci growing anaerobically in the urethra or cervix, where tissue damage and inflammation may introduce low concentrations of serum into the diseased area. It is possible that the presence of some anaerobically induced or altered outer membrane protein(s) could modify the antigenic structure of the outer membrane and cause this slight decrease in serum sensitivity.

Gonococci are sialylated within neutrophils in urethral pus from males with gonorrhea.[12,23] If we assume that these gonococci were sialylated before they were phagocytized, our observations indicate that such intracellular sialylated gonococci must have been opsonized before their ingestion; if they were not opsonized, they would then be unable to associate with neutrophils. These combined observations also suggest that the concentration of complement components in the urethra is by definition functional and sufficient for opsonization. On the other hand, some gonococci may not be sufficiently sialylated when they are outside neutrophils; thus, they would be phagocytized by neutrophils and may become sialylated once inside neutrophils. Our newest studies indicate that sialylated gonococci are killed to the same extent as are nonsialylated gonococci by granule extracts, that is, by the contents of human neutrophil phagolysosomes. Thus, the chances for survival of most intracellular gonococci apparently are slim. However, this conclusion is far from being soundly proven!

In our adherence studies, but not in the phagocytic killing studies, we used neutrophils stimulated with the chemotactic peptide fmlp. Farrell and Rest[33] showed that human peripheral blood neutrophils bind substantially more Opa⁺ gonococci after incubation with any of a number of potent neutrophil-stimulating agents, including the tripeptide fmlp, the calcium ionophore A23187, and the co-carcinogen phorbol myristate acetate (PMA).[33] We concluded from these observations that neutrophil Opa receptors (as yet incompletely identified) are located within the membranes of specific granules and are being brought to the cytoplasmic membrane surface upon activation of neutrophils.[39] Exudate neutrophils, such as neutrophils found in the urethra or cervix during gonorrhea, are naturally activated in that during diapedesis and chemotaxis, they are induced to degranulate (release) some or all of their specific granule contents. Therefore, the use of activated neutrophils in our adherence assays probably more accurately reflects gonococcus-neutrophil interactions occurring during gonorrhea, for example, within the urethra or cervix *in vivo,* than does the use of resting (unstimulated) neutrophils.

A very simple but important observation is that CMP-NANA effects are dose dependent. Thus, sialylation of gonococcal LOS is not an all-or-nothing phenomenon, *in vitro* or *in vivo*; it follows that the biologic responses of sialylated gonococci are also graded. We assume that the 5 μg/ml CMP-NANA that we used to confer maximal sialylation of anaerobic gonococci and to maximally inhibit biologic functions (and the 50 μg/ml CMP-NANA we used for aerobic gonococci) is substantially higher than the amounts of CMP-NANA actually found in gonorrhea pus; this is not known. What may be occurring in the microenvironment of the urethra or cervix during acute gonorrhea is a competition between the number of gonococci, gonococcal growth rate, limited availability of CMP-NANA, release of sialidase-like enzymes by neutrophils, limited availability of oxygen, and other conditions as yet unstudied. All of these things to one degree or another have an effect on the ability of gonococci to be sialylated by CMP-NANA and to be killed by serum components and neutrophils. The dynamics of sialylation and desialylation of gonococci *in vivo* is terribly complex and remains to be determined.

How could sialylation of LOS affect the function of Opa proteins so dramatically? The sialic acid could be causing a change in overall charge in the microenvironment of individual Opa proteins, causing the affinity of Opa proteins for their receptor(s) to be decreased, or, perhaps the change in charge caused by the addition of sialic acid causes a conformational change in the surface-exposed portions of Opa proteins, thus decreasing or abrogating their ability to bind their receptor(s). It is also possible that the fully sialylated LOS acts as a type of capsule or negatively charged halo surrounding the gonococcus, preventing its close association with the negatively charged neutrophil surface. Perhaps sialylation of LOS alters LOS structure, which in turn interacts with Opa proteins in such a way as to decrease their affinity for receptor(s). It remains possible that gonococcal outer membrane components other than LOS are being affected by growth in CMP-NANA, but they have not yet been detected. None of these possibilities is mutually exclusive. Regardless of which mechanism is actually functioning *in vivo,* our idea of how Opa proteins function as virulence factors in gonorrhea must be reassessed.

SUMMARY

N. gonorrhoeae initiates infection by adhering to and invading columnar epithelial cells. Over time these activities often induce inflammation, with the influx of neutrophils and serum into the urethral lumen, cervical os, conjunctiva, and the like. At least some of these infected niches contain CMP-NANA (cytidine monophospho-*N*-acetyl neuraminic acid, also called CMP-sialic), contain sialylated gonococci, and are relatively or strictly anaerobic due to neutrophil and gonococcal metabolism and to the site of disease, that is, the peritoneal cavity. Gonococci thus encounter environmental conditions, reagents, and substrates in the human body that are not normally present *in vitro.* Knapp and Clark[24] were the first to successfully grow gonococci anaerobically in an easily reproducible system, allowing researchers to begin to investigate *in vitro* the effects of anaerobiosis on gonococcal virulence traits. As a result of a series of elegant and in depth studies, Smith and Parsons and their colleagues showed that growth in CMP-NANA confers on the gonococcus a high degree of phenotypic (readily reversible) serum resistance and that CMP-NANA is available *in vivo* at sites of gonococcal infection and disease; gonococci become covalently coated with sialic acid and they become serum resistant (reviewed in refs. 8–10). Given that gonococci growing in the absence of oxygen or in the presence of CMP-NANA probably more closely resemble gonococci growing inside the human host, we studied several possible virulence traits of gonococci cultivated under these conditions.

We first observed that anaerobic growth (in the absence of CMP-NANA) increases gonococcal resistance to killing by low (but not high) concentrations of normal human serum. We also asked whether anaerobic growth affected gonococcal association with host cells. Contrary to the effects on serum killing, anaerobic growth (in the absence of CMP-NANA) does not appear to affect the ability of gonococci (expressing certain adhesive outer membrane proteins called Opa proteins) to bind to and enter human epithelial cell lines or to bind to or resist killing by human neutrophils. The results from studies investigating the modulatory role of CMP-NANA were more striking. Growth in CMP-NANA dramatically inhibits the adherence of Opa⁺ gonococci to human neutrophils. It does not, however, appear to significantly decrease their sensitivity to phagocytic killing or to *in vitro* killing by lysosomal contents (aqueous extracts of human neutrophil granules). Perhaps most impressive of all were results obtained when these two *in vivo* conditions, namely, anaerobiosis and CMP-

NANA, were combined; we found that anaerobic growth acts synergistically with low concentrations of CMP-NANA to cause high level serum resistance. Thus, gonococci have evolved multiple mechanisms to take advantage of a complex *in vivo* milieu to increase their resistance to several host defenses.

We delved a little more deeply into the anaerobiosis–CMP-NANA axis. Gonococci can express several different lipooligosaccharide (LOS) molecules simultaneously. We observed that compared to aerobic gonococci, anaerobic gonococci express more of the LOS molecule that acts as the acceptor for sialic acid from CMP-sialic acid. Similarly, triton X-100 extracts of anaerobic gonococci contain about four times more sialyltransferase (STase) activity (the enzyme that transfers sialic acid to gonococcal LOS from CMP-sialic acid) than do extracts of aerobic gonococci. One way that anaerobiosis may modulate bacterial gene activity is by affecting DNA supercoiling. We have begun to investigate this in the gonococcus and have observed that the major, 4.1-kbp cryptic plasmid isolated from anaerobic gonococci is more negatively supercoiled than is the same plasmid isolated from aerobic gonococci. Thus, we are getting our first clues as to the molecular mechanisms by which gonococci may modulate some of their virulence determinants *in vivo.* These data indicate that anaerobic conditions or the presence of CMP-NANA, that is, conditions encountered by gonococci *in vivo,* may lead to altered LOS biosynthesis and to increased STase activity in the gonococcus and that these changes modulate gonococcal resistance to killing by normal human serum and human neutrophils.

ACKNOWLEDGMENTS

We thank Timothy Mietzner and Brendon Wahlberg, the University of Pittsburgh School of Medicine, for discussing with us methods for determining the degree of gonococcal DNA supercoiling.

REFERENCES

1. BRITIGAN, B. E., M. S. COHEN & P. F. SPARLING. 1985. N. Engl. J. Med. **312:** 1683–1694.
2. CASEY, S. G., D. R. VEALE & H. SMITH. 1979. J. Gen. Microbiol. **113:** 395–398.
3. CASEY, S. G., D. R. VEALE & H. SMITH. 1980. FEMS Microbiol. Lett. **8:** 97–100.
4. PARSONS, N. J., A. A. KWAASI, P. V. PATEL, C. A. NAIRN & H. SMITH. 1986. J. Gen. Microbiol. **132:** 3277–3287.
5. FISCHER, S. H. & R. F. REST. 1988. Infect. Immun. **56:** 1574–1579.
6. SHAFER, W. M. & R. F. REST. 1989. Ann. Rev. Microbiol. **43:** 121–145.
7. VIRJI, M. & J. E. HECKELS. 1986. J. Gen. Microbiol. **132:** 503–512.
8. SMITH, H. 1990. J. Gen. Microbiol. **136:** 377–393.
9. SMITH, H. 1991. Proc. Roy. Soc. London, B: Biol. Sci. **246:** 97–105.
10. SMITH, H., J. A. COLE & N. J. PARSONS. 1992. FEMS Microbiol. Lett. **79:** 287–292.
11. WARD, M. E., P. J. WATT & A. A. GLYNN. 1970. Nature (Lond.) **227:** 382–384.
12. MANDRELL, R. E., A. J. LESSE, J. V. SUGAI, M. SHERO, J. McL. GRIFFISS, J. A. COLE, N. J. PARSONS, H. SMITH, S. A. MORSE & M. A. APICELLA. 1990. J. Exp. Med. **171:** 1649–1664.
13. KING, G. & J. SWANSON. 1978. Infect. Immun. **21:** 575–584.

14. LAMBDEN, P. R., J. E. HECKELS, L. T. JAMES & P. J. WATT. 1979. J. Gen. Microbiol. **114:** 305–312.
15. REST, R. F., S. H. FISCHER, Z. Z. INGHAM & J. F. JONES. 1982. Infect. Immun. **36:** 737–744.
16. SWANSON, J. 1982. Infect. Immun. **37:** 359–368.
17. WATT, P. J. & M. E. WARD. 1980. Adherence of *Neisseria gonorrhoeae* and other *Neisseria* species to mammalian cells. *In* Bacterial Adherence. E. H. Beachey, ed.: 253–288. Chapman and Hall. New York.
18. CONNELL, T. D., D. SHAFFER & J. G. CANNON. 1990. Molec. Microbiol. **4:** 439–449.
19. STERN, A., M. BROWN, P. NICKEL & T. F. MEYER. 1986. Cell **47:** 61–71.
20. BARRITT, D. S., R. S. SCHWALBE, D. G. KLAPPER & J. G. CANNON. 1987. Infect. Immun. **55:** 2026–2031.
21. CONNELL, T. D., W. L. BLACK, T. H. KAWULA, D. S. BARRITT, J. F. DEMPSEY, K. KNERNELAND, JR., A. STEPHENSON, S. S. SCHEPART, B. L. MURPHY & J. G. CANNON. 1988. Molec. Microbiol. **2:** 227–236.
22. GIBBS, C., R. HAAS & T. F. MEYER. 1988. Microb. Pathog. **4:** 393–399.
23. APICELLA, M. A., R. E. MANDRELL, M. SHERO, M. E. WILSON, J. McL. GRIFFISS, G. F. BROOKS, C. LAMMEL, J. F. BREEN & P. A. RICE. 1990. J. Infect. Dis. **162:** 506–512.
24. KNAPP, J. S. & V. L. CLARK. 1984. Infect. Immun. **46:** 176–181.
25. CLARK, V. L., L. A. CAMPBELL, D. A. PALERMO, T. M. EVANS & K. W. KLIMPEL. 1987. Infect. Immun. **55:** 1359–1364.
26. CLARK, V. L., J. S. KNAPP, S. THOMPSON & K. W. KLIMPEL. 1988. Microb. Pathog. **5:** 381–390.
27. KEEVIL, C. W., N. C. MAJOR, D. B. DAVIES & A. ROBINSON. 1986. J. Gen. Microbiol. **132:** 3289–3302.
28. ELKINS, C. & R. F. REST. 1990. Infect. Immun. **58:** 1078–1084.
29. ROCK, J. P. & R. F. REST. 1988. J. Gen. Microbiol. **134:** 509–519.
30. FRANGIPANE, J. V. & R. F. REST. 1993. Infect. Immun. **61:** 1657–1666.
31. REST, R. F. & J. V. FRANGIPANE. 1992. Infect. Immun. **60:** 989–997.
32. FRANGIPANE, J. V. & R. F. REST. 1992. Infect. Immun. **60:** 1793–1799.
33. FARRELL, C. F. & R. F. REST. 1990. Infect. Immun. **58:** 2777–2784.
34. HITCHCOCK, P. J. 1984. Infect. Immun. **46:** 202–212.
35. DARVEAU, R. P. & R. E. W. HANCOCK. 1983. J. Bacteriol. **155:** 831–838.
36. LESSE, A. J., A. A. CAMPAGNARI, W. E. BITTNER & M. A. APICELLA. 1990. J. Immunol. Methods **126:** 109–117.
37. REST, R. F. 1970. Infect. Immun. **25:** 574–579.
38. KIM, J. J., D. ZHOU, R. E. MANDRELL & J. M. GRIFFISS. 1992. Infect. Immun. **60:** 4439–4442.
39. FARRELL, C. F., F. L. NAIDS & R. F. REST. 1991. Identification of a human neutrophil receptor for gonococcal outer membrane protein PII. M. *In Neisseriae* 1990. Achtman *et al.,* eds.: 580–584. Walter de Gruyter. Berlin.

Molecular and Cellular Mechanisms of Tissue Invasion by *Shigella flexneri*[a]

ARTURO ZYCHLINSKY,[b] JUANA J. PERDOMO,[c] AND
PHILIPPE J. SANSONETTI[b,d]

[b]*Unité de Pathogénie Microbienne Moléculaire*
INSERM U199 and
[c]*Station Centrale de Microscopie Electronique*
Institut Pasteur
28 rue du Dr. Roux
75724 Paris, Cedex 15, France

Diarrhea is one of the main problems of public health in the world. An estimated 5 million children aged less than 5 years die annually worldwide of diarrheal diseases.[1] Shigellae are one of the most important etiologic agents of these diseases,[2] causing a severe form of bloody diarrhea called dysentery. In developing countries, *Shigella flexneri* is most prevalent, but *Shigella sonnei* and *Shigella boydii* are sometimes isolated. *Shigella dysenteriae* is not very common but can cause devastating epidemics.[3,4]

Shigella is a very virulent microorganism. In clinical trials an inoculum of 10 to 100 virulent bacteria is sufficient to cause dysentery. The syndrome caused by shigellae consists of painful abdominal cramps, nausea, fever, tenesmus, and frequently blood[3] and mucus in the stools. These symptoms reflect the invasion of the colonic submucosa by shigella. Histopathologic analysis of the colon of patients with shigellosis reveals destruction of the epithelium, mucosal erosion, and the typical signs of inflammation including infiltration and exudation of polymorphonuclear (PMN) cells, edema, and cellular infiltration into the lamina propria.[5–7]

A crucial property in the pathogenesis of bacillary dysentery is the microorganism's capacity to invade eukaryotic cells. After phagocytosis, shigella is capable of breaking the phagocytic vacuole and escaping into the cytoplasm of the cell. Electron microscopic analysis and subcellular localization using specific drugs indicate that a few minutes after the bacterium is phagocytized by the cell it destroys the membrane of the vacuole that contains it and is liberated into the cytoplasm of the host cell.[3,8]

S. flexneri invasiveness and pathogenesis are encoded in a 220-kb plasmid. Strains that have been cured of this plasmid are completely nonpathogenic. The molecular biology of shigella's pathogenicity has recently been analyzed in great detail. Through cosmid vector cloning analysis the invasion capability of *S. flexneri* has been localized

[a] A.Z. was supported by an EMBO fellowship.
[d] To whom correspondence should be addressed.

to 31 kb in the pathogenicity plasmid.[9] This 31-kb region codes for many closely linked genes, including the invasion plasmid antigen (*ipa*), membrane expression of invasion plasmid antigens (*mxi*), and surface presentation of invasion plasmid antigen (*spa*) genes as well as other, independently expressed genes. The *ipa* genes encode the IpaA, IpaB, IpaC, and IpaD polypeptides which are the dominant antigens in the humoral response to shigellosis. Transposon insertion and deletion mutagenesis has demonstrated that *ipaB, ipaC,* and *ipaD* genes, which belong to the same transcriptional unit, are essential for vacuolar escape and the ability to provoke keratoconjunctivitis in experimental animals.[10–12] Both the *mxi* and *spa* genes code for the secretion apparatus to release other plasmid proteins.[13–15] The plasmid also codes for *icsA,* a gene essential for intracellular and intercellular movement.[16]

Detailed knowledge of the molecular components of shigella pathogenicity permits the study of the bacterial-host interaction at the cellular and organismal level. One astounding feature of shigella infections is that, although very few bacteria can cause dysentery in humans, this microorganism is completely nonpathogenic for experimental animals[3,4] except certain primates. Paradoxically, *in vitro, S. flexneri* can efficiently invade all vertebrate cells tested so far. Thus, shigella pathogenicity has to be analyzed using cell culture of both explanted cells and established cell lines as well as *in vivo* models such as the rabbit ligated ileal loop assay and the Serény test.[4,17] Rabbits are not sensitive to shigellae, but injection of the bacterial pathogen into the lumen of ligated ileal loops closely mimics the pathophysiology observed in experimental human and monkey infections. The Serény test is based on the capability of pathogenic shigellae to induce a purulent keratoconjunctivitis in guinea pigs when inoculated directly into the conjunctiva. Here we propose a new model for the invasion by *S. flexneri* of the colonic submucosa and the initiation of inflammation based on recent findings from *in vitro* models.

BACTERIAL PASSAGE FROM THE LUMEN TO THE COLONIC SUBMUCOSA

Mounier *et al.*[18] showed that *S. flexneri* is only capable of invading epithelial cells through the basolateral membrane. This study investigated the invasion by shigella of the human colonic epithelial cell line Caco-2. This cell line is able to establish a confluent epithelial monolayer where cells are differentiated and polarized with an apical brush border. Therefore, the apical face of a Caco-2 monolayer resembles the epithelial surface that a bacterium encounters when it reaches the intestine. When Caco-2 cells are infected with *S. flexneri,* only a few bacteria interact with the apical surface of cells, and they are incapable of invading them. When the epithelial monolayer is treated with agents that disrupt the intercellular junctions, the cells are efficiently infected. These data suggest that *S. flexneri* cannot directly infect epithelial cells in intact epithelia and that during a natural infection the bacteria reach both the submucosa and the epithelium through a different port of entry. These results correlate with observations at the electron microscopic level of infected rabbit ileal loop assays. When epithelia were observed shortly after infection, no bacteria were detectable inside the epithelial cells (Perdomo and Sansonetti, unpublished observation). Shigellae appear to be unique in their selectivity for the basolateral membrane.

Other enteric pathogens, such as salmonellae, can invade cells through both the apical and the basolateral membranes.[19]

M cells are specialized cells that develop only in the epithelia over lymphoid tissue associated with the mucosa.[20] These cells nonselectively transport intact antigens from the lumen into the lymphoid tissue and deliver them in the appropriate microenvironment to ensure a mucosal immune response. M cells are differentiated from other enterocytes by their characteristic morphology, the specific binding capacity of their apical membrane, and their lack of some digestive enzymes. Several enteric pathogens, including reovirus, poliovirus, retroviruses as well as the bacterial pathogens salmonellae and yersiniae, use M cells as a transepithelial pathway. M cells also transport shigella into the lymphoid tissue.[21] Recent observations both in the rabbit ligated ileal loop model as well as in biopsies of experimentally infected monkeys indicate that the pioneer entry of *S. flexneri* into the submucosa is via M cells[21] (Perdomo *et al.*, manuscript in preparation).

The absence of epithelial cell infection, together with the observation of shigellae in M cells at early points after infection, strongly suggests that *S. flexneri* reaches the submucosa of the colon via the M cell. After M-cell transcytosis the microorganism is delivered into follicular structures. There, shigella encounters both the cells that will present the bacterial antigens to generate a mucosal immune response[20,22,23] and the first line of natural immune defense, namely, the resident tissue macrophages.[24,25] These cells are equipped with a vast antimicrobial arsenal. Most microorganisms that come in contact with this cell are killed. Pathogenic bacteria have evolved different mechanisms to survive the hostile environment of microphages. Some species, such as *Legionella pneumophila* and *Mycobacterium tuberculosis,* inhibit the fusion of lysosomes to the phagocytic vacuole. Other microorganisms, such as *Coxiella burnetii,* are not damaged by the phagolysosome environment.[19] As yet another alternative strategy, shigella avoids being killed by the macrophage by triggering the macrophage's suicide program.[26]

S. flexneri INDUCES MACROPHAGE APOPTOSIS

Necrosis and apoptosis are the two forms of cell death characterized so far. Necrosis is a passive process, which occurs when a cell dies because of physical alteration, as, for example, in complement-mediated killing. In contrast, apoptosis, or programmed cell death, calls for active participation of the cell in its own death, implying induction of a genetic program in reaction to a specific stimulus. Apoptotic cell death has classically been described during normal embryonic development and differentiation, in tumor regression, and during growth factor deprivation.[27,28]

The first enterobacterial species that was shown to induce apoptosis is *S. flexneri.* We reported recently that the mechanism of cytotoxicity by which *S. flexneri* kills macrophages[29] is induction of programmed cell death.[26] This was determined by the two main characteristics of apoptosis: fragmentation of the cell's DNA to multimers of about 200 bp which correspond to the size of a nucleosome, and the distinctive ultrastructural morphology in which the cytoplasm is heavily vacuolized and the chromatin is intensely condensed.

Apoptosis is induced when either a membrane or a cytoplasmic receptor binds the appropriate ligand which provokes the generation of second messengers.[27,28] Both an increase in the concentration of intracellular calcium[30,31] and cAMP[32,33] have been implicated. Eventually the genes necessary for cell death are expressed and the cell dies. Very few eukaryotic genes are known to be involved in apoptosis. On the one hand, expression of the tumor suppressor gene *p53* is apparently sufficient to commit a cell to undergo apoptosis. Also, expression of the oncogenes *c-myc* and *c-fos* is required, but probably insufficient to induce apoptosis. On the other hand, the onco-gene *bcl-2* can block the process of programmed cell death.[34]

Shigella can only cause damage if it escapes from the phagolysosome into the cytoplasm of the cell. Thus, it is likely that *S. flexneri* does not induce apoptosis by binding to a receptor. There are at least three possible pathways for this bacterium to induced macrophage apoptosis: (1) generating second messengers that signal the cell to activate an apoptotic program, (2) secreting bacterial factors that are directly cytotoxic to the cells, and (3) destroying a host factor that constantly inhibits a constitutive program for apoptosis.[35] Further investigations will hopefully lead us to understand the molecular details of shigella's relationship to the macrophage.

During an infectious process, in addition to their microbicidal activity, macro-phages have a crucial role in signaling to other cells the presence of an invasive agent and the generation of inflammation.[36] As response to a variety of stimuli, macrophages can express three of the most important inflammatory cytokines: in-terleukin-1 (IL-1), IL-6, and tumor necrosis factor (TNFα). IL-6 and TNFα are transcribed, translated, and secreted as soon as the cell is stimulated, while IL-1 is accumulated in the cytosol. The two forms of IL-1 are IL-1α and IL-1β. These two forms bind to the same receptors and have undistinguishable biologic activity. Both forms of IL-1 are synthesized in a precursor form as polypeptides of 35 kD which are proteolytically cleaved by specific proteases to the mature form of 17.5 kD. Both the precursor and the mature form of IL-1α, but only the mature form of IL-1β, are biologically active. The immature polypeptides of IL-1 are synthesized and accumulated in the cytosol of macrophages. The mature, proteolytically treated form is found exclusively in tissue culture supernatants. Neither form of IL-1 has a secretion signal sequence and is released via a classic secretory pathway.[36] One of the possible mechanisms for this cytokine release is as a consequence of apoptosis.[37]

To determine if macrophage apoptosis plays a role in the initiation of inflammation we studied the release of inflammatory cytokines by infected macrophages *in vitro*. As a model system we tested cytokine release of lipopolysaccharide (LPS)-stimulated murine peritoneal macrophages infected with *S. flexneri*. These cells contain pools of IL-1 and probably reflect the activation state of colonic macrophages.[24,25,38–40] We showed that large amounts of IL-1, but not IL-6 or TNFα, are released by stimulated peritoneal macrophages infected with wild-type *S. flexneri,* but not with a noninvasive derivative. Time course experiments of cytokine release demonstrated that IL-1 is present in the supernatant of infected cells as early as 15 minutes after infection. IL-1 release, assayed either by its biologic activity or antigenically in an ELISA assay, happens before macrophage integrity is compromised. The supernatants of LPS-stimulated macrophages infected with shigella contain IL-1α only in its precursor form, which is biologically active. IL-1β is present in both its precursor and its mature forms. Taken together, these results strongly suggest that IL-1 is released early in apoptosis and that release is an active process and not the result of leakage of intracellular stores of cytokine when the integrity of the plasma membrane is compromised.[41]

Bacteria induced apoptosis of macrophages might play an active role *in vivo* by eliciting an early inflammatory response in epithelial tissues. Release of IL-1 would be the first signal to initiate the inflammatory process. This signal is likely amplified by the induction of the production of other inflammatory cytokines like IL-1, IL-6, IL-8, and TNFα by other cells such as noninfected macrophages, endothelial and epithelial cells.[42,43]

Interestingly, shigella appears to induce apoptosis exclusively in macrophages. Epithelioid and fibroblastoid cells infected *in vitro* with *S. flexneri* can support significant intracellular bacterial growth while appearing healthy (Zychlinsky and Sansonetti, unpublished observation). These cells eventually die by necrosis, presumably through nonspecific mechanisms due to the heavy bacterial load in their cytoplasm. Furthermore, infection of HeLa cells with shigella does not lead to host cell DNA fragmentation (Zychlinsky and Sansonetti, unpublished observation). Preliminary experiments in our lab show that explanted human PMN are not susceptible to *S. flexneri* cytotoxicity and show no morphologic signs of apoptosis (Zychlinsky, Perdomo, and Sansonetti, unpublished observation). However, the very short life span of explanted PMN makes definitive experiments of induction of DNA fragmentation difficult to perform.

PMN CELLS TRANSMIGRATE INTO THE LUMEN OF THE COLON AND FACILITATE *S. flexneri* INVASION

An important characteristic of shigellosis is that in later stages of the infection, a very extensive inflammatory reaction and tissue destruction is found far beyond Peyer's patches in the rabbit ligated ileal loop model and lymphoid solitary nodules in biopsies of humans and monkeys.[4,44] In these late stages bacteria are also found in epithelial cells. These data suggest that other secondary sites of bacterial entry exist besides the M cell.

It is therefore tempting to hypothesize that the early inflammatory reaction induced by the release of IL-1 by apoptotic macrophages provokes edema and the extravasation of PMN cells. Polymorphonuclear cells[36] have a strong chemotactic activity towards gram-negative bacteria and migrate to the lumen of the colon. The transmigration of PMN cells would destroy the epithelial cell barrier, providing secondary invasion sites for shigella and allowing the bacteria access to the basolateral membrane of colonocytes. Novel *in vitro* data strongly support this model.[45] Perdomo *et al.*[45] showed that PMN cells migrate through the epithelium in response to the presence of shigella in the apical side of colonocytes. This migration disrupts intercellular junctions and opens a paracellular pathway for bacteria to reach the basolateral side of epithelial cells.

The migration of PMN cells was tested using the T-84 cell line. This cell line derives from a lung cancer metastasis of a human colonic carcinoma, and if it is grown on permeable supports, the cells are polarized, present numerous microvilli on their apical side, and develop tight junctions.[46] The structure of the T-84 epithelium is reminiscent of that of intestinal crypt cells, and this system has been used to study chemotactic substances that induce the transmigration of neutrophils across epithelia.[47] When T-84 cells were allowed to differentiate and form intercellular junctions for either 3 or 8 days, 3-day cells formed looser junctions than did 8-day cells. The different maturation time mimics the degree of differentiation of cells of the colonic crypt and the upper part of the Lieberkühn gland, respectively. When PMN cells were placed in the basolateral side of the epithelium and bacteria on the apical side, both the wild-type strain of *S. flexneri* and a plasmid-cured, nonpathogenic derivative provoked the transmigration of neutrophils across a 3-day-old T-84 monolayer. However, only the wild-type strains efficiently invaded the epithelial cells. The 8-day-old cells did not allow significant PMN cell transmigration or epithelial cell infection. In control experiments in which only bacteria were added to the apical side without PMN cells in the system, no significant invasion of T-84 cells occurred. Taken together these results clearly indicate that *S. flexneri,* like other enterobacteria, can induce transmigration of PMN cells and that destruction of the epithelial barrier provides bacteria with access to the basolateral membrane of 3-day-old cells. Release of oxygen radicals as well as proteolytic enzymes, such as elastase, metalloproteases, and serine proteases, by PMN cells could destroy the epithelium through a "bystander" effect, providing even greater access for bacteria to infect the basolateral membrane of epithelial cells.[48]

Transmigration requires the adhesion of PMN cells to epithelial cells. The interaction between these two cells is specific and is mediated by the integrins CD11a/CD18 (LFA I) and CD11b/CD18 (Mac 1).[49] Monoclonal antibodies against CD18 can neutralize PMN cell transmigration. The importance of PMN in the invasion of shigella has been confirmed in experiments in the rabbit ligated ileal loop assay. In recent experiments (Perdomo *et al.,* manuscript in preparation), rabbits were preloaded with monoclonal antibodies against CD18 before ligating the ileal loops and infecting them with wild-type shigella. Under these conditions there was very strong inhibition of inflammation and almost no bacterial invasion. These results confirm that bacterial passage through the epithelial barrier depends on transmigration of PMN cells and consequent destruction of epithelial cell junctions. Thus, bacterial entry through M cells, infection and induction of apoptosis on resident tissue macrophages, and consequent release of IL-1 would permit the extravasation of PMN cells. These cells are able to transmigrate into the lumen of the colon and, in turn, allow passage of more bacteria into the submucosa and the basolateral epithelial membrane.

INTRACELLULAR MOVEMENT AND SHIGELLOSIS

Shigellae do not have flagella and therefore are immobile bacteria. *S. flexneri* manipulates the host-cell cytoskeleton to move around the cytoplasm and from cell to cell.[50] In *in vitro* infected cells, short filaments of actin bundle up towards one pole of each intracellular bacterium. The actin filaments form a tail that can be several micrometers long and contain actin-binding proteins. This actin tail forms on one pole of the bacterium and makes it move.[50]

The intracellular cell spread *icsA* (*virG*) locus responsible for *S. flexneri* intracellular movement was identified through transposon mutagenesis analysis and is localized to the pathogenicity plasmid.[16] *icsA* mutants are invasive, but once in the cytoplasm

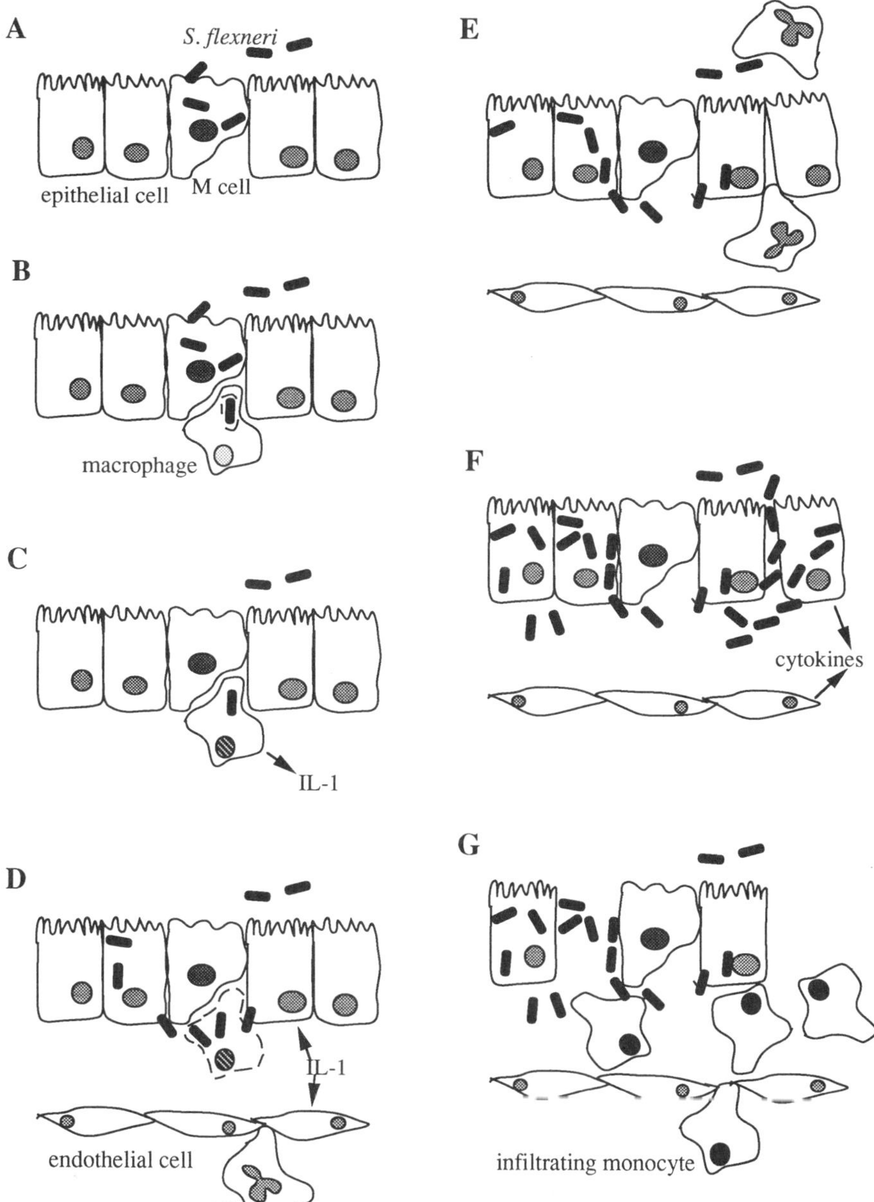

FIGURE 1. Model for initiation of shigellosis in the colon. (**A**). Transcytosis of *S. flexneri* through M cells from the lumen into the submucosa of the colon. (**B**) Infection of resident tissue macrophages and onset of apoptosis. (**C**) Release of IL-1. (**D**) Dissemination of *S. flexneri* through the epithelium and lamina propria and initiation of inflammation. (**E**) Extravasation of polymorphonuclear cells and rupture of epithelial barrier. (**F**) Massive bacterial entry through the intercellular space and production of cytokines by epithelial and endothelial cells. (**G**) Destruction of epithelial layer, entry of monocytes, and frank inflammation.

they do not move, do not form an actin tail, and are incapable of spreading to adjacent cells.[16] These mutants, however, are capable of inducing apoptosis in macrophages (Zychlinsky and Sansonetti, unpublished observation). IcsA is a surface protein with ATPase activity and it is localized to only one pole of the bacterium.[51] This protein can be phosphorylated by a cAMP-dependent protein kinase and the host cell apparently can control bacterial movement by phosphorylating or dephosphorylating IcsA.[52]

The pathogenicity of an *icsA* mutant was tested on macaque monkeys and evaluated by both endoscopy and histopathology.[44] By contrast, in monkeys infected with the wild-type parental strain, the *icsA* mutants caused only transient emission of slightly dysenteric stools and mild clinical symptoms. This mutant caused a few scattered abscesses with nodular morphology or limited bloody ulcerations. In biopsies, these infectious foci showed superficial alterations of the mucosa over lymphoid nodules, or with ulcerations there was destruction of the mucosal surface, again over lymphoid nodules, that became exposed to the colonic lumen.

The mild symptoms seen in monkeys infected with the *icsA* mutant indicate that intracellular movement as well as cell-to-cell spread play a crucial role in the development of full-fledged shigellosis. The fact that the few abscesses caused by this mutant localized to lymphoid nodules indicates again that shigella penetrates the submucosa via M cells. *In vitro,* the *icsA* mutant induces apoptosis; therefore, it is likely that IL-1 is released, but this has to be tested *in vivo.* Taken together, these data suggest that even if *S. flexneri* reaches the submucosa and is capable of initiating an inflammatory response, intracellular movement is essential to generate the massive bacterial infection that results in serious inflammation and culminates in dysentery.

The importance of intercellular spread in shigellosis is also exemplified by the function of another pathogenicity-plasmid gene, *icsB.*[53] This gene is essential for allowing passage from one epithelial infected cell to the cytoplasm of the next cell, but it is not necessary for macrophage cytotoxicity (Zychlinsky and Sansonetti, unpublished observation). A mutant in *icsB* does not provoke keratoconjunctivitis in guinea pigs, suggesting that cell-to-cell spread by itself is essential for pathogenicity. Future studies in infected animals will determine if, as foreseen, *icsA* and *icsB* mutants cause a similar infection in monkeys.

CONCLUDING REMARKS

The absence of a manageable animal model for *S. flexneri* infections makes the direct study of the pathophysiology of shigellosis difficult. Combining information from many diverse sources such as infection of tissue cultured cells, organotypic animal models, and histopathology from experimentally infected monkeys and patients, we propose a model for the initiation of shigellosis. FIGURE 1 shows the proposed sequence of events. First, *S. flexneri* makes contact with M cells in the colon and is transcytosed from the lumen into the submucosa (FIG. 1A). M cells deliver bacteria directly into lymphoid nodules. These nodules are densely populated by resident tissue macrophages which are infected by shigella (FIG. 1B). Infection by *S. flexneri* induces macrophage apoptosis with the concomitant release of IL-1 (FIG. 1C). Shigella starts disseminating through the epithelium and the lamina propria. The IL-1 liberated by macrophages starts an inflammatory response. There is extravasation of PMN cells from the circulation into the submucosa (FIG. 1D). Polymorphonuclear cells are chemoattracted into the lumen of the colon, and transmigration disrupts the integrity of the epithelial barrier (FIG. 1E). *S. flexneri* massively infects epithelial cells through the basolateral membrane. Bacterial products induce the production of more cytokines which potentiates the inflammation (FIG. 1F). In the final stage very serious inflammation occurs with destruction of the epithelium and entry of monocytes into the tissue. This model may provide guidelines for future research and vaccine development.

SUMMARY

Shigella flexneri, a member of the family of enterobacteriaceae, causes bacillary dysentery by invading the human colonic mucosa and provoking a very intense inflammation. Recent *in vitro* data allow us to integrate different phenomena into a model of the infectious process during shigellosis. *In vivo,* bacteria appear to enter the submucosa via the M cells, specialized cells that cover the follicular structures of the intestinal mucosa. Once inside the submucosa, shigellae encounter resident tissue macrophages, which are infected, and apoptosis is rapidly induced. During programmed cell death the inflammatory cytokine interleukin-1 (IL 1) is released. Interleukin-1 triggers an inflammatory reaction characterized by extravasation of polymorphonuclear (PMN) cells. The inflammation is probably potentiated by the production of other cytokines by epithelial, endothelial, and PMN cells. Polymorphonuclear cells migrate through the epithelium into the lumen of the colon, destabilizing the integrity of the epithelial barrier. The damaged epithelium allows massive entry of bacteria into the submucosa. Further colonization of the epithelium aggravates inflammation, which in turn causes extensive tissue destruction. Both the *in vitro* and *in vivo* results that support this model are discussed.

REFERENCES

1.　BARUA, D. 1981. Diarrhea as a global problem and the WHO program for its control. *In* Acute Enteric Infections in Children. New Prospects for Treatment and Prevention. T. Holme, J. Holmgren, M. H. Merson & R. Möllby, eds.: 1–6. Elsevier/North-Holland Biomedical Press. Amsterdam.

2.　SANYAL, S. C. 1981. Epidemiological importance of diarrheal agents in India. *In* Acute Enteric Infections in Children. New Prospects for Treatment and Prevention. T. Holme, J Holmgren, M. H. Merson & R. Möllby, eds.: 149–157. Elsevier/North-Holland Biomedical Press. Amsterdam.

3.　MAURELLI, A. T. & P. J. SANSONETTI. 1988. Genetic determinants of Shigella pathogenicity. Ann. Rev. Microbiol. **42:** 127–150.

4.　LINDBERG, A. A. & T. PÁL. 1993. Strategies for development of potential candidate *Shigella* vaccines. Vaccine **11:** 168–179.

5.　ANAND, B. S., V. MALHORTA, S. K. BHATTACHARYA, P. DATTA, D. SEN, M. K. BHATTACHARYA, P. P. MUKHERJEE & S. C. PAL. 1986. Rectal histology in acute bacillary dysentery. Gastroenterology 90: 654–660.

6.　LABREC, E. H., H. SCHNEIDER, T. J. MAGNANI & S. B. FORMAL. 1964. Epithelial cell penetration as an essential step in the pathogenesis of bacillary dysentery. J. Bacteriol. **88:** 1503–1518.

7. MATHAN, M. M. & V. I. MATHAN. 1991. Morphology of rectal mucosa of patients with shigellosis. Rev. Infect. Dis. **13**(suppl. 4): S314–318.

8. FINLAY, B. B. AND S. FALKOW. 1988. Comparison of the invasion strategies used by *Salmonella cholera-suis, Shigella flexneri* and *Yersinia enterocolitica* to enter cultured animal cells: Endosome acidification is not required for bacterial invasion or intracellular replication. Biochimie **70**: 1089–1099

9. MAURELLI, A. T., B. BAUDRY, H. D'HAUTEVILLE, T. L. HALE & P. J. SANSONETTI. 1985. Cloning of plasmid DNA sequences involved in invasion of HeLa cells by *Shigella flexneri*. Infect. Immun. **49**: 164–171.

10. SASAKAWA, C., K. KAMATA, T. SAKAI, S. MAKINO, M. YAMADA, N. OKADA & M. YOSHI-KAWA. 1988. Virulence-associated genetic regions comprising 31 kilobases of the 230-kilobase plasmid in *Shigella flexneri* 2A. J. Bacteriol. **170**: 2480–2484.

11. HIGH, N., J. MOUNIER, M. C. PREVOST & P. J. SANSONETTI. 1992. IpaB of *Shigella flexneri* causes entry into epithelial cells and escape from the phagocytic vacuole. EMBO J. **11**: 1991–1999.

12. MÉNARD, R., P. J. SANSONETTI & C. PARSOT. 1993. Nonpolar mutagenesis of the *ipa* genes defines IpaB, IpaC, and IpaD as effectors of *Shigella flexneri* entry into epithelial cells. J. Bacteriol. **175**: 5899–5906.

13. ANDREWS, G. P., A. E. HROMOCKYJ, C. COKER & A. T. MAURELLI. 1991. Two novel virulence loci, mxiA and mxiB, in *Shigella flexneri* 2A facilitate excretion of invasion plasmid antigens. Infect. Immun. **59**: 1997–2005.

14. ALLAOUI, A., P. J. SANSONETTI & C. PARSOT. 1992. MxiJ, a lipoprotein involved in secretion of Shigella Ipa invasins, is homologous to YscJ, a secretion factor of the Yersinia Yop proteins. J. Bacteriol. **174**: 7661–7669.

15. ALLAOUI, A., P. J. SANSONETTI & C. PARSOT. 1993. MxiD: An outer membrane protein necessary for the secretion of the *Shigella flexneri* Ipa invasins. Mol. Microbiol. **7**: 59–68.

16. BERNARDINI, M. L., J. MOUNIER, H. D'HAUTEVILLE, M. COQUIS-RONDON & P. J. SANSO-NETTI. 1989. Identification of *icsA*, a plasmid locus of *Shigella flexneri* that governs bacterial intra and intercellular spread through interaction with F-actin. Proc. Natl. Acad. Sci. USA **86**: 3867–3871.

17. SERÉNY, B. 1955. Experimental *Shigella* keratoconjunctivitis. Acta Microbiol. Acad. Sci. Hung **2**: 293–296.

18. MOUNIER, J., T. VASSELON, R. HELLIO, M. LESOURD & P. J. SANSONETTI. 1992. *Shigella flexneri* enters human colonic Caco-2 epithelial cells through the basolateral pole. Infect. Immun. **60**: 237–248.

19. FALKOW, S., R. R. ISBERG & D. A. PORTNOY. 1992. The interaction of bacteria with mammalian cell. Ann. Rev. Cell. Biol. **8**: 333–363.

20. KRAEHENBUHL, J.-P. & M. R. NEUTRA. 1992. Molecular and cellular basis of immune protection of mucosal surfaces. Physiol. Rev. **72**: 853–879.

21. WASSEF, J. S., D. F. KEREN & J. L. MAILLOUX. 1989. Role of M cells in initial antigen uptake and in ulcer formation in rabbit intestinal loop model of shigellosis. Infect. Immun. **57**: 858–863.

22. LIU, L. M. & G. G. MACPHERSON. 1993. Antigen acquisition by dendritic cells: Intestinal dendritic cell acquire antigen administered orally and can prime naive T cells *in vivo*. J. Exp. Med. **177**: 1299–1307.

23. PAVLI, P., D. A. HUME, E. VAN DEN POL & W. F. DOE. 1993. Dendritic cells, the major antigen-presenting cells of the human colonic lamina propria. Immunology **78**: 132–141.

24. SOESTAYO, M., J. BIEWENGA, G. KRAAL & T. SMINIA. 1990. The localization of macro-phages subsets and dendritic cells in the gastrointestinal tract of the mouse with special

reference to the presence of high endothelial venules. An immuno- and enzyme-histochemical study. Cell Tissue Res. **259:** 587-593.

25. JARRY, A., M. ROBASZKIEWICZ, N. BROUSSE & F. POTET. 1989. Immune cells associated with M cells in the follicle-associated epithelium of Peyer's patches in the rat. Cell Tissue Res. **255:** 293-298.

26. ZYCHLINSKY, A., M. C. PREVOST & P. J. SANSONETTI. 1992. *Shigella flexneri* induces apoptosis in infected macrophages. Nature **358:** 167-169.

27. ARENDS, M. J. & A. H. WYLLIE. 1991. Apoptosis: Mechanisms and roles in pathology. Int. Rev. Exp. Pathol. **32:** 223-254.

28. ELLIS, R. E., J. YUAN & H. R. HORVITZ. 1991. Mechanisms and functions of cell death. Annu. Rev. Cell Biol. **7:** 663-698.

29. CLERC, P. L., A. RYTER, J. MOUNIER & P. J. SANSONETTI. 1987. Plasmid-mediated early killing of eucaryotic cells by *Shigella flexneri* as studied by infection of J774 macrophages. Infect. Immun. **55:** 521-527.

30. CARON-LESLIE, L.-M.M. & J. A. CIDLOWSKI. 1991. Similar actions of glucocorticoids and calcium on the regulation of apoptosis in S49 cells. Mol. Endocrinol. **5:** 1169-1179.

31. OJCIUS, D. M., A. ZYCHLINSKY, L. M. ZHENG & J. D.-E. YOUNG. 1991. Ionophore-induced apoptosis. Role of DNA fragmentation and calcium fluxes. Exp. Cell Res. **197:** 43-49.

32. MCCONKEY, D. J., S. ORRENIUS, S. OKRET & M. JONDAL. 1993. Cyclic AMP potentiates glucocorticoid-induced endogenous endonuclease activation in thymocytes. FASEB J. **7:** 580-585.

33. VINTERMYR, O. K., B. J. GJERTSEN, M. LANOTTE & S. O. DOSKELAND. 1993. Microinjected catalytic subunit of cAMP-dependent protein kinase induces apoptosis in myeloid leukemia (IPC-81) cells. Exp. Cell Res. **206:** 157-161.

34. FREEMAN, R. S., S. ESTUS, K. HORIGOME & E. M. J. JOHNSON. 1993. Cell death genes in invertebrates and (maybe) vertebrates. Curr. Opinion Neurobiol. **3:** 25-31.

35. ZYCHLINSKY, A. 1993. Programmed cell death in infectious diseases. Trends Microbiol. **1:** 114-117.

36. DINARELLO, C. A. 1992. Role of interleukin-1 and tumor necrosis factor in systemic responses to infection and inflammation. *In* Inflammation, basic principles and clinical correlates. J. I. Gallin, I. M. Goldstein & R. Snyderman, eds.: 211-232. Raven Press. New York.

37. HOGQUIST, K. A., M. A. NETT, E. R. URANUE & D. D. CHAPLIN. 1991. Interleukin-1 is processed and released during apoptosis. Proc. Natl. Acad. Sci. USA **88:** 8485-8489.

38. YOUNGMAN, K. R., P. L. SIMON, G. A. WEST, F. COMINELLI, D. RACHMILEWITZ, J. S. KLEIN & C. FIOCCHI. 1993. Localization of intestinal interleukin 1 activity and protein and gene expression to lamina propria cells. Gastroeneterology **104:** 749-758.

39. MAHIDA, Y. R., S. PATEL, P. GIONCHETTI, D. VAUX & D. P. JEWELL. 1989. Macrophage subpopulations in lamina propria of normal and inflamed colon and terminal ileum. Gut **30:** 826-834.

40. MAHIDA, Y. R., K. WU & D. P. JEWELL. 1989. Enhanced production of interleukin-1β by mononuclear cells isolated from mucosa with active ulcerative colitis of Crohn's disease. Gut **30:** 835-838.

41. ZYCHLINSKY, A., C. FITTING, J.-M. CAVAILLON & P. J. SANSONETTI. 1993. Interleukin-1 is released by macrophages during *Shigella flexneri* induced apoptosis. Submitted.

42. AGACE, W., S. HEDGES, U. ANDERSSON, J. ANDERSSON, M. CESKA & C. SVANBORG. 1993. Selective cytokine production by epithelial cells following exposure to *Escherichia coli*. Infect. Immun. **61:** 602-609.

43. NAKAMURA, H., K. YOSHIMURA, H. A. JAFFE & R. G. CRYSTAL. 1991. Interleukin-8 gene expression in human bronchial epithelial cells. J. Biol. Chem. **266:** 19611-19617.

44. SANSONETTI, P. J., J. ARONDEL, A. FONTAINE, H. D'HAUTEVILLE & M. L. BERNARDINI. 1991. *OmpB* (osmo-regulation) and *icsA* (cell to cell spread) mutants of *Shigella flexneri*: Vaccine candidates and probes to study the pathogenesis of shigellosis. Vaccine **9:** 416–422.

45. PERDOMO, J. J., P. GOUNON & P. J. SANSONETTI. 1994. Polymorphonuclear leucocyte transmigration promotes invasion of colonic epithelial monolayer by *Shigella flexneri*. J. Clin. Invest. **93:** 633–643.

46. MCROBERTS, J. A. & K. E. BARRETT. 1989. Hormone-regulated ion transport in T84 colonic cells. *In* Functional Epithelial Cells in Culture.: 235–265. Alan R. Liss. Inc. New York.

47. COLGAN, S. P., C. A. PARKOS, C. DELP, M. A. ARNAOUT & J. L. MADARA. 1993. Neutrophil migration across cultured intestinal epithelium monolayers is modulated by epithelial exposure to IFN-γ in a highly polarized fashion. J. Cell Biol. **120:** 785–798.

48. WEISS, S. J. 1989. Tissue destruction by neutrophils. N. Engl. J. Med. **320:** 365–376.

49. PARKOS, C. A., C. DELP, M. A. ARNAOUT & J. L. MADARA. 1991. Neutrophil migration across a cultured intestinal epithelium. Dependence on a CD11b/CD18-mediated event and enhanced efficiency in physiological direction. J. Clin. Invest. **88:** 1605–1612.

50. PRÉVOST, M. C., M. LESOURD, M. ARPIN, F. VERNEL, J. MOUNIER, R. HELLIO & P. J. SANSONETTI. 1992. Unipolar reorganization of F-actin layer at bacterial division and bundling of actin filaments by plastin correlate with movement of *Shigella flexneri* within HeLa cells. Infect. Immun. **60:** 4088–4099.

51. GOLDBERG, M. B., O. BÂRZU, C. PARSOT & P. J. SANSONETTI. 1993. Unipolar localization and ATPase activity of IcsA, a *Shigella flexneri* protein involved in intracellular movement. J. Bacteriol. **175:** 2189–2196.

52. D'HAUTEVILLE, H. & P. J. SANSONETTI. 1992. Phosphorylation of IcsA by cAMP-dependent protein kinase and its effects on intercellular spread of *Shigella flexneri*. Mol. Microbiol. **6:** 833–841.

53. ALLAOUI, A., J. MOUNIER, M. C. PRÉVOST, P. J. SANSONETTI & C. PARSOT. 1992. *icsB*: A *Shigella flexneri* virulence gene necessary for the lysis of protrusions during intercellular spread. Mol. Microbiol. **6:** 1605–1616.

Antiidiotype Antibodies As Surrogates for Polysaccharide Vaccines

M. A. JULIE WESTERINK,[a]
ANTHONY A. CAMPAGNARI,[b] PETER GIARDINA,[b]
AND MICHAEL A. APICELLA[c,d]

[a]Medical College of Ohio
Toledo, Ohio 43699-0008

[b]SUNY at Buffalo
Buffalo, New York 14215

[c]University of Iowa College of Medicine
Iowa City, Iowa 52242

Polysaccharide antigens have been the bane of developers of bacterial vaccines. For most of the preventable infections of childhood (*Haemophilus influenzae* type b meningitis,[1] *Streptococcus pneumoniae* meningitis and middle ear infections,[2] and *Neisserria meningitidis* meningitis and sepsis,[3] to name but a few) the capsular polysaccharide surrounding these organisms is a prime target for protective antibodies. Successful vaccines have been developed using polysaccharides in adults, but these antigens must be modified by protein conjugation for use in children.[4,5] The reason is that the rules governing the immune response to these antigens differ significantly from those of protein antigens. These polysaccharides are T-independent antigens.[6] They fail to stimulate a memory response and to undergo affinity maturation.[7] Most importantly, the response to them develops late in ontogeny,[8] and humans below the age of 2 fail to generate a sustained protective response after immunization.

Efforts to overcome neonatal unresponsiveness to polysaccharide antigens have resulted in vaccines in which the polysaccharide capsular antigens are changed into functional T-cell-dependent antigens by coupling the polysaccharide to an immunogenic thymus-dependent carrier.[5] An alternative strategy for the conversion of the thymus-independent polysaccharide into a thymus-dependent polysaccharide into a thymus-dependent immunogen is the development of the surrogate image of the polysaccharide in the combining site of an antiidiotype antibody.[9] This latter technique is based on the immune regulatory network theory of Jerne that defines the immune system as a web of interacting idiotopes.[10] Antibodies carry idiotopes, which are regions in or near the antigen recognition sites. Idiotypes are capable of acting as antigens and of stimulating antibody production. Idiotype vaccines are proteins and therefore may act as T-dependent antigens. McNamara *et al.*[11] and Stein and Soderstrom[12] showed the usefulness of antiidiotype vaccines by inducing and priming for

---

[d]Address for correspondence: Michael A. Apicella, MD, Professor and Head, Department of Microbiology, BSB3-404, University of Iowa College of Medicine, Iowa City, Iowa 52242.

protective antibodies against encapsulated organisms. Our laboratory has been developing antiidiotype antibodies as surrogates for meningococcal capsular polysaccharides. The ultimate goal of our efforts is the development of an anticapsular peptide vaccine that is based on the composition and configuration of the antigen recognition site of the antiidiotype antibody. Recently, Pride and co-workers,[13] showed the feasibility of this approach for protein antigens. On the basis of sequence analysis of the CDR regions of an antiidiotype antibody that is a surrogate for an HBsAg epitope, they identified a peptide that generated an anti HBsAg response, primed for *in vitro* proliferative T-cell responses to HBsAg and stimulated *in vitro* human CD_4 cells that had been primed by previous HBsAg infection.[13]

In this manuscript, we describe studies which confirm that the antiidiotype antibody 6F9, whose antigen recognition site is a surrogate of the meningococcal capsular C polysaccharide antigen,[14,15] is a T-dependent antigen that will generate a memory response in neonatal mice.

MATERIALS AND METHODS

Bacterial Strains. N. *meningitidis* serogroup C strain 35E was obtained from our own collection. It was stored frozen at $-70°C$ in glycinerated Mueller-Hinton broth, reconstituted and grown on supplemented CG agar (Difco Laboratories, Detroit, Michigan) in 5% CO_2 at 37°C overnight, and suspended in sterile phosphate-buffered saline solution (PBS) to the desired number of colonies per milliliter.

Animals. BALB/c mice were obtained from West Seneca Laboratories, West Seneca, New York. The animals were bred at the animal facility of the Clinical Center of SUNY at Buffalo. Adult mice were immunized at 4-6 weeks of age.

Meningococcal C Polysaccharide. Vaccine quality group C meningococcal C polysaccharide (MCP) was a gift from Dr. Philip Vella, Merck Sharp and Dohme Research Laboratories (West Point, Pennsylvania).

Monoclonal Antiidiotype Antibodies. The development of the monoclonal antiidiotype antibody 6F9 was described previously. Large quantities of 6F9 (IgG2b), free of other contaminating proteins, were obtained by growing the hybridoma cells in protein-free hybridoma medium (Gibco Laboratories, Grand Island, New York). The antibodies were purified by affinity chromatography using protein A conjugated to Sepharose (Pharmacia, Uppsala, Sweden).

Immunizations. Adult BALB/c mice 4-6 weeks of age were immunized intraperitoneally with an optimal immunizing dose of 6F9 (100 μg) or MCP (5 μg) diluted in 250 μl of sterile PBS. The control group of mice were immunized with PBS alone. Neonatal mice were primed intraperitoneally within 24 hours of birth with an optimal dose of 6F9 (25 μg) or MCP (1 μg) in 50 μl of sterile PBS. The control group of mice were immunized with PBS.

Challenge Experiments. To enhance susceptibility to meningococcal infection all mice received 1 mg/g intraperitoneally of iron dextran 1 week prior to the live challenge study.[16] To determine the LD_{50} unimmunized BALB/c mice were challenged intraperitoneally with 10^3-10^5 (10^4 cfu) of strain 35E. The mice were bled from the tail vein under sterile conditions at 4, 8, 24, and 48 hours after challenge and serial dilutions of the blood were cultured on supplemented CG agar plates to determine the degree of bacteremia. All survivors were sacrificed and bled 3 days after the challenge date, and sera were tested for anti-MCP antibodies.

ELISA Analysis. Purified capsular polysaccharide was diluted in carbonate buffer, pH 9.6, to a final concentration of 10 μg/ml. The wells of 96-well polyvinyl plates (Linbro/Titertek, Flow Laboratories, McLean, Virginia) were coated with 100 μl of polysaccharide in buffer and incubated for 1 hour at 37°C and then overnight at 4°C. Plates were washed three times with 0.01 M PBS-0.05% Tween 20. The plates were blocked for 1 hour with 3% gelatin at 37°C and washed. Serial dilutions of serum starting at 1 : 10 to 1 : 320 were prepared, and 100 ml was added per well. Plates were incubated for 1 hour at 37°C and washed three times. The plates were incubated with anti-mouse IgG or IgM peroxidase-labeled conjugate (Kirkengaard and Perry Laboratories, Gaithersburg, Maryland), washed three times, and developed with 100 μl of substrate buffer containing 0.02% *o*-phenylene diamine (Sigma Chemical, St Louis, Missouri). The absorbance was read with the electroimmunoassay reader (Bio-tek Instrument, Burlington, Vermont). Each serum sample was analyzed in duplicate. The mean of all values per group of mice is present in the results. Each assay was standardized using a pool of normal mouse sera as the negative control and a pool of sera from adult BALB/c mice immunized with 6F9 as the positive controls.

Statistics. Statistical analysis was performed using an Apple-Macintosh SE computer with a STAT View 512+ program. Analysis of variance (ANOVA) was used to determine differences between groups. The Fisher PLSD was used for post-hoc ANOVA comparison, with p value of less than 0.01 considered significant.

RESULTS AND DISCUSSION

In previous studies in our laboratory we were able to successfully develop a site-associated antiidiotype $AB_{2\beta}$ that was a surrogate antigen for the *N. meningitidis* serogroup C polysaccharide.[14,15] We demonstrated that this anti-id could inhibit a monoclonal antibody specific for the serogroup C polysaccharide, which was capable of producing anti-antiidiotype antibodies in BALB/c mice that had identical binding characteristics as the monoclonal antibody used to develop the anti-id.[14,15] In the presence of complement, the AB_3 was also bactericidal for *N. meningitidis* serogroup C strains.[14,15] These studies also showed that immunization with the anti-id in rabbits led to the development of anticapsular antibodies.

In this paper we describe studies which demonstrate that the anti-id 6F9 can be used as a successful vaccine in BALB/c mice. Previous investigators had shown that iron dextran loaded mice had a markedly increased susceptibility to intraperitoneal challenge with *N. meningitidis.*[16] We decided to establish this model in our laboratory and determine if this model could be used to evaluate the anti-id 6F9 as a vaccine for prevention of mortality in BALB/c mice. In our initial experiments, we found no evidence of increased susceptibility of iron dextran loaded BALB/c mice to the majority of the *N. meningitidis* strain we tested. One strain, *N. meningitidis* serogroup C strain 35E, proved to be virulent in the model system. The LD_{50} for strain 35E was defined in BALB/c mice. The mice received 1 mg/g body weight of iron dextran 1 week prior to the challenge to enhance susceptibility to infection. Three groups of mice received either 10^4, 10^5, or 10^6 cfu. There were 10 mice in each group. The

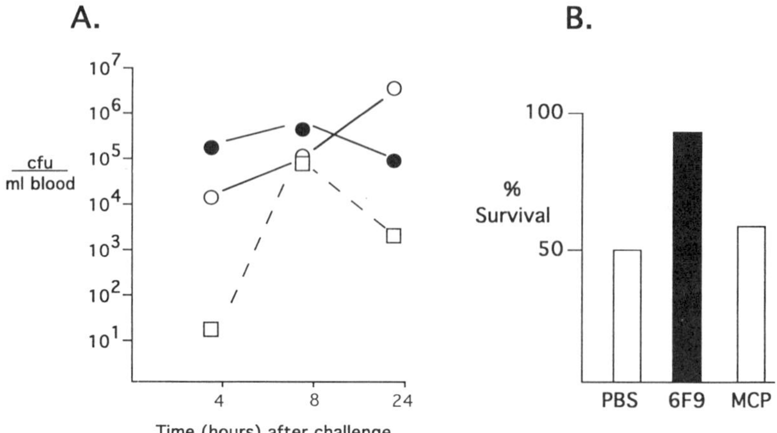

FIGURE 1. (**A**) The colony-forming units per milliliter of blood at 4, 8, and 24 hours after challenge with 10 LD_{50} of *N. meningitidis* serogroup C strain 35E in iron-dextran-treated adult BALB/c mice immunized with PBS (O), MCP (□), or anti-id 6F9 (●). Ten mice were studied in each group. (**B**) The percentage of survival 48 hours after challenge with 10 LD_{50} of *N. meningitidis* serogroup C strain 35E in iron-dextran-treated BALB/c mice immunized with PBS (O), MCP (□), or anti-id 6F9 (■).

mice either died within 48 hours or recovered. The LD_{50} was determined to be 10^3 cfu per mouse.

Once the LD_{50} had been determined, we set up a series of experiments to determine if we could protect adult BALB/c mice against this challenge. In previous studies, we showed that there is an optimal immunizing dose for antiidiotype 6F9. For adult mice this was shown to 100 μg/mouse. In these experiments, mice were immunized with the optimal dose of MCP, 6F9, or PBS at 4 weeks of age. There were 10 mice in each group. The mice received iron dextran and were challenged with $10 \times LD_{50}$ of strain 35E. The mice were bled from the tail vein and colony-forming units determined serially at 4, 8, and 24 hours after challenge. The unimmunized mice had a 50% survival and all survivors had a high level of bacteremia at 24 hours (2.4 $\times 10^6$ cfu). Mice immunized with 6F9 had a survival rate of 100% and a significantly reduced level of bacteremia at 24 hours (1×10^3). Mice immunized with MCP had an 80% survival rate and the group had a mean bacteremia at 24 hours of 5×10^4 cfu. These studies showed that the anti-id 6F9 was as effective as MCP in preventing mortality in BALB/c mice when challenged with *N. meningitidis* serogroup C strain 35E after the mice were iron dextran loaded. In addition, the mice immunized with 6F9 cleared their bacteremia sooner and had lower levels of bacteremia than did the MCP immunized mice (FIG. 1). These studies indicated that the 6F9 could be used too as a vaccine to prevent mortality to experimental meningococcal sepsis.

Our primary goal in this project since its inception was to determine if anti-ids to the capsular polysaccharides would function as T-dependent antigens. Specifically we were interested in determining if we could overcome the tolerance of neonates to immunization with the C polysaccharide capsule. Inasmuch as children are the principal group at risk for meningococcal meningitis and sepsis, we felt that our experimental model should include the ability to protect and develop evidence of a memory response in newborn animals. We established a breeding colony of BALB/c mice and established a series of challenge experiments in newborn mice. Previous studies in our laboratory have shown that newborn BALB/c mice are tolerant to immunization with the meningococcal A and C polysaccharide for 24–48 hours after birth. We had also previously determined that the optimal immunizing dose of 6F9 for newborn mice was 25 μg/mouse. Mice were primed within 24 hours of birth with MCP, 6F9, or PBS and immunized at 4 weeks of age with MCP, 6F9, or PBS. The mice were then treated with iron dextran and challenged at 5 weeks of age with $10 \times LD_{50}$. Control mice had a survival rate of 50% and all the survivors were bacteremic at 24 hours. Mice primed and immunized with MCP had a survival rate of 100%. In all, bacteremia had cleared by 24 hours. Mice primed and immunized with 6F9 also had a 100% survival. In this group bacteremia cleared by 8 hours. This is significantly faster than the MCP primed and immunized group. Mice primed with MCP and immunized with 6F9 were comparable to the MCP primed and immunized group, whereas mice primed with 6F9 and immunized with MCP were comparable to the 6F9 primed and immunized group. The MCP IgG ELISA in the 6F9 primed groups showed similar titer elevations which were significantly greater than control. This experiment did not completely answer the question we had raised. A memory response was suggested based on the ability of the 6F9 primed and immunized mice to more rapidly clear their bacteremia when compared to the MCP primed and immunized mice. The MCP primed and immunized mice were protected, but our previous studies showed that anti-IgM MCP response is peaking by 5 days in these mice and we believed that the 4-week immunizing dose was the source of protection.

To explore this question more closely, BALB/c mice were primed with MCP, 6F9, or PBS within 24 hours of birth. At 4 weeks of age, the mice received iron dextran and were challenged with $10 \times LD_{50}$ at 5 weeks of age. Mice primed with 6F9 had a significantly higher survival rate than did the control group (FIG. 2). All mice were bacteremic at 24 hours, and the 6F9 primed mice had a significantly increased anti-MCP titer. The mice primed with MCP had a 60% survival which was not significantly different from that of the controls. No anti-MCP IgG titers were present in the serum of the MCP-primed mice. An experiment was also performed in which mice primed at 24 hours after birth were immunized 8 days later and challenged at 5 weeks after iron dextran. These studies demonstrated that both the MCP and 6F9 immunized mice had 100% survival. The principal difference between the MCP and 6F9 groups was the ability of the 6F9 group to clear bacteremia by 8 hours (9 of 10). This compared to the MCP-immunized group in which all mice remained bacteremic at 24 hours.

It has been established that anti-idiotypes may serve as an alternative means of inducing neutralizing antibody or priming neonatal animals against various bacterial, viral, and parasitic infections.[9,11,12] We previously demonstrated that 6F9, the surrogate of the meningococcal C polysaccharide, is capable of inducing a T-dependent antibody response in neonatal and adult mice. It does not necessarily follow that the antibody response induced by 6F9 confers protection against meningococcal C serogroup disease. Vakil, Briles, and Kearney demonstrated that mice primed within 24 hours

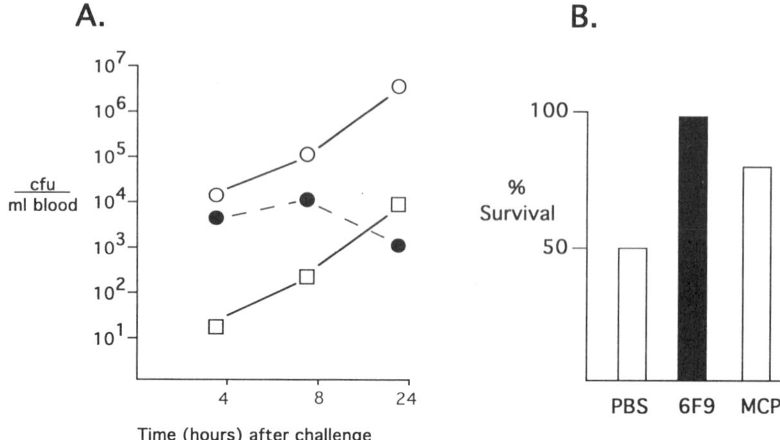

FIGURE 2. (A) The colony-forming units per milliliter of blood at 4, 8, and 24 hours after challenge at 5 weeks of age with 10 LD_{50} of *N. meningitidis* serogroup C strain 35E in iron-dextran–treated BALB/c neonatal mice immunized less than 24 hours after birth. Mice were immunized with PBS (O), MCP (□), and anti-id 6F9 (●). Ten mice were studied in each group. (B) The percentage survival 48 hours after challenge with 10 LD_{50} of *N. meningitidis* serogroup C strain 35E in iron-dextran–treated BALB/c mice immunized as neonates with PBS (□), MCP (□), or anti-id 6F9 (■).

of birth with pneumococci and vaccinated at 6 weeks of age generated an anti-PC response.[17] This response was not protective against infection, and these mice failed to respond at $\alpha1$-3 dextran. This indicates that major alterations in the immune system had occurred. It is essential to demonstrate not only the production of specific antigen-directed antibody by an anti-id but also the protective nature of these anti-idiotype–induced antibodies.

In a series of live challenge experiments, we showed that mice immunized with the monoclonal anti-id 6F9 were protected against meningococcal group C infection, resulting in 100% survival and markedly reduced levels of bacteremia at 24 hours. Similar results were obtained by immunization with MCP. This is not unexpected, as we have demonstrated a significant anti-MCP IgG antibody response following live challenge. This is not surprising because an IgG antibody response is not seen until 2–3 weeks following immunization with a T-dependent antigen.

Priming neonatal mice within 24 hours of birth and immunizing at either 8 days or 4 weeks of age with either MCP or 6F9 result in 100% protection against meningococcal infection. Mice primed with anti-id cleared the bacteremia significantly faster and demonstrated a significantly higher anti-MCP IgG titer than did mice primed with MCP. We demonstrated that neonatal mice primed with 6F9 within 8 days of birth show a low level anti-MCP IgG response, but a significant anti-MCP IgG response after secondary immunization.[15] We have now shown that neonatal mice immunized with 6F9 within 24 hours of birth demonstrate a similar secondary anti-MCP IgG response following live challenge. Finally, we demonstrated that priming without immunization with anti-idiotype leads to protective immunity whereas priming with MCP without immunization fails to protect against infection. These data suggest that priming with the anti-idiotype 6F9 results in the formation of either long-lived B or T memory cells which expand on exposure to live meningococci. The immune response triggered by 6F9 seems to be more efficient than the response seen by priming or immunization with nominal antigen, MCP. Our results concur with the finding of other investigators that priming with anti-idiotypes can stimulate expression of silent B-cell clones, induce a protective response upon subsequent immunization against a lethal dose of *Escherichia coli,* and alter the response to high molecular weight polysaccharide from mainly IgM to an enhanced IgG1 response.[12] In addition, we showed that in contrast to the finding described by Vakil *et al.,*[17] the antibody response induced by priming and/or immunizing with MCP or the anti-idiotype resulted in an anti-MCP antibody response which offered protective immunity. It is clear that the risk of inducing nonprotective antibody in an immature system is a distinct possibility and will need to be carefully investigated in different antigen systems.

SUMMARY

In past studies we demonstrated that monoclonal antibody 6F9 is a surrogate image of the meningococcal C capsular polysaccharide. These studies indicated that immunization with this anti-id resulted in a T-dependent antibody response. In the studies reported in this paper, we show that the response which is elicited is protective.

Using a model of meningococcal infection in BALB/c mice in which the animals are rendered susceptible with iron dextran, we studied the ability of this anti-id to protect adult mice against challenge. These studies encompassed the ability of 6F9 to prime neonatal mice and provide them with protection to later challenge. Adult BALB/c mice immunized with 6F9 had a 100% survival and a significantly reduced level of bacteremia at 24 hours. Neonatal mice primed within 24 hours of birth and immunized at 4 weeks of age with 6F9 had a 100% survival and cleared their bacteremia by 8 hours. Neonatal mice primed with 6F9 and challenged at 5 weeks had a 90% survival. These data indicate that anti-id 6F9 is a surrogate antigen for the meningococcal C polysaccharide and is capable of inducing protective immunity in immunologically mature as well as immature animals.

REFERENCES

1. MOXON, E. R. 1990. *Haemophilus influenzae. In* Principles and Practices of Infectious Diseases. G. L. Mandell, R. G. Douglas & J. E. Bennett, Eds. Churchill Livingston. New York.

2. MUFSON, M. A. 1990. Streptococcus pneumoniae. *In* Principles and Practices of Infectious Diseases. G. L. Mandell, R. G. Douglas & J. E. Bennett, Eds. Churchill Livingston. New York.

3. APICELLA, M. A. 1990. *Neisseria meningitidis. In* Principles and Practices of Infectious Diseases. G. L. Mandell, R. G. Douglas & J. E. Bennett, Eds. Churchill Livingston. New York.

4. ARTENSTEIN, M. S., R. GOLD, J. G. ZIMMERLY *et al.* 1970. Prevention of meningococcal disease by group C polysaccharide vaccine. N. Engl. J. Med. **282:** 417–420.

5. GREENBERG, D. P., C. M. VADHEIM, N. BORDENAVE, L. ZIONTZ, P. CHRISTENSON, S. H. WALTERMAN & J. I. WARD. 1991. Protective efficacy of *Haemophilus influenzae* type b polysaccharide and conjugate vaccine in children 18 months of age or older. JAMA **265:** 987–992.

6. MOSIER, D. E., N. M. ZALVIDAS, E. GOLDINGS *et al.* 1977. Formation of antibody in the newborn mouse: Study of T-cell independent antibody response, J. Infect. Dis. **136:** S14–19.

7. GOLD, R. & M. L. LEPROW. 1975. Clinical evaluation of Group A and C meningococcal polysaccharide vaccines in infants. J. Clin. Invest. **56:** 1536–1547.

8. KAYHTY, H., V. KARANKO, H. PETOLA *et al.* 1984. Serum antibodies after immunization with *H. influenzae* type b capsular polysaccharide and responses to reimmunization: No evidence of immunologic tolerance or memory. Pediatrics **74:** 857–865.

9. KIEBER-EMMONS, T., R. E. WARD, S. RAYCHAUDHURI *et al.* 1986. Rationale design and application of idiotype vaccines. Int. Rev. Immunol. **1:** 1–26.

10. JERNE, N. K. 1974. Toward a network theory of the immune system. Ann. Immunol. (Paris) **125:** 373–389.

11. MCNAMARA, M., R. E. WARD & H. KOEHLER. 1984. Monoclonal idiotype vaccine against *Streptococcus pneumoniae* infection. Science **226:** 1325–1326.

12. STEIN, K. E. & T. SODERSTROM. 1984. Neonatal administration of idiotype or anti-idiotype primes for protection against *E. coli* K13 infection in mice. J. Exp. Med. **160:** 1001–1011.

13. PRIDE, M. W., H. SHI, J. M. ANCHIN *et al.* 1992. Molecular mimicry of hepatitis B surface antigen by an anti-idiotype synthetic peptide. Proc. Natl. Acad. Sci. USA **89:** 11900–11904.

14. WESTERINK, M. A. J., P. C. GIARDINA, A. A. CAMPAGNARI & M. A. APICELLA, 1990. The thymus dependent nature of the murine antibody response to a monoclonal anti-idiotype antibody to the *Neisseria meningitidis* serogroup C capsular polysaccharide. Microb. Pathog. **8:** 411–419.

15. WESTERINK, M. A. J., A. A. CAMPAGNARI, M. A. WIRTH & M. A. APICELLA. 1988. Development and characterization of an anti-idiotope antibody to the capsular polysaccharide of *Neisseria meningitidis* group C. Infect. Immun. **56:** 1101–1106.

16. CALVER, G. A., C. P. KENNY & G. LAVERGNE. 1976. Iron as a replacement for mucin in the establishment of meningococcal infection in mice. Can. J. Microbiol. **22:** 832–838.

17. VAKIL, M., D. E. BRILES & J. F. KEARNEY. 1991. Antigen independent selection of T15 idiotype during B-cell ontogeny in mice. Dev. Immunol. **1:** 203–212.

Oral Vaccine Models: Multiple Delivery Systems Employing Tetanus Toxoid[a]

RAYMOND J. JACKSON,[c] HERMAN F. STAATS,[c]
JIANGCHUN XU-AMANO,[d] ICHIRO TAKAHASHI,[c]
HIROSHI KIYONO,[b] MICHAEL E. HUDSON,[e]
RICHARD M. GILLEY,[e] STEVEN N. CHATFIELD,[f]
AND JERRY R. McGHEE [c]

*Departments of [b]Oral Biology and [c]Microbiology
Immunobiology Vaccine Center
and the Mucosal Immunization Research Group
University of Alabama at Birmingham Medical Center
Birmingham, Alabama 35294*

*[d]Department of Immunology
DNAX Research Institute
901 California Avenue
Palo Alto, California 94304*

*[e]Vaccine and Oral Formulations Section
Southern Research Institute
Birmingham, Alabama 35255*

*[f]Medeva Group Research
Vaccine Research Unit
Department of Biochemistry
Imperial College of Science, Technology and Medicine
London, SW7, UK*

The advances in molecular biology, biotechnology, and immunology in recent years have prompted the Expanded Program on Immunization to target no less than 19 diseases for vaccine development in the next decade.[1,2] Of the commonly administered vaccines, only one, the Sabin trivalent polio vaccine, is given by the oral route. The prospect of developing oral vaccines for prevention of disease is advantageous from a number of viewpoints. Aside from convenience, elimination of needles and syringes and, consequently, trained personnel would lower costs and permit more widespread and facile dissemination of oral vaccines in developing countries. Vaccines have traditionally been administered parentally to evoke protective antibody and cell-mediated immunity in systemic lymphoid tissues and the bloodstream. Only relatively

[a]This work was supported by U.S. Public Health Service Contract AI 15128 for the UAB Mucosal Immunization Research Group.

217

recently has it been appreciated that most pathogens are acquired through mucosal surfaces (i.e., respiratory, gastrointestinal, and urogenital tracts) and that immune responses at these sites are protective. (For recent reviews see refs. 3 and 4.) Moreover, systemic administration of vaccine is a poor inducer of mucosal immunity, and therefore the systemic and mucosal immune systems are generally considered separate compartments. However, certain antigen delivery systems (to be described) applied at mucosal surfaces are capable of stimulation of immune responses in both systemic and mucosal compartments.

The mucosal immune system differs in several basic aspects from the more widely studied systemic immune system. The major antibody isotype found at mucosal sites and in external secretions is secretory IgA (S-IgA), predominantly in dimeric form, whereas the principal isotype found in the peripheral blood and in tissue spaces is IgG. The vast mucosal surface area, estimated at over 400 m^2 in humans, produces 5 g of IgA daily and represents 60% of all Ig isotypes produced.[5,6] A unique feature of mucosal surfaces is the presence of specialized lymphoid tissues where antigens are encountered and processed and initial responses induced (inductive sites) and of other effector regions rich in IgA-producing plasma cells.[7-9] The major inductive sites in the gastrointestinal tract are Peyer's patches, whereas the lamina propria regions serve as the primary effector sites.

The anatomy of Peyer's patch includes a dome region consisting of macrophages, lymphocytes, and plasma cells. This region is protected from the luminal environment by epithelial cells, which include a subpopulation that is termed microfold or follicle associated epithelial cells.[10-12] These cells transport intact antigens, including bacteria and viruses, from the lumen to the interior of this lymphoid tissue. Peyer's patch contains germinal centers with surface IgA-positive (sIgA$^+$) B cells and parafollicular areas rich in mature T cells and antigen-presenting cells. Following antigen processing and B-cell triggering, the precursor IgA cells mature in mesenteric lymph nodes and, via the thoracic duct, enter the blood circulation. At their final destination, the lamina propria, these precursor B cells undergo terminal differentiation into IgA-secreting plasma cells under the influence of locally produced cytokines.[13,14]

Antigen-specific B-cell responses to protein delivered to mucosal surfaces or administered parentally depend on a group of lymphocytes termed T (thymus-derived) helper cells. Two subsets of Th cells were recently identified based on distinctive patterns of cytokines (interleukins [IL]) produced following antigen stimulation.[15,16] Th1 type cells selectively secrete IL-2, gamma interferon (IFN-γ), and tumor necrosis factor β (TNF-β). This subset is preferentially involved in cell-mediated immunity and therefore would be the preferred subset for protection against intracellular pathogens. In addition, the cytokine IFN-γ has been demonstrated to induce B cells to secrete IgG$_{2a}$ and thus also provides some B-cell help. In contrast, the Th2 subset produces IL-4, IL-5, IL-6, and IL-10. IL-4 may have autocrine properties and is known to significantly enhance IgG$_1$ and IgE secretion by B cells, while IL-5 and IL-6 were demonstrated to enhance surface IgA$^+$ Peyer's patch B cells to secrete IgA.[17,18] Some degree of regulation exists between the two subsets, and polarization in response to an antigen in terms of dominant Th1 or Th2 subsets has been reported.[19,20]

In evaluating responses to oral vaccines it would thus be crucial to evaluate not only antibody isotype levels but also the isotype subclasses produced and finally the cytokine profiles of antigen-stimulated Th cells to classify the pattern as Th1 or Th2 type responses. Rational design of vaccines may hinge on the stimulation of the Th2 subset for evoking S-IgA antibodies at the mucosal surfaces for protective immunity to soluble antigens such as toxins and noninvasive pathogens, while activation of cell-mediated immune responses (Th1 subset) may be required for eliminating intracellular bacteria and viruses. In the case of oral vaccines in which adjuvants, packaging the antigen in inert vehicles such as microspheres or in recombinant vectors such as bacteria or viruses, may be employed to optimize a response, one should be cognizant of the ability of the vector, packaging agent, or adjuvant to influence the isotypes, isotype subclasses, and Th cell responses induced (see *Results* section).

We employed the well-characterized soluble protein vaccine tetanus toxoid (TT) as a model oral protein vaccine using three distinct delivery systems in mice. The initial system utilized oral TT immunization with or without the mucosal adjuvant cholera toxin (CT), the second delivery system consisted of TT encapsulated in poly-L-lactide-co-glycolide microspheres, and finally mice were orally immunized with recombinant *Salmonella typhimurium* expressing the C fragment of tetanus toxin. In each of these studies we evaluated levels of antigen-specific antibody isotype responses in serum and in fecal extracts as representative of the systemic and mucosal immune responses, respectively. In addition, IgG subclasses were assayed in serum as an indication of the type of Th cell response obtained (elevated IgG_1, Th2 type, *vs* IgG_{2a}, Th1 type). We also examined the cytokine profiles of Peyer's patch and spleen $CD4^+$ T cells by cytokine-specific ELISPOT assays during peak antibody production in the oral delivery system employing CT as an adjuvant. These assays are planned for the microencapsulated and recombinant *Salmonella* delivery systems. It should be emphasized that an elevated serum IgG subclass, that is, IgG_{2a}, indicative of a Th1-type systemic response may not reflect the Th cell responses in mucosal tissue. A dichotomy may exist between the two compartments in terms of the antigen-specific Th cell-type induced which may involve presentation of antigen and other signals to the T cell by various antigen-presenting cells (i.e., macrophages, dendritic, or B cells).[21,22]

ORAL IMMUNIZATION WITH TETANUS TOXOID AND ADJUVANT

In our initial series of studies we employed TT with and without the mucosal adjuvant cholera toxin (CT). Most soluble proteins when given by the oral route induce poor and short-lived antibody responses. Administration of large doses of protein by this route may even result in unresponsiveness to systemic immunization, a condition termed oral tolerance.[23] Exceptions to this phenomenon are both CT and the heat-labile enterotoxin (LT) produced by *Escherichia coli*. Both toxins are potent immunogens and both exhibit adjuvant activity when coadministered with soluble proteins.[24,25]

The initial studies using soluble TT with CT as an adjuvant were designed to formulate an immunization protocol to optimize both systemic and mucosal antibody responses to TT. We also monitored antibody responses to CT as this protein is one of the most potent mucosal immunogens known. Thus, antibody titers to CT would serve as a relative indication of the potency of titers obtained against TT. ELISA

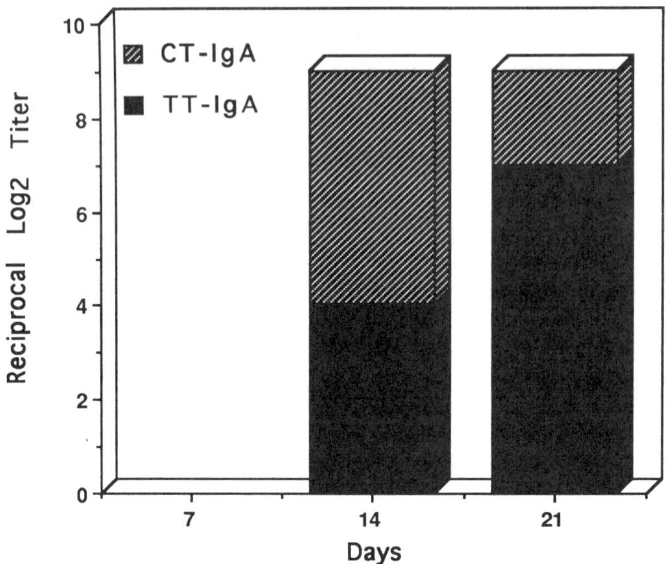

FIGURE 1. Time course of antigen-specific mucosal IgA responses to CT and TT. C57BL/ 6 mice were orally intubated with 250 μg of TT and 10 μg of CT on days 0, 7, and 14. Fecal extracts were assayed by ELISA endpoint titrations at the time points shown.[26]

assays were employed to determine the endpoint titers. Mice were intubated with a blunt feeding needle on days 0, 7, and 14 (standard immunization procedure). Dose response experiments established that 10 μg of CT coadministered with 250 μg of TT gave optimal antigen-specific anti-TT mucosal IgA and serum IgG responses on day 21 (data not shown).

Mucosal Antibody Responses

FIGURE 1 depicts the time course of mucosal responses to both TT and CT as reflected by antibody titers in fecal extracts. The IgA anti-CT titers reached 1:512 by day 14 and remained constant at day 21. Lower levels of anti-CT IgG were also present.

The fecal anti-TT specific IgA antibody titers were initially detected by day 14 and rose to a titer of 1:128 by day 21. Thus, oral administration of 10 μg of CT with TT resulted in a significant mucosal adjuvant effect as 250 μg of TT given alone did not give rise to detectable fecal anti-TT-specific antibody titers (not shown).

Analysis of Antibody-Secreting Cells

To ensure that the IgA antibody titers found in fecal extracts reflected locally produced S-IgA and not serum-derived IgA excreted in bile, animals immunized

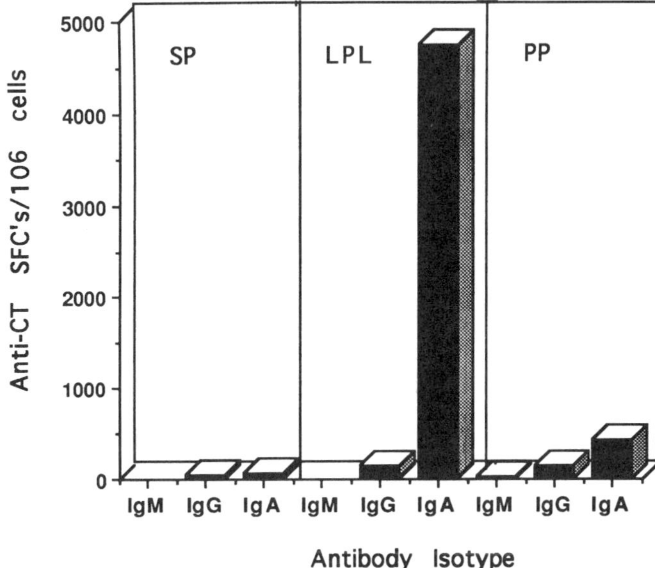

FIGURE 2. Anti-CT-secreting antibody-producing cells from spleen, Peyer's patch, and lamina propria. Orally immunized mice were sacrificed on day 21 and single cell preparations were isolated from each tissue. Antigen-specific IgM, IgG, and IgA cells were enumerated by an ELISPOT assay.[26]

with 250 μg TT and 10 μg CT or with 250 μg TT only were sacrificed at peak fecal IgA titers (day 21). Lymphocytes were isolated from spleen, Peyer's patch, and lamina propria and antigen-specific antibody-secreting cells analyzed by the ELISPOT technique. FIGURE 2 illustrates the results obtained when CT-specific antibody-secreting cells (spot forming cells [SFC]) were enumerated. A large number of IgA spot forming cells were found in lymphocytes isolated from the lamina propria. An average of approximately 4,700 CT-specific IgA-secreting cells were observed per 10^6 cells in three experiments. Considerably fewer spot forming cells were found in Peyer's patch or spleen. These results are consistent with the lamina propria's role as a mucosal effector site. The analysis of TT-specific spot forming cells from mice immunized with 250 μg TT and 10 μg of CT is shown in FIGURE 3. Again, large numbers of anti-TT-specific IgA-secreting cells were isolated from the lamina propria (1,200 per 10^6 cells). The number of antigen-specific CT- and TT-secreting cells generally reflected the IgA ELISA titers found in fecal extracts. When similar experiments were performed with mice orally immunized with 250 μg of TT only, <100 spot forming cells per 10^6 cells were observed, thus correlating with the failure to detect significant fecal IgA antibody titers in mice immunized without CT as an adjuvant. The foregoing results provide strong evidence that the antigen-specific CT and TT IgA antibodies monitored in fecal extracts are derived from activated B cells located in the lamina propria of the gut.

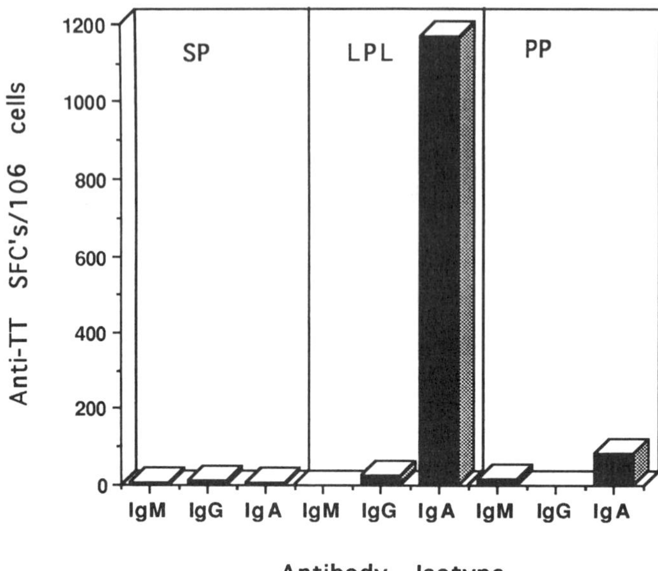

FIGURE 3. ELISPOT assay of TT-specific antibody-secreting cells. Assays were performed as described in FIGURE 2.[26]

Systemic Antibody Responses

Mice immunized by the standard protocol were analyzed for systemic responses as reflected by serum antigen-specific antibody titers. FIGURE 4 presents the time course of serum anti-TT and anti-CT responses. All three major antibody isotypes (IgM, IgG, and IgA) were present at various levels in serum. CT-specific IgG antibody levels (FIG. 4A) were first detected 7 days following immunization and rose to a titer of >1 : 1,000,000 by day 21. A transient IgM response was noted on day 14 (not shown). Serum CT-specific IgA (FIG. 4B) was observed on day 14 and reached a titer of 1 : 32,000 by day 21.

Serum IgG anti-TT titers peaked at day 14 (1 : 260,000) (FIG. 4A) and remained relatively constant at day 21. The IgM anti-TT response was transitory (not shown), and an IgA anti-TT response of 1 : 4,000 was evident on day 21 (FIG. 4B). Mice orally immunized with 250 μg of TT without CT as adjuvant exhibited no IgM or IgA anti-TT antibody and a weak IgG serum response (1 : 2,000) detected only on day 21 (not shown). Thus, CT also served as an adjuvant for eliciting systemic responses to TT as well as inducing mucosal responses. In this regard, when dose response studies were performed, as little as 10 μg of TT along with 10 μg of CT induced an anti-TT serum IgG response of 1 : 32,000 on day 21. This demonstrates that generation of a significant systemic response to TT when given with CT as an adjuvant required considerably less protein than was necessary to evoke a mucosal immune response.

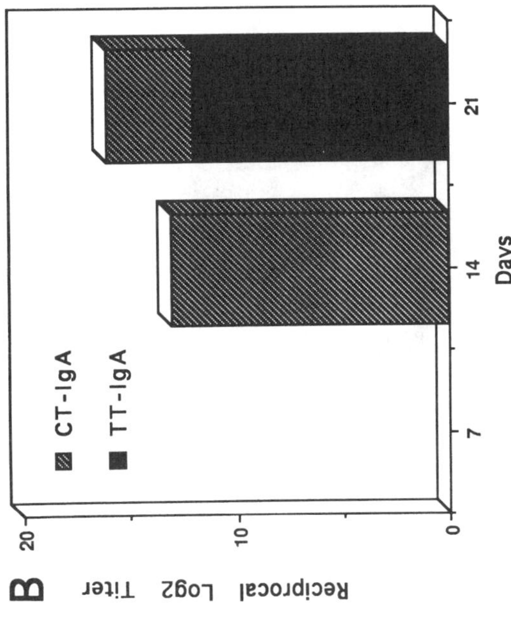

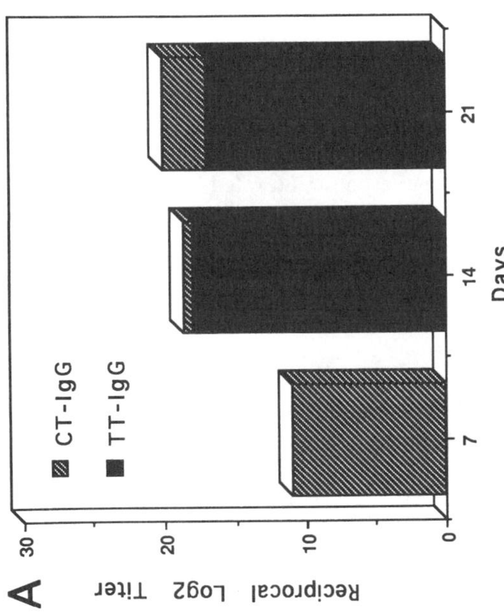

FIGURE 4. (A) Time course of serum anti-CT and anti-TT-specific IgG responses. (B) Serum anti-CT and TT-specific IgA responses.[26]

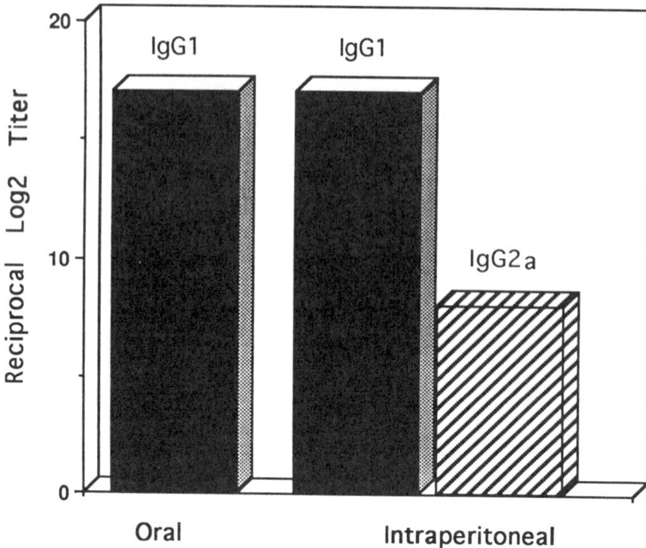

FIGURE 5. Anti-TT serum IgG subclasses elicited following oral or intraperitoneal immunization with TT and CT as an adjuvant. Mice were orally immunized with 250 μg of TT and 10 μg of CT on days 0, 7, and 14 or immunized with 10 μg of TT and 200 μg of CT on day 0 and 14 intraperitoneally. Anti-TT–specific IgG subclass assays were performed on day 21.

It was of interest to examine the antigen-specific IgG subclasses induced when TT was given orally with CT. Since route of antigen administration may influence the Th cell subsets induced, we also immunized mice interperitoneally with 10 μg TT and 200 ng CT and analyzed for IgG subclasses. Mice given TT + CT orally produced the IgG_1 anti-TT subclass exclusively. Mice injected intraperitoneally also responded with predominantly antigen-specific IgG_1, although low levels of IgG_{2a} were observed (FIG. 5). The results suggested that either route induced elevated IL-4 levels, typical of a Th2 type response. Elevated IL-4 levels are also associated with murine and human polyclonal IgE production.[16] We examined total IgE production in mice orally immunized with 250 μg TT and 10 μg CT and demonstrated that this immunization protocol induces large increases in serum IgE levels characteristic of strong Th2-type responses (not shown).

Oral Immunization Provides Protective Antibodies

To determine whether oral immunization provided protective immunity, we challenged mice orally immunized with 250 μg of TT and 10 μg of CT as well as control mice with 100 minimum lethal doses of standard tetanus toxin (Lot T-1) kindly supplied by Drs. J. Halpern and W. Habig (Food and Drug Administration). As shown in TABLE 1, protective immunity was achieved with the standard oral immunization protocol when mice were challenged on day 21. No evidence of paralysis was observed in any of the mice orally immunized with TT and CT.

T Helper (Th) Cell Responses in Mice Orally Immunized with TT and CT

In parallel with the antibody studies we directly investigated the characteristics of the Th cell responses required for antigen-specific TT or CT antibody production. Mice were immunized orally with the standard protocol and sacrificed on day 21. Peyer's patch and spleen were removed and CD4[+] T cells (>99% purity) isolated as described previously.[28] Initially we determined the various parameters required for optimum antigen-specific T-cell proliferation. T cells were cultured in 96-well Corning microplates with RPMI 1640 supplemented with nonessential amino acids, sodium pyruvate, HEPES, penicillin, streptomycin, gentamicin, and 10% fetal calf serum at 10^5 cells/well. In addition, IL-2 (10 U/ ml), T-cell-depleted irradiated (3,000 rad) splenic feeder cells, and antigen were added and cultures incubated for 1, 3, or 6 days at 37 °C in 5% CO_2. Six hours prior to harvest, 0.5 μC of [^{3}H] thymidine was added. Proliferation was assessed by scintillation counting and expressed as a stimulation index (CPM-experimental/CPM-control). Soluble TT and CT-B were found to be rather poor inducers of proliferation, and for this reason we employed a modified method[29] of adsorbing these proteins to Polybead®-hydroxylate microspheres (1.0 μm; Polysciences Inc., Warrington, Pennsylvania). This procedure routinely yielded 0.5 μg of TT or CT-B adsorbed per 10^8 beads. Various bead-to-T-cell ratios were tested, and incubation varied for 1, 3, or 6 days. Optimal proliferative responses were obtained at an antigen-coated bead-to-T-cell ratio of 10 : 1 for both TT and CT-B coated beads after 6 days in culture. Stimulation indexes (E/C) of 40 to 60 were obtained with CD4[+] T cells isolated from Peyer's patch and spleen (data not shown). Controls consisted of cells only or incubation with the unrelated antigens keyhole limpet hemocyanin or diphtheria toxoid adsorbed to beads (E/C indexes of 2 or less). Having established conditions under which significant antigen-stimulated T-cell proliferation occurred, we examined the cytokine profiles of antigen-stimulated T cells by employing cytokine-specific ELISPOT assays.[30,31] FIGURE 6 illustrates the cytokine profiles obtained with T cells from Peyer's patch and spleen following oral immunization and cultured for 6 days in the presence of antigen-coated beads. IFN-γ and IL-2 ELISPOT assays were employed as indicative of a Th1-type profile,

TABLE 1. Oral Immunization with Tetanus Toxoid (TT) and Cholera Toxin (CT) Provides Protective Immunity to Tetanus Toxin[a]

Dose of Antigen (μg)	Reciprocal Log$_2$ Serum Anti-TT IgG Titer	Number of Mice Surviving at 96 Hours (4 per group)
CT (10)	0	0
TT (250)	11	0
TT (250) + CT (10)	17	4

[a] Naive mice were employed to establish the minimum lethal dose (MLD) of tetanus toxin (1 μg). Mice were orally immunized on days 0, 7, and 14 with CT, TT, or TT and CT. All groups were challenged subcutaneously with 100 MLDs of toxin on day 21.

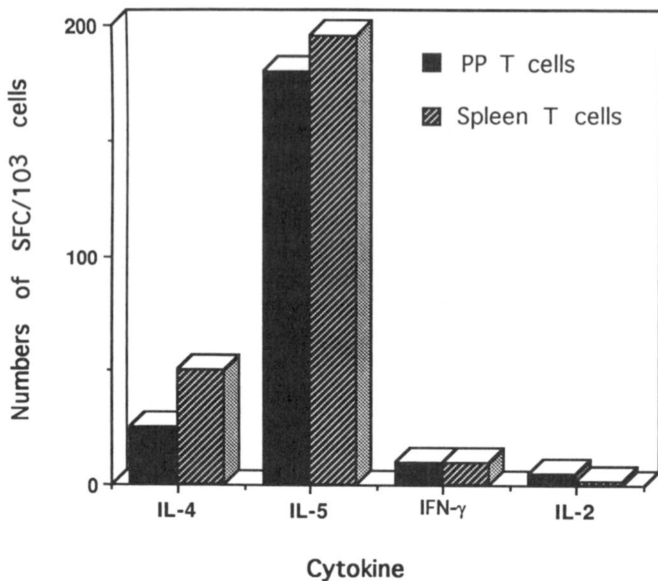

FIGURE 6. Cytokine profile of spleen and Peyer's patch T cells from mice orally immunized with TT and CT. The cytokine profile was determined by cytokine-specific ELISPOT assays after stimulation of purified CD4+ T cells *in vitro* with TT-coated beads. A bead-to-T-cell ratio of 10 : 1 was employed and assays were performed after 6 days in culture.[27]

while IL-4 and IL-5 ELISPOT assays were used as representative of a Th2-type response. Clearly, in both Peyer's patch and spleen, the number of T cells secreting IL-4 and IL-5 far outnumbered those secreting Th1-type cytokines throughout the culture period.

To confirm the ELISPOT data, both Northern blot analysis and reverse transcriptase-polymerase chain reaction (RT-PCR) experiments were performed. Cytokine-specific mRNA expression was assessed in Northern blot analyses with specific cDNA probes for IL-2, IFN-γ, IL-4, and IL-5. The results of these mRNA analyses correlated well with the ELISPOT assay. No mRNA or RT-PCR products for either IL-2 or IFN-γ were detected in mice orally immunized with TT plus CT following stimulation in an *in vitro* assay employing TT-coated latex microspheres. In contrast, both methods confirmed message for IL-4 and IL-5 in purified CD4+ T cells from Peyer's patch and spleen. The data suggest that in mice orally immunized with TT and CT, a strong Th2-type response occurred both systemically (spleen) and in the intestinal mucosa (Peyer's patch).

The cytokine profiles from Peyer's patch T cells of mice orally immunized with TT only and TT plus CT are presented in FIGURE 7. Although low in number, Peyer's patch CD4+ T cells from mice immunized with TT only presented a Th2-type profile. This profile was considerably skewed in favor of the Th2-profile in mice immunized with TT and CT as adjuvant. This suggests that the adjuvant effect of CT involves stimulation of TT-responsive Th2-type cells. The molecular mechanism(s) for this

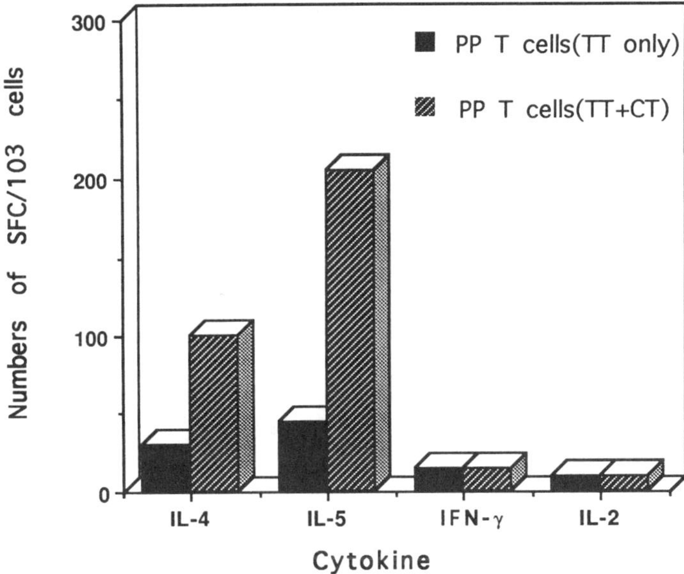

FIGURE 7. The adjuvant CT stimulates TT-specific CD4[+] T cells in Peyer's patch. T cells from mice orally immunized with TT and CT or TT only were isolated on day 21 and stimulated for 6 days *in vitro* with TT adsorbed beads. The cytokine profile revealed that CT enhances the Th2-type TT-specific T-cell populations.[27]

upregulation remains to be elucidated. However, it seems clear that skewing to antigen-specific Th2 cells *in vivo* would constitute a major route whereby an immune response is generated to coadministered proteins when CT is employed as an adjuvant. The high-serum IgG_1 anti-TT titers, the rise in serum IgE levels, the elevated fecal anti-TT IgA titers, ELISPOT LPL IgA data, and cytokine patterns of antigen-stimulated CD4[+] T cells from both Peyer's patch and spleen are all consistent with oral immunization employing CT as an adjuvant inducing a strong anti-TT–specific Th2-type response in both the mucosal and the systemic immune compartments.

T Helper Cell Responses in Systemically Immunized Mice

To determine whether the route of administration influenced Th cell responses, mice were immunized intraperitoneally with 10 μg of TT with and without 1 μg of CT on day 0 or day 14 (primary and secondary immunizations, respectively). Mice were killed 1 week following immunization. Spleen CD4[+] T cells were cultured for 6 days, and the numbers of cytokine-secreting cells evaluated by cytokine-specific ELISPOT assays. FIGURE 8 illustrates these results. In contrast to oral immunization, interperitoneal immunization resulted in high frequencies of both Th1- and Th2-type cells in spleen. At the time points chosen to evaluate cytokine production (i.e., 1 week after primary or secondary immunizations) no distinct T-cell subset pattern

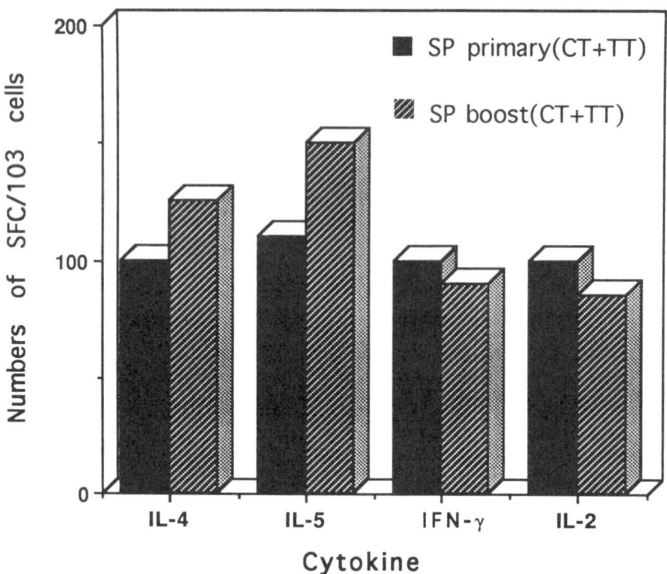

FIGURE 8. Systemic immunization with TT and CT promotes induction of both Th1- and Th2-type TT-specific T cells in spleen. Mice were systemically immunized with TT and CT and CD4+ T cells isolated from spleen 1 week following primary or secondary immunization. The cells were cultured *in vitro* with TT-coated beads for 6 days and the cytokine-secreting cells were enumerated by ELISPOT assays.[27]

was evident. These results argue that the adjuvant effect of systemically delivered CT does not discriminate between subsets. Yet, the IgG subclass analysis (to be described) revealed a predominant IgG_1 serum response with considerably lower IgG_{2a} titers, indicative of Th2-type responses. The known redundancy, synergism, and antagonism within the complex cytokine network[15,16] suggests that cyokines other than those detected in the ELISPOT assay may influence IgG subclass responses. It is also uncertain how antigen-presenting cells or other accessory cells influence T-cell cytokine patterns or regulate Ig isotype selection. Clearly, our knowledge of the cytokine network and cellular regulation of immune responses is far from complete.

MICROSPHERES AS AN ORAL DELIVERY SYSTEM FOR TETANUS TOXOID

Our research efforts evaluating microspheres and live attenuated vectors (in the following section) for use as oral vaccines are ongoing, and current data are less extensive than is the soluble TT and CT adjuvant model just described.

Soluble proteins encapsulated in 50 : 50 poly D-L-lactide-co-glycolide microspheres delivered systemically and orally were previously demonstrated to stimulate both the systemic and mucosal immune systems.[32] In collaboration with Southern

Research Institute we are investigating the parameters required for efficient encapsulation of TT and monitoring the immune responses both systemically and in mucosal sites. Microspheres composed of poly D-L-lactide-co-glycocide are an attractive delivery vehicle for the following reasons: (1) they are nonimmunogenic, (2) they decompose nonenzymatically and release antigen based on their lactide-to-glycolide ratio and therefore preparations may contain relatively quick releasing populations together with more sustained antigen-releasing populations, (3) microspheres are nontoxic and degrade into the normal metabolites lactic and glycolic acids, and (4) encapsulation provides antigen protection from low stomach pH and the multitude of proteases encountered in the gastrointestinal tract when antigen is administered orally.

Microsphere preparations containing TT were routinely analyzed for antigen content (core loading), *in vitro* protein release characteristics, particle size distribution, and total recovery of TT. *In vitro* release characteristics were determined by the addition of microspheres into 2 ml of 0.1N HCl. After 2 hours at 37°C the microspheres were harvested and the HCl solution was replaced with 0.05 M phosphate buffer, pH 6.8. Incubation was continued, buffer replaced at 6, 24, and 48 hours, and protein content assayed by conventional methods. *In vitro* release of protein ranged from 4% to 26% of total protein and varied with form of toxoid (i.e., soluble or lyophilized) and buffer composition used during encapsulation. The majority of preparations released less than 10% of total entrapped proteins in the *in vitro* assay. The size distribution of particles was analyzed employing a Malvern Particle Size Analyzer (Malvern Instruments, Malvern, England) and data were expressed as volume distributions by microsphere diameter. Most preparations exhibited greater than 85% of particles in a range of $1-10$ μm.

The microencapsulation process requires the use of organic solvent (we have primarily employed ethyl acetate) and thus may affect the antigenicity of certain proteins. We have, therefore, as a type of control, injected mice subcutaneously to determine retention of antigenicity. The endpoint titers obtained following subcutaneous injection also serve as a reference for evaluation of systemic responses to the same preparation of orally administered microspheres.

When a typical batch of TT microspheres containing approximately 100 μg of antigen was injected subcutaneously, serum IgG titers of approximately 1 : 30,000 were obtained 4 weeks following immunization. Mice were boosted at 6 weeks with an identical dose of microspheres, and serum IgG endpoint titers rose to several million. Fecal extracts from these mice, as expected, failed to reveal any detectable mucosal anti-TT-specific responses. Mice orally immunized with the same dose of microspheres failed to elicit a primary response. However, following two additional boosts, serum anti-TT-specific IgG levels reached endpoint titers comparable to those obtained with orally administered soluble TT and CT. Antigen-specific serum IgM or IgA was not detected. Although a weak transient mucosal IgA response was noted 4 weeks following the initial boost, no significant anti-TT IgA titers were observed following a second boost. In parallel with these studies, we orally immunized mice with the same lot of TT containing microspheres and 10 μg of exogenous CT. Somewhat surprisingly we found anti-TT-specific IgG responses 2 weeks after the initial immunization and after boosting, anti-TT IgG and IgA levels comparable to levels obtained following three oral immunizations with soluble TT and CT. However, significant mucosal IgA and anti-TT responses required a third immunization with microspheres, and anti-TT IgA responses were seen transiently 3 to 4 weeks following the boost. These results clearly indicate that CT serves as an adjuvant when given with microspheres. While we previously showed that low concentrations (10 μg) of soluble TT when given orally with CT induced serum IgG anti-TT titers of 1 : 32,000 following three oral immunizations, the microsphere preparation employed in these studies released less than 5% of the antigen content in *in vitro* studies over a 48-hour period. Given the limited time frame in which CT is capable of serving as an adjuvant for coadministered soluble proteins[33] and the half-life of 50 : 50 poly-D-L-lactide-co-glycolide microspheres, it seems unlikely that a small initial "burst" phase and release of antigen could account for these results. Alternatively, CT may act by increasing the permeability of the gut, thereby increasing uptake of microspheres from the gastrointestinal tract. We are currently encapsulating known adjuvants into microspheres with antigen in an effort to enhance both systemic and mucosal immune responses.

ORAL IMMUNIZATION WITH RECOMBINANT *S. typhimurium* EXPRESSING THE TOX-C FRAGMENT

A third oral antigen delivery system that we are investigating in collaboration with Dr. S. Chatfield of Medeva Group Research, Vaccine Research Unit, Imperial College of Science and Technology, London, UK, is a live vector expressing the Tox-C fragment of tetanus toxoid.[34] Two recombinant strains were constructed by Dr. Chatfield's group from the attenuated *Aro A, Aro D* parent strain BRD 509. BRD 753 contains the plasmid pTET85 which controls fragment C expression from the *tac* promoter, and expression is constitutive since the organism lacks the *lac I* repressor gene. A second construct, BRD 847, contains the pTET *nir* 15 plasmid, and Tox-C expression is controlled by the anaerobically inducible *nir* B promoter.

BALB/c and C57BL/6 mice were orally immunized with 10^{12} colony-forming units (cfus) of BRD 509, BRD 753, and BRD 847 and boosted orally on day 29 with 5×10^9 cfus. Mice were monitored for both serum and mucosal anti-TT antibody responses at weekly intervals. By day 35 serum IgG antibody levels in both strains of mice intubated with BRD 847 had titers comparable to those of mice receiving soluble TT and the adjuvant CT. Strain BRD 753 induced much lower titers, whereas the parent strain of BRD 509 did not induce detectable antibody.

Mucosal IgA titers against fragment C in BALB/c mice were low, and a weak response was detected only on day 35. In contrast, C57BL/6 mice exhibited a relatively strong mucosal IgA response by day 28 which was maintained through day 42. We do not understand the disparity in inducing mucosal IgA responses in BALB/c *versus* 57BL/6 mice, although it may be related to the intrinsic protective mechanisms of the two strains of mice. Invasion through Peyer's patch into the mesenteric lymph nodes and thus into the bloodstream through the thoracic duct may be more rapid in BALB/c mice, whereas in C57BL/6 mice the mucosal tissues may tend to limit invasion and thus are exposed to higher levels of antigen. Enumeration of colony-forming units at various time intervals following infection in Peyer's patches and other tissues may provide some clues as to the rapidity of infection in the two mouse strains.

TABLE 2. IgG Subclass Distribution Induced by Various Tetanus Toxoid (TT) Oral Delivery Systems[a]

IgG Subclass	TT + CT	TT Microspheres	TT Microspheres + CT	*Salmonella* Tox-C
			Delivery Systems	
IgG_1	100%	>99%	>99%	3%
IgG_2	ND	<1%	<1%	97%

ABBREVIATIONS: CT = cholera toxin; ND = not detected.
[a] Values expressed as approximate percentage of total anti-TT IgG at peak responses.

SUMMARY

We have not yet directly examined the Th cell responses induced by using *Salmonella/* BRD 847 as a vector nor have we performed these experiments following immunization with microspheres. However, production of high serum levels of antigen-specific IgG_1 may be indicative of a Th2-type response, whereas high serum levels of IgG_{2a} may reflect a Th1-type response. An important issue in using various oral delivery systems is whether the system(s) employed affects the Th cell response to the same antigen. We therefore analyzed the serum antigen-specific IgG subclasses induced in each of the model systems we studied. TABLE 2 presents these results. Clearly, oral administration of soluble TT with CT as an adjuvant induced an IgG_1 subclass, and encapsulation of TT within microspheres had no effect on this Th2-type response. On the other hand, oral immunization with live *Salmonella* expressing fragment C of tetanus toxin induced a strong IgG_{2a} subclass response indicative of a Th1-type response. It should be noted that protection against a lethal TT challenge was afforded by elevated levels of both anti-TT IgG_1 and IgG_{2a} subclasses.[26,34] We intend to examine the cytokine profiles in spleen $CD4^+$ T cells from mice immunized with microspheres or *Salmonella* following *in vitro* antigen stimulation to confirm the T helper type responses suggested by the IgG subclass data.

It will also be important to examine the cytokine patterns induced in Peyer's patch $CD4^+$ T cells following immunization of C57BL/6 with *Salmonella*/BRD 847. Whereas analysis of the serum IgG subclass profile indicated a strong IgG_{2a} response and thus a systemic Th1-type pattern, this vector also induced a good mucosal IgA response. If our current hypothesis concerning S-IgA production is correct,[28] we would expect a predominant Th2-type profile in $CD4^+$ T cells from Peyer's patch in these mice. Such a result would emphasize the bifurcation of T-cell responses in the systemic *versus* the mucosal immune environments.

The data obtained to date suggest that adjuvants and various vehicle delivery systems may influence the induction of distinct T helper cell subsets to a specific antigen. The unique cytokine arrays produced by these T-cell subsets influence the immune responses in terms of systemic Ig subclasses produced, cell-mediated immune responses, and the production of mucosal S-IgA antibodies. Although additional studies are necessary, the manipulation of T-cell subsets employing adjuvants, antigen packaging, or perhaps even the addition of individual cytokines to various formulations holds significant promise for optimizing immune responses to orally administered vaccines.

ACKNOWLEDGMENT

We thank Julia Hagle for typing this paper.

REFERENCES

1. INSTITUTE OF MEDICINE. 1986. New Vaccine Development Establishing Priorities. Vol. 2. National Academy Press. Washington, DC.
2. ROBBINS, A., P. FREEMAN & K. R. POWELL. 1993. International childhood vaccine initiative. Pediatr. Infect. Dis. J. **12:** 523–527.
3. MCGHEE, J. R. & H. KIYONO. 1993. New perspectives in vaccine development: Mucosal immunity to infections. Infectious Agents and Disease, in press.
4. HOLMGREN, J., C. CZERKINSKY, N. LYCKE & A. SVENNERHOLM. 1992. Mucosal immunity: Implications for vaccine development. Immunobiology **184:** 157–159.
5. CONLEY, M. E. & D. L. DELACROIX. 1987. Intravascular and mucosal immunoglobulin A: Two separate but related systems of immune defense? Ann. Intern. Med. **106:** 892–899.
6. MESTECKY, J. & J. R. MCGHEE. 1987. Immunoglobulin A (IgA): Molecular and cellular interactions involved in IgA biosynthesis and immune response. Adv. Immunol. **40:** 153–245.
7. CRAIG, S. W. & J. J. CEBRA. 1974. Peyer's patches: An enriched source of precursors for IgA-producing immunocytes in the rabbit. J. Exp. Med. **134:** 188–200.
8. LEBMAN, D. A., P. M. GRIFFIN & J. J. CEBRA. 1987. Relationship between expression of IgA by Peyer's patch cells and functional IgA memory cells. J. Exp. Med. **166:** 1405–1418.
9. MCGHEE, J. R., J. MESTECKY, C. O. ELSON & H. KIYONO. 1989. Regulation of IgA synthesis and immune response by T cells and interleukins. J. Clin. Immunol. **9:** 175–199.
10. OWEN, R. L. & P. NEMANIC. 1978. Antigen processing structures of the mammalian intestinal tract: An SEM study of lymphoepithelial organs. Scanning Electron Microsc. **2:** 367–378.
11. NEUTRA, M. R., T. L. PHILLIPS, E. L. MAYER & D. J. FISHKIND. 1987. Transport of membrane-bound macromolecules by M cells in follicle-associated epithelium of rabbit Peyer's patch. Cell Tissue Res. **247:** 537–546.
12. PAPPO, J. & T. H. ERMAK. 1989. Uptake and translocation of fluorescent latex particles by rabbit Peyer's patch follicle epithelium: A quantitative model for M cell uptake. Clin. Exp. Immunol. **76:** 144–148.
13. GOWANS, J. L. & E. J. KNIGHT. 1964. The route of re-circulation of lymphocytes in the rat. Proc. R. Soc. Lond. B. Biol. Sci. **159:** 257–282.
14. MCDERMOTT, M. & J. BIENENSTOCK. 1979. Evidence for a common mucosal immunologic system. I. Migration of B immunoblasts into intestinal, respiratory and genital tissues. J. Immunol. **122:** 1892–1898.
15. MOSMANN, T. R. & R. L. COFFMAN. 1989. Th1 and Th2 cells: Different patterns of lymphokine secretion lead to different functional properties. Annu. Rev. Immunol. **7:** 145–173.

16. FINKLEMAN, F. D., J. HOLMES, I. M. KATONA, J. F. URBAN, JR.. M. P. BECKMANN, L. S. PARK, K. A. SCHOOLEY, R. L. COFFMAN, T. R. MOSMANN & W. E. PAUL. 1990. Lymphokine control of *in vivo* immunoglobulin isotype selection. Annu. Rev. Immunol. **8:** 303-333.

17. BEAGLEY K. W., J. H. ELDRIDGE, H. KIYONO, M. P. EVERSON, W. J. KOOPMAN, T. HONJO & J. R. McGHEE. 1988. Recombinant murine IL-5 induces high rate IgA synthesis in cycling IgA positive Peyer's patch B cells. J. Immunol. **141:** 2035-2042.

18. BEAGLEY, K. W., J. H. ELDRIDGE, F. LEE, H. KIYONO, M. P. EVERSON, W. J. KOOPMAN, T. HIRANO, T. KISHIMOTO & J. R. McGHEE. 1989. Interleukins and IgA synthesis. Human and murine interleukin 6 induce high rate IgA secretion in IgA-committed B cells. J. Exp. Med. **169:** 2133-2148.

19. PARRONCHI, P., M. DE CARLI, R. MANETTI, C. SIMONELLIE, S. SAMPOGNARO, M. PICCINNI, M. DONATELLA, E. MAGGI, G. DELPRETE & S. ROMAGNANI. 1992. IL-4 and IFN (α and γ) exert opposite regulatory effects on the development of cytolytic potential by Th1 or Th2 human T cell clones. J. Immunol. **149:** 2977-2983.

20. SCOTT, P. 1991. IFN-γ modulates the early development of the Th1 and Th2 responses in murine model of cutaneous leishmaniasis. J. Immunol. **147:** 3149-3155.

21. WEAVER, C. T., C. M. HAWRYLOWICZ & E. R. URANUE. 1988. T helper cell subsets require the expression of distinct costimulatory signals by antigen presenting cells. Proc. Natl. Acad. Sci. USA **85:** 8181-8185.

22. SPALDING, D., S. WILLIAMSON, W. KOOPMAN & J. R. McGHEE. 1984. Preferential induction of polyclonal IgA secretion by murine Peyer's patch dendritic cell-T cell mixtures. J. Exp. Med. **160:** 941-946.

23. TOMASI, T. B., JR. 1980. Oral tolerance. Transplantation **29:** 353-356.

24. ELSON, C. O. & W. EALDING. 1984. Cholera toxin feeding did not induce oral tolerance in mice and abrogated oral tolerance to an unrelated protein antigen. J. Immunol. **133:** 2892-2897.

25. CLEMENTS, J. D., N. M. HARTZOG & F. L. LYON. 1988. Adjuvant activity of *Escherichia coli* heat-labile enterotoxin and effect on the induction of oral tolerance in mice to unrelated protein antigens. Vaccine **6:** 269-277.

26. JACKSON, R. J., K. FUJIHASHI, J. XU-AMANO, H. KIYONO, C. O. ELSON & J. R. McGHEE. 1993. Optimizing oral vaccines: Induction of systemic and mucosal B cell and antibody responses to tetanus toxoid by use of cholera toxin as adjuvant. Infect. Immun. **61:** 4272-4279.

27. XU-AMANO, J., H. KIYONO, R. J. JACKSON, H. F. STAATS, K. FUJIHASHI, P. D. BURROWS, C. O. ELSON, S. PILLAI & J. R. McGHEE. 1993. Helper T cell subsets for immunoglobulin A responses: Oral immunization with tetanus toxoid and cholera toxin as adjuvant selectively induces Th2 cells in mucosa-associated tissues. J. Exp. Med. **168:** 1309-1320.

28. XU-AMANO, J. W., K. AICHER, T. TAGUCHI, H. KIYONO & J. R. McGHEE. 1992. Selective induction of Th2 cells in murine Peyer's patches by oral immunization. Intern. Immunol. **4:** 433-445.

29. WU, J. Y., C. H. RIGGIN, J. R. SEALS, C. I. MURPHY & M. J. NEWMAN. 1991. *In vitro* measurements of antigen-specific cell-mediated immune responses using recombinant HIV-1 proteins adsorbed to latex microspheres. J. Immunol. Methods **143:** 1-9.

30. TAGUCHI, T., J. R. McGHEE, R. L. COFFMAN, K. W. BEAGLEY, J. H. ELDRIDGE, K. TAKATSU & H. KIYONO. 1990. Detection of individual mouse splenic T cells producing IFN-γ and IL-5 using the enzyme-linked immunospot (ELISPOT) assay. J. Immunol. Methods **128:** 65-72.

31. FUJIHASHI, K., J. R. McGHEE, K. W. BEAGLEY & H. KIYONO. 1993. Cytokine specific ELISPOT assay: Single cell analysis of IL-2, IL-4, and IL-6 producing cells. J. Immunol. Methods **160:** 181-189.

32. ELDRIDGE, J. H., C. J. HAMMOND, J. A. MEULKBROEK, J. K. STASS, R. M. GILLEY & T. R. TICE. 1990. Controlled vaccine release in the gut-associated lymphoid tissues. I. Orally administered biodegradable microspheres target the Peyer's patches. J. Controlled Release **11:** 205-214.

33. DERTZBAUGH, M. T. & C. O. ELSON. 1991. Cholera toxin as a mucosal adjuvant. *In* Topics in Vaccine Adjuvant Research. D. R. Spriggs & W. C. Koff, Eds.: 119-131. CRC Press. Boca Raton, FL.

34. CHATFIELD, S. N., I. G. CHARLES, A. J. MAKOFF, M. D. OXER, G. DOUGAN, D. PICKARD, D. SLATER & N. F. FAIRWEATHER. 1992. Use of the nirB promoter to direct the stable expression of heterologous antigens in *Salmonella* oral vaccine strains: Development of a single-dose oral tetanus vaccine. Biotechnology **10:** 888-892.

Clinical Use of Hematopoietic Growth Factors for Control of Infections after High-Dose Chemotherapy

JAMES M. FELSER

Cytokine Development Unit
Sandoz Pharmaceuticals Corporation
East Hanover, New Jersey 07936

Myelosuppression, particularly neutropenia, is a major dose-limiting side effect of many of the cytotoxic chemotherapeutic drugs that are used in clinical practice. Despite dramatic improvements in cancer management, the mortality rate among patients with documented infections (in particular, gram-negative bacteremia) remains at approximately 10%.[1] The risk of infection is directly related to the severity and duration of neutropenia; as the absolute neutrophil count drops below 500/μL, the risk of infection increases; when the absolute neutrophil count is less than 100/μL, both the incidence of severe infection and the mortality rate are increased.[2] To reduce severe neutropenia and decrease the risk of life-threatening infections, the prescribed dose of chemotherapy is usually reduced and/or chemotherapy is delayed.

The administration of cytotoxic drugs in dose-intensive regimens represents an effort to improve response rates in patients with potentially curable malignancies. However, the use of such regimens had been limited by increased morbidity associated with severe bone marrow suppression and abnormalities in cellular and humoral immune defense mechanisms.

The management of bone marrow toxicity associated with high-dose, potentially curative chemotherapy has benefited from advances in the clinical use of hematopoietic growth factors, bone marrow transplantation, and/or peripheral blood progenitor cell transplantation. Increasingly, hematopoietic growth factors are being evaluated and used not only to accelerate the recovery of myelopoiesis following high-dose chemotherapy in cancer patients, but also to permit the dose escalation of chemotherapy.

THE HEMATOPOIETIC CASCADE AND HEMATOPOIETIC GROWTH FACTORS

The bone marrow compartment contains blood cells in various stages of development. These cells include pluripotent stem cells as well as relatively undifferentiated

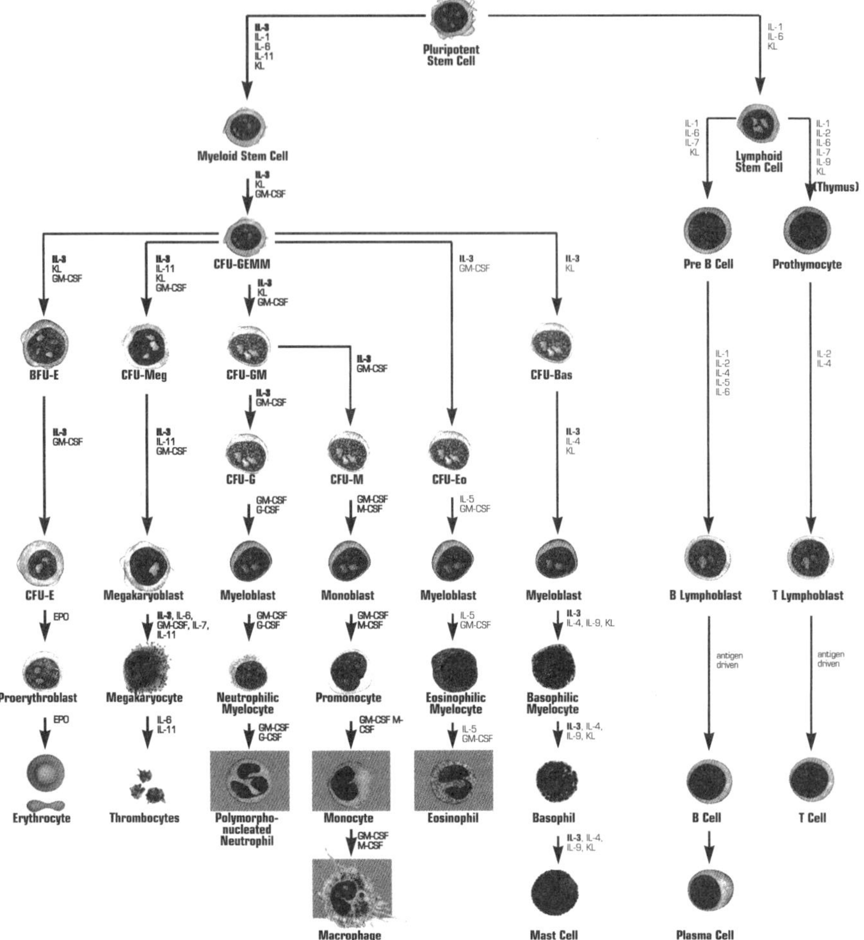

FIGURE 1. The hematopoietic cascade.

multilineage progenitor cells that are the precursors for the cells of myeloid, lymphoid, and megakaryocytic lineages (FIG. 1).

The differentiation and proliferation of both myeloid and lymphoid progenitor cells as well as many of the functions of mature blood cells are under the regulation of hematopoietic growth factors.

With the advent of recombinant DNA technology, growth factors have become available for preclinical and clinical investigations. Growth factors that have demonstrated clinical efficacy include erythropoietin, granulocyte colony-stimulating factor (G-CSF), and granulocyte-macrophage colony-stimulating factor (GM-CSF). Growth factors that are under clinical development include interleukin-3 (IL-3) and interleukin-6 (IL-6).

TABLE 1. Biologic Effects of GM-CSF on Mature Myeloid Cell Functions[a]

Neutrophils	*Mononuclear Phagocytes*
Prolonged *in vitro* survival	Enhanced cytotoxicity
Increased expression of adhesion proteins	Enhanced intracellular killing
Membrane ruffling	Increased phagocytosis
Decreased random migration	Potentiation of antigen processing
Increased chemotaxis	Increased HIV replication
Increased protein synthesis	*Eosinophils*
Priming for enhanced oxidative metabolism	Prolonged *in vitro* survival
Priming for increased release of arachidonic acid and leukotriene β_4	Increased antibody-dependent cytotoxicity
Priming for degranulation, PAF production	Priming for increased leukotriene C_4 release
Enhanced phagocytosis and intracellular killing	
Enhanced antibody-dependent cytotoxicity	

[a] Reprinted with permission from Glaspy and Golde.[6]

G-CSF, GM-CSF, AND IL-3

Effect on Regulation of Hematopoiesis

G-CSF preferentially stimulates the development of neutrophils from committed granulocytic progenitor cells.[3] GM-CSF preferentially induces the growth and development of neutrophil and monocyte/macrophage progenitor cells. GM-CSF also acts synergistically with other factors to stimulate blast colony-forming units (CFU-blasts), colony-forming units – granulocyte, erythrocyte, monocyte, and megakaryocyte (CFU-GEMMs), and eosinophils.[3] IL-3, a relatively early-acting growth factor, directly stimulates proliferation and development of pluripotent stem cells, multilineage myeloid progenitor cells, and megakaryocytes.[4,5]

Effect on Mature Cell Function

The activity of G-CSF is restricted to neutrophils, enhancing both cytotoxicity and phagocytosis. The effects of G-CSF are generally of smaller magnitude than are those of GM-CSF. GM-CSF, in addition to stimulating cytotoxic and phagocytic responses in neutrophils, also plays an important role in host defense by inducing inflammatory and immune responses of monocytes and macrophages. Some of the functions enhanced include antigen presentation, chemotaxis, adherence, phagocytosis, oxidative metabolism, and microbicidal activity against bacteria as well as fungi such as candida and aspergillus. The biologic effects of GM-CSF are summarized in TABLE 1.[6] IL-3, which is primarily active in the early stages of hematopoiesis, does not affect mature neutrophil function, but IL-3 does increase the cytotoxic and phagocytic activity of eosinophils.[6]

In theory, the respective functions of hematopoietic growth factors suggest that the combination of early- and late-acting growth factors, particularly when they are administered sequentially, may be the most efficient way to restore mature blood-forming cells after myelosuppressive chemotherapy.

CLINICAL STUDIES USING RECOMBINANT HUMAN G-CSF AND GM-CSF

For both G-CSF and GM-CSF, reduction in the duration of neutropenia, infectious episodes, number of days of intravenous antibiotic usage, and duration of hospitalization after chemotherapy has now been demonstrated in several clinical trials. G-CSF increases neutrophil counts in patients with advanced neoplasms, thus reducing the magnitude of chemotherapy-induced neutropenia.[1,7] G-CSF has also been reported to enhance neutrophil recovery following high-dose chemotherapy and autologous bone marrow transplantation.[8]

Similarly, the administration of GM-CSF to patients with advanced sarcoma before and after cytotoxic chemotherapy accelerated the recovery of neutrophils and reduced the period of neutropenia.[9] Additionally, the use of GM-CSF has been shown to be beneficial in the autologous bone marrow transplantation setting.[10,11] In a study of 128 patients with lymphoid malignancies after autologous bone marrow transplantation, GM-CSF significantly reduced the interval of profound granulocytopenia compared with placebo.[10] Although the incidence of fever was similar in GM-CSF and placebo-treated patients, significant decreases in the incidence of documented infections, duration of antimicrobial therapy, and duration of hospitalization after transplantation were reported. Of interest, streptococcal bacteremia, usually associated with indwelling catheters, was the only documented bacterial infection in patients receiving GM-CSF; additionally, two patients had candida infections. By contrast, patients receiving placebo had infections involving several different organisms including fusobacterium, corynebacterium, staphylococcus, and legionella in addition to streptococcus. Furthermore, two control patients had disseminated aspergillosis and two patients had candida fungemia.[10]

With the widespread clinical use of G-CSF and GM-CSF, these cytokines alone are recognized as efficacious in ameliorating neutropenia and thus reducing the predisposition for infection in cancer patients. However, it has also become apparent that recovery from thrombocytopenia has not been affected by these growth factors; the treatment of thrombocytopenia still relies on the administration of platelet transfusions.

CLINICAL STUDIES USING RECOMBINANT HUMAN IL-3 ALONE

The hematologic activity of IL-3 has been investigated in phase I/II clinical studies. When administered as a single agent, IL-3 has shown clear but inconsistent biologic activity in patients with normal or myelosuppressed hematologic function.

TABLE 2. Biologic Effect of IL-3 after Autologous Bone Marrow Transplantation in Lymphoma Patients Compared with Historical Data[a]

	Placebo	GM-CSF	IL-3
No. of patients	63	65	16
Day ANC $\geq$100/μL	15	14	12
Day ANC $\geq$1000/μL	33	26	23
Day of platelet transfusion independence	29	26	26
Infection (days 0–28)	19%	3%	12%

ABBREVIATION: ANC = absolute neutrophil count.

[a] From Nemunaitis *et al.*[15]

In patients with normal hematopoietic function, IL-3 induced a multilineage response, including increased numbers of circulating leukocytes, platelets, and reticulocytes.[12] When administered to patients with cancer or bone marrow failure states, IL-3 showed activity in restoring multilineage hematopoietic function in some patients and variably reduced the neutropenia and thrombocytopenia associated with chemotherapy-induced myelotoxicity.[12–14]

To evaluate the effects of IL-3 in a more dose-intensive chemotherapy setting, Nemunaitis *et al.*[15] studied IL-3 alone in patients with lymphoid malignancies who received autologous bone marrow transplantation after myeloablative chemotherapy. The hematologic activity of IL-3 was compared to historical data from lymphoma patients who underwent autologous bone marrow transplantation and received either GM-CSF or placebo.[10]

In patients who received IL-3, recovery of neutrophils to an absolute neutrophil count >100/μL occurred earlier than in the historical cohort that received GM-CSF. The time to platelet transfusion independence in IL-3-treated patients, although shorter than in the placebo cohort, was similar to that in the GM-CSF-treated group (TABLE 2).

CYTOKINE COMBINATIONS

When administered as single agents, most cytokines have shown either limited or variable biologic activity. However, the use of cytokines in combination has the potential to expand the range of responding hematopoietic cell populations. Recent studies suggest that cytokine combinations may be clinically important after myeloablative chemotherapy when both neutropenia and thrombocytopenia may be dose-limiting toxicities. For example, the use of early-acting cytokines such as IL-3 combined with late-acting factors such as GM-CSF has theoretical advantages; the early-acting growth factor expands the pool of hematopoietic progenitor cells, whereas the late-acting growth factor induces the proliferation and differentiation of mature blood cells.

CLINICAL STUDIES WITH IL-3 AND GM-CSF

A phase I/II study in patients with refractory lymphoma was conducted to evaluate the effects of the sequential use of IL-3 and GM-CSF on hematopoietic recovery after ABMT.[16] IL-3, at dosages of 2.5 or 5 μg/kg/day, was administered subcutaneously for 5 or 10 days followed by GM-CSF (250 μg/m^2 per day) until a sustained absolute neutrophil count $\geq$1,500/μL was obtained. Preliminary data suggest that IL-3 and GM-CSF are reasonably well tolerated in this setting. Additionally, a sustained absolute neutrophil count of $\geq$1,000/μL was noted at a median of 12.5 days (range 11–26), and a sustained platelet count of $\geq$20,000/μL was seen at a median of 11.5 days (range 5–22).[16] These data suggest that the cytokine combination may be superior to GM-CSF with respect to platelet engraftment.

FUTURE PROSPECTS OF COLONY-STIMULATING FACTORS

As dose escalation of chemotherapy becomes more widely practiced, the role of cytokines will become increasingly important. Combinations of cytokines provide a flexible approach to expand the range of hematopoietic response to meet individual needs. Combining IL-3 with G-CSF or GM-CSF permits the expansion of progenitor cells as well as neutrophils and/or monocytes to augment host defense. To optimize platelet response, one approach that is being investigated is to combine IL-3 with IL-6, to potentiate the thrombopoietic effect of IL-6. In preclinical studies using a primate model system, the sequential combination of IL-3 and IL-6 has already demonstrated a synergistic effect on platelet production.[17] Using such combination therapies to overcome the myelotoxic effects of chemotherapy may provide the means to escalate the dose of chemotherapeutic drugs in order to achieve better tumor response rates in cancer patients.

CONCLUSIONS

1. Although GM-CSF and G-CSF are clinically useful in accelerating recovery from neutropenia and thus reducing the risk of infection, they have not been overly beneficial in treating or preventing thrombocytopenia.

2. In high-dose chemotherapy settings in which bone marrow recovery may be prolonged, treatment with early- and late-acting hematopoietic growth factors may provide the optimal strategy for expansion of progenitor cells and amelioration of the complications from both neutropenia and thrombocytopenia.

3. Preliminary phase I/II clinical data suggest that sequentially administered IL-3 and GM-CSF accelerate recovery from both neutropenia and thrombocytopenia in lymphoma patients who receive myeloablative chemotherapy followed by autologous bone marrow transplantation. Phase III investigations are ongoing in this clinical setting.

SUMMARY

Hematopoietic growth factors are being used to accelerate the recovery of myelopoiesis following high-dose chemotherapy in cancer patients. G-CSF and GM-CSF reduce the duration of neutropenia following chemotherapy. Rapid restoration of neutrophils has been associated with reduced incidence of neutropenic fever and documented infections and fewer days of intravenous antibiotics and hospitalization.

Recent studies suggest that combinations of cytokines may further expand the hematopoietic cell populations, which may be particularly useful following myeloablative chemotherapy, when thrombocytopenia may be a dose-limiting toxicity. For example, IL-3, which stimulates early progenitor cells, has definite but inconsistent effects on increasing neutrophil and platelet counts. However, in combination with later-acting cytokines (e.g., GM-CSF and IL-6), recovery from both thrombocytopenia and neutropenia is accelerated. As dose escalation of chemotherapy becomes more widely practiced, the role of cytokine combinations will become increasingly important.

REFERENCES

1. CRAWFORD, J., H. OZER, R. STOLLER, D. JOHNSON, G. LYMAN, I. TABBARA, M. KRIS, J. GROUS, V. PICOZZI, G. RAUSCH, R. SMITH, W. GRADISHAR, A. YAHANDA, M. VINCENT, M. STEWART & J. GLASPY. 1991. Reduction by granulocyte colony-stimulating factor of fever and neutropenia induced by chemotherapy in patients with small-cell lung cancer. N. Engl. J. Med. **325:** 164– 170.

2. BODEY, G. P., M. BUCKLEY, Y. S. SATHE & E. J. FREIREICH. 1966. Quantitative relationships between circulating leukocytes and infection in patients with acute leukemia. Ann. Intern. Med. **64:** 328–340.

3. CLARK, S. C. & R. KAMEN. 1987. The human hematopoietic colony-stimulating factors. Science **236:** 1229–1237.

4. VALENT, P., K. GEISSLER, C. SILLABER, K. LECHNER & P. BETTELHEIM. 1990. Why clinicians should be interested in interleukin-3. Blut **61:** 338–345.

5. GROOPMAN, J. E., J. M. MOLINA & D. T. SCADDEN. 1989. Hematopoietic growth factors: Biology and clinical applications. N. Engl. J. Med. **321:** 1449–1459.

6. GLASPY, J. A. & D. W. GOLDE. 1990. The colony-stimulating factors: Biology and clinical use. Oncology **4:** 25–34.

7. PETTENGELL, R., H. GURNEY, J. A. RADFORD, D. P. DEAKIN, R. JAMES, P. M. WILKINSON, K. KANE, J. BENTLEY & D. CROWTHER. 1992. Granulocyte colony-stimulating factor to prevent dose-limiting neutropenia in non-Hodgkin's lymphoma: A randomized controlled trial. Blood **80:** 1430–1436.

8. SHERIDAN, W. P., G. MORSTYN, M. WOLF, A. DODDS, J. LUSK, D. MAHER, J. E. LAYTON, M. D. GREEN, L. SOUZA & R. M. FOX. 1989. Granulocyte colony-stimulating factor and neutrophil recovery after high-dose chemotherapy and autologous bone marrow transplantation. Lancet **2:** 891–895.

9. ANTMAN, K. S., J. D. GRIFFIN, A. ELIAS, M. A. SOCINSKI, L. RYAN, S. A. CANNISTRA, D. OETTE, M. WHITLEY, E. FREI, III & L. E. SCHNIPPER. 1988. Effect of recombinant human granulocyte-macrophage colony-stimulating factor on chemotherapy-induced myelosuppression. N. Engl. J. Med. **319:** 593–598.

10. NEMUNAITIS, J., S. N. RABINOWE, J. W. SINGER, P. J. BIERMAN, J. M. VOSE, A. S. FREEDMAN, N. ONETTO, S. GILLIS, D. OETTE, M. GOLD, C. D. BUCKNER, J. A. HANSEN, J. RITZ, F. R. APPELBAUM, J. O. ARMITAGE & L. M. NADLER. 1991. Recombinant granulocyte-macrophage colony-stimulating factor after autologous bone marrow transplantation for lymphoid cancer. N. Engl. J. Med. **324:** 1773–1778.

11. GULATI, S. C. & C. L. BENNETT. 1992. Granulocyte-macrophage colony-stimulating factor (GM-CSF) as adjunct therapy in relapsed Hodgkin's disease. Ann. Intern. Med. **116:** 177-182.

12. HOELZER, D., G. SEIPELT & A. GANSER. 1991. Interleukin-3 alone and in combination with GM-CSF in the treatment of patients with neoplastic disease. Semin. Hematol. **28**(suppl 2): 17-24.

13. GANSER, A., A. LINDEMANN, G. SEIPELT, O. G. OTTMANN, F. HERRMANN, M. EDER, J. FRISCH, G. SCHULZ, R. MERTELSMANN & D. HOELZER. 1991. Clinical effects of recombinant human interleukin-3. Am. J. Clin. Oncol. **14**(suppl 1): S51-S63.

14. GANSER, A., G. SEIPELT, A. LINDEMANN, O. G. OTTMANN, S. FALK, M. EDER, F. HERRMANN, R. BECHER, K. HÖFFKEN, T. BÜCHNER, M. KLAUSMANN, J. FRISCH, G. SCHULZ, R. MERTELSMANN & D. HOELZER. 1990. Effects of recombinant human interleukin-3 in patients with myelodysplastic syndromes. Blood **76:** 455-462.

15. NEMUNAITIS, J., C. D. BUCKNER, F. R. APPELBAUM, K. LILLEBY, S. WOLFF, P. BIERMAN, A. KESSINGER, D. RESTA, M. CAMPION, D. C. YOUNG, Z. ZEIGLER, C. ROSENFELD, R. K. SHADDUCK & J. W. SINGER. 1992. Phase I trial with recombinant human interleukin-3 (rhIL-3) in patients with lymphoid cancer undergoing autologous bone marrow transplantation (ABMT). Abstract 331. Blood **80**(suppl 1): 85a.

16. FAY, J., S. BERNSTEIN, R. HERZIG, H. LAZARUS, L. PIÑEIRO, R. COLLINS, G. HERZIG, J. DICESARE & J. FELSER. 1992. A phase I study of sequential rhIL-3 (SDZ ILE 964) and rhGM-CSF (Leucomax) following autologous bone marrow transplantation therapy for lymphoma (Abstract 334). Blood **80**(suppl 1): 86a.

17. GEISSLER, K., P. VALENT, P. BETTELHEIM, C. SILLABER, B. WAGNER, P. KYRLE, W. HINTERBERGER, K. LECHNER, E. LIEHL & P. MAYER. 1992. *In vivo* synergism of recombinant human interleukin-3 and recombinant human interleukin-6 on thrombopoiesis in primates. Blood **79:** 1155-1160.

Recolonization Therapy with Nonadhesive *Escherichia coli* for Treatment of Inflammatory Bowel Disease

MICHAEL L. McCANN,[a] RICHARD S. ABRAMS,[b] AND
ROBERT P. NELSON, Jr. [c]

[a]*Department of Clinical Immunology*
Kaiser Permanente
12301 Snow Rd.
Cleveland, Ohio 44130

[b]*Grant Hospital*
43 East Ohio St.
Chicago, Illinois 60611

[c]*Department of Immunology*
University of South Florida
All Children's Hospital
801 Sixth St. South
St. Petersburg, Florida 33701

The etiology of inflammatory bowel disease is not known. Immunogenic adhesive *Escherichia coli* proteins were recently identified in the feces of patients with ulcerative colitis but not controls.[1] Antibacterial therapy is associated with temporary remission in patients with Crohn's disease and ulcerative colitis.[2] We postulate that coliform antigens elicit immunologic responses in genetically susceptible individuals which cross-react with colonic epithelium and that replacement of resident flora may result in disease remission. Murine bowel coliform recolonization is difficult unless the anaerobic component is replaced. We treated selected patients with inflammatory bowel disease with antibiotics and replacement bacteria with variable results.[3,4] One patient (AP) in a sustained 4-year remission continued to take daily *Lactobacillus acidophilus* supplement, and the stool repeatedly grew the replacement Pingel strain as the predominate gram-negative coliform at 6, 12, 24, and 36 months posttreatment. His pre- and posttreatment biopsy specimens are shown in FIGURE 1.

Two other patients who experienced long-term remissions prompted changes in our regimen to include the following: (1) parenteral antibiotics; (2) longer pretreatment time; (3) use of multiple species of nonpathogenic *E. coli;* (4) addition of anaerobes; and (5) continued bacterial replacement.

Between 1990 and 1993, seven more patients were treated, one with Crohn's disease and six with ulcerative colitis. (TABLE 1). Patients who had severe or long-standing disease (6 of 7 patients; duration of illness 3–15 years) with complications from conventional therapy were selected. All were prepared according to a decontami-

243

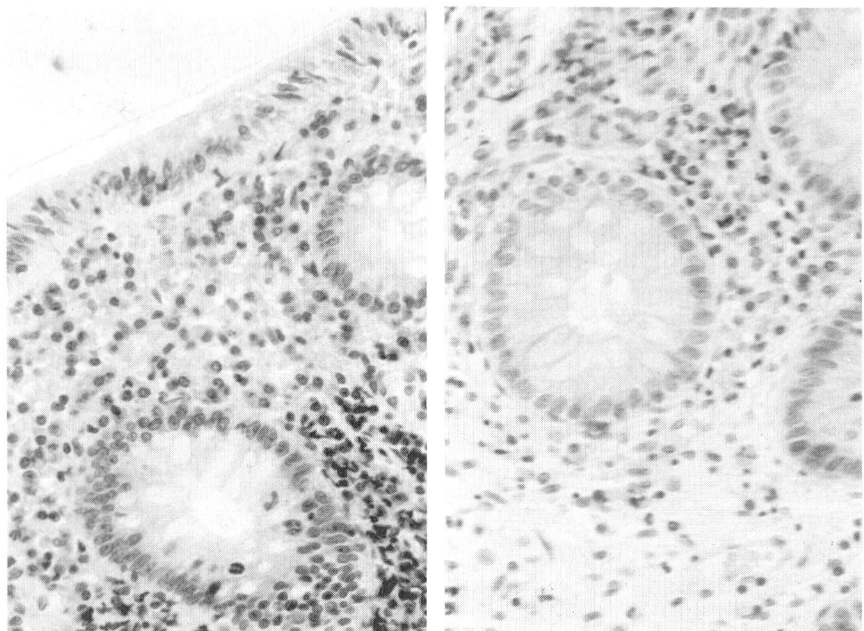

FIGURE 1. Biopsy of colon before (*left*) and after (*right*) treatment. This 73-year-old man was diagnosed with ulcerative colitis refractory to steroid and sulfasalazine therapy. The hemorrhagic and cellular infiltrate with crypt abscesses resolved completely. He remains in complete remission with normal endoscopy and biopsy 4 years after treatment. (Referral was courtesy of Dr. Steven Hanauer, University of Chicago.)

nation protocol previously described[3,4] with 72 hours of antibacterial and antifungal antibiotics. Asulfidine and corticosteroids were discontinued. Biopsies were obtained before and 6 months after treatment. The two most recent patients (RG and AV) have sustained complete remissions. By contrast to the earlier patients in whom transient recolonization was associated with remission followed by relapse, these two patients sustained complete remissions and both were permanently recolonized by the donor Pingel *E. coli.*

CONCLUSION

A subset of patients with inflammatory bowel disease who are successfully recolonized with nonadhesive *E. coli* achieved complete, sustained, drug-free remissions. We have named this method "reflorastation." Rather than whole organisms, the epitopes which are pathogenic may be only one part of the organism, such as the adhesins, among a whole group of different *Enterobacteriaceae.* Reflorastation is not only a method that has the potential to identify these putative etiologic antigens

TABLE 1. Results of Inflammatory Bowel Disease Reflorastation Therapy (1990–1993)

Patient	Age (yr)/Sex	Diagnosis	Results
EL	31/F	UC	6 wk remission, then relapse[a]
JA	9/M	UC	9 mo remission, then relapse[b]
MC	24/F	UC	6 mo remission, then relapse[a]
RS	27/M	CD	1 yr clinical remission[c]
JR	40/M	UC	Failure; colectomy
RG	10/F	UC	Complete remission, sustained >1 yr[d]
AV	6/M	UC	Remission, then relapse[e]
AP	73/M	UC/CD	Complete remission, sustained >4 yr

ABBREVIATIONS: CD = Crohn's disease; UC = ulcerative colitis.

[a] Colonization with donor coliform was not sustained

[b] Relapsed twice. After the second treatment, 6-month follow-up biopsy was normal.

[c] Did not return for 6-month posttreatment biopsy.

[d] Six-month posttreatment biopsy was normal. She continues to take *E. coli* (Nissel 1917 strain, Mutaflor, Ardeypharm Co.), *L. acidophilus (DDS-1 strain),* and *B. bifidum* (Malyoth strain, Bifido Factor, Natren Co.) twice daily. Pingel *E. coli,* which was not continued after the first week, nevertheless continues to predominate in aerobic coliform cultures of the feces.

[e] Treated on September 1, 1993 with parenteral ceftriaxone, oral gentamycin, mycostatin, diflucan, vancomycin, and cefuroxime for 72 hours. Mycostatin was continued during recolonization. After treatment all antimicrobials, sulfasalazine, and corticosteroids were discontinued, Pingel *E. coli* and *L. acidophilus* was replaced 4× daily for 72 hours, then 2× daily for 1 week. Nissel *E. coli, L. acidophilus,* and *B. bifidum* continue to be replaced 2× daily. Posttreatment stool grows Pingel *E. coli* as the predominant strain. All organisms were incubated in amino acid hydrolysate (Pregestimil) and given in a dose of $>5 \times 10^8$ organisms/dose. There were no side effects to treatment.

but also a clinical method to induce long-term remissions without the use of toxic drugs.

REFERENCES

1. LOBO, A., P. HAWKEY, J. ROTHWELL & A. AXON. 1992. The adhesin of ulcerative colitis associated *E. coli* differs genetically and phenotypically from that of enteropathogenic *E. coli.* Gastroenterology **102:** A 654.

2. BURKE, D. A., S. A. CLAYDEN, M. F. DIXON, A. T. R. AXON, D. JOHNSTON & R. W. LACEY. 1988. A follow-up study of adjunctive oral tobramycin therapy in acute ulcerative colitis (UC). Gastroenterology **94:** A55.

3. McCANN, M. L., R. GREINWALD, U. SONNENBORN, R. NELSON & R. GOOD. 1992. Long-lasting remissions of inflammatory bowel disease produced by sustained colonization with non-pathogenic *E. coli.* J. Allergy Clin. Immunol. **89:** 290.

4. McCANN, M. L. 1992. Reflorastation: A method to treat autoimmune diseases associated with enteric antigens. 2. Interdisziplinares Symposium, Darmflora in Symbiose with Pathogenitat, March 5–7. Attendorn, Germany. Der Internist Beilage **33:** 10.

The Molecular Response of *Escherichia coli* to the Short Chain Organic Acid Butyrate[a]

DENNIS E. GUILFOYLE[b,c] AND
IRVIN N. HIRSHFIELD [b,d]

[b]*Department of Biological Sciences*
St. John's University
8000 Utopia Parkway
Jamaica, New York 11439

[c]*Food & Drug Administration*
North East Regional Laboratory
Brooklyn, New York 11232

It is well known that in the mammalian colon, short chain organic acids (SCOAs), particularly acetic, propionic, and butyric acid, are generated by fermentation of carbohydrates by the resident anaerobes. The level of *Enterobacteriaceae,* such as *Escherichia coli,* in the colon is apparently regulated, at least in part, by SCOAs. It is established that acetate and butyrate with pKas of 4.8 and 4.9, respectively, can inhibit the growth of *E. coli* at a mildly acidic pH (5.5). This is due in large part to the ability of the protonated form of these acids to permeate the cytoplasmic membrane of the bacterium and to dissociate to lower the internal pH.

The mode of action of SCOAs on microorganisms has been intensively investigated, but little is known of the molecular response of bacteria to these compounds. We set out to identify gene products of *E. coli* that are induced by 0.1% (11 mM) butyrate added to a culture grown to log phase at 37°C in a morpholineethanesulfonic (MES)-buffered minimal medium supplemented with amino acids, vitamins, and bases (SMM) at pH 5.5. Through two-dimensional gel electrophoresis, we detected 13 polypeptides whose synthesis was enhanced by butyrate. Six of these were identified from the gene-protein database[1] or independently.[2,3] They are LysU, an inducible lysyl-tRNA synthetase,[4] HtpG, and ClpB (HtpM) and F68.5, which are alternative translational products of the *clpB* gene.[3] These four are classified as heat shock proteins.[3,5] Additionally, Adi, inducible arginine decarboxylase, and lipoamide acetyltransferase were induced. LysU, HtpG, ClpB, and Adi were previously shown to be synthesized in response to external acid pH stress at pH 5.3, but in cells grown in highly enriched broth to early stationary phase.[6]

[a]This work was supported in part through a SARAP fellowship awarded to Dennis E. Guilfoyle by the Office of Regulatory Affairs, FDA.

[d]Address for correspondence: Dr. Irvin N. Hirshfield, Department of Biological Sciences, St. John's University, 8000 Utopia Parkway, Jamaica, NY 11439.

TABLE 1. Effect of 0.1% Butyrate on Beta-Galactosidase Activity in the *adi* : :*lac* Fusion Strain GNB7145 Grown in Different Media at pH 5.5 or 6.5[a]

Medium[b] + Butyrate	Beta-Galactosidase Activity (Miller Units)						Induction Ratio (induced/uninduced)
	0 Time	Post 10'	Post 30'	Post 90'	Post 120'	Post 150'	
Min, pH 5.5	16 (5.5)[c]	ND	20.6 (5.35)	23 (5.22)	ND	1.8 (5.2)	1.4
SMM, pH 6.5	20 (6.4)	ND	61 (6.35)	110 (6.22)	93 (6.15)	ND	5.5
SMM, pH 5.5	44.8 (5.63)	ND	74 (5.56)	213 (5.53)	ND	324 (5.49)	7.3
Falkow, pH 6.5	10.7 (6.58)	123 (6.57)	271 (6.55)	585 (6.40)	ND	ND	54.7
Falkow, pH 5.5	263 (5.54)	288 (5.54)	411 (5.54)	465 (5.50)	ND	ND	1.8

ABBREVIATIONS: BA = butyric acid; Min = minimal; SMM = supplemented minimal; ND = not done.

[a] *E. coli* GNB7145 was cultured at 37±1°C, aerobically, shaken at 200 rpm until an optical density of 0.1 at 580 nm was reached, and then 0.1% butyrate was added at 0 time.

[b] All media were buffered with 100 mM morpholineethanesulfonic acid (MES).

[c] pH values of the culture at time of sampling.

Since Adi was induced, we used the *adi* : : *lac* fusion strain GNB 7145[7] as a barometer to examine the influence of 0.1% butyrate at pH 5.5 and 6.5 on *adi* expression in cells grown in a variety of media (TABLE 1). These results corroborate the data from two-dimensional gel electrophoresis in showing that *adi* expression is stimulated by butyrate. In Falkow medium, butyrate enhances *adi* expression markedly better at pH 6.5 than at pH 5.5. This is paradoxical because less acid should permeate the cell at pH 6.5.

Our finding that butyrate induces proteins that may be involved in acid habituation[6,8] raises the question of whether *Enterobacteriaceae* in the colon could be rendered more acid resistant by exposure to SCOAs produced by resident anaerobes. Future work will address whether or not the response of genes to SCOAs is due to a flux in internal pH.

REFERENCES

1. VANBOGELEN, R. A., P. SANCAR, R. L. CLARK, J. A. BOGAN & F. C. NEIDHARDT. 1992. Electrophoresis **13:** 1014-1054.
2. HASSANI, M., M. V. SALUTA, G. N. BENNETT & I. N. HIRSHFIELD. 1991. J. Bacteriol. **173:** 1965- 1970.
3. SQUIRES, C. L., S. PEDERSEN, B. M. ROSS & C. SQUIRES. 1991. J. Bacteriol. **173:** 4254- 4262.
4. HIRSHFIELD, I. N., P. L. BLOCH, R. A. VANBOGELEN & F. C. NEIDHARDT. 1981. J. Bacteriol. **146:** 345-351.
5. NEIDHARDT, F. C. & R. A. VANBOGELEN. 1987. *In* F. C. Neidhardt, J. L. Ingraham, K. B. Low, B. Magasnik, M. Schaecter & H. E. Umbarger, eds. *Escherichia coli* and *Salmonella typhimurium:* Cellular and Molecular Biology. American Society for Microbiology, Washington, DC.
6. HASSANI, M., D. PINCUS, G. N. BENNETT & I. N. HIRSHFIELD. 1992. Appl. Environ. Microbiol. **58:** 2704-2707.
7. AUGER, E. A., K. E. REDDING, T. PLUMB, L. C. CHILDS, S.-Y. MENG, & G. N. BENNETT. 1989. Mol. Microbiol. **3:** 1-12.
8. HEYDE, M. & R. PORTALIER. 1990. FEMS Microbiol. Lett. **69:** 19-26.

Identification of Porcine Respiratory Tract Mucus Proteins Binding Lipopolysaccharides of *Actinobacillus pleuropneumoniae*[a]

MYRIAM BÉLANGER, DANIEL DUBREUIL, AND
MARIO JACQUES

Département de pathologie et microbiologie
Faculté de médecine vétérinaire
Université de Montréal
C.P. 5000
Saint-Hyacinthe (Québec), Canada J2S 7C6

Bacterial adherence is the first step in the colonization of the mucosal surfaces of the host.[1] Bacteria adhere to cells via adhesins, which have the potential to interact specifically with receptors on the epithelial cell surfaces.[2] Many putative receptors are located on the epithelial cell surface and in the overlaying mucus layer. Respiratory mucosal surfaces are bathed by mucus gel, and some bacteria appear to show affinity for this mucus layer. *Pasteurella multocida,* a member of the *Pasteurellaceae* family

TABLE 1. Surface Properties and Adherence to Mucus of *A. pleuropneumoniae* Isolates and Reference Strains

Isolate	Serotype	Thickness of Capsule[a]	Hydrophobicity[b]	Congo Red Binding	Adherence to Mucus
4074	1	+++	−	−	++
Q87-586	1	+++	−	−	++
FMV87-682	1	+++	−	−	++
87-4118-88	1	++	−	−	++
4226	2	++	−	−	++
84-4397	2	+	+	+	+++
Q87-981	2	+	+	+	++++
JG-141	2	++	−	−	++

[a] As estimated by electron microscopy after immunostabilization and ruthenium red staining.

[b] As determined by a salt aggregation test: $(-) = \geq 4$ M; $(+) = \leq 0.05$ M.

[a] This work was supported in part by grants from NSERC (A3428) and the Association Pulmonaire du Québec. Myriam Bélanger is the recipient of a studentship from UniMédia and from MRC.

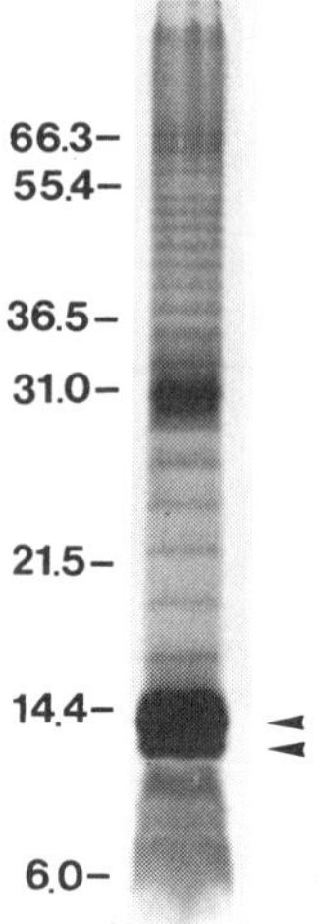

FIGURE 1. Silver-stained SDS-PAGE profile of the fraction obtained after affinity chromatography on a Detoxi-Gel column. Complexes of *A. pleuropneumoniae* 4226 LPS and mucus components retained by the column showed a smooth LPS profile with two additional major bands of approximately 10 and 11 kD (*arrows*). Molecular mass markers (in kilodaltons) are indicated on the *left*.

and a swine respiratory pathogen implicated in atrophic rhinitis,[3] adhered to respiratory tract mucus.[4] Preliminary characterization identified low molecular mass proteinaceous components as potential mucus receptors for *P. multocida*.[4] Recently, we demonstrated that another member of *Pasteurellaceae* and the causative agent of porcine pleuropneumonia, *Actinobacillus pleuropneumoniae*,[5] also showed affinity for porcine respiratory tract mucus and that its lipopolysaccharides (LPS) were involved.[6]

The affinity for porcine respiratory tract mucus of isolates of the *Pasteurellaceae* family and of some unrelated gram-negative bacteria was examined. Affinity for porcine respiratory tract mucus was not a property shared by all *Pasteurellaceae* isolates tested. Furthermore, affinity for porcine mucus was not unique to the *Pasteurellaceae* group and did not seem to be restricted to bacteria originating from pigs. However, bacteria not associated with respiratory tract infections demonstrated less adherence to mucus than did bacteria associated with respiratory tract infections.

Different surface properties of *A. pleuropneumoniae* isolates in relation with their adherence to mucus were examined (TABLE 1). The capsular layer seemed to mask the adhesin and interfered with adherence to mucus. Two poorly capsulated isolates, which had a more hydrophobic surface and bound congo red, were also heavily labeled by gold particles coated with polymyxin which is known to interact with the lipid A-core region of LPS, and adhered strongly to respiratory tract mucus. Results obtained in this study indicate that LPS is indeed more accessible at the surface of less capsulated cells.

To identify the receptor(s) recognized by the lipopolysaccharidic adhesin of *A. pleuropneumoniae*, we used a Detoxi-Gel column which specifically binds LPS. We preincubated mucus and purified LPS, and separated the LPS-mucus complexes by affinity chromatography. After elution, we observed two major additional bands of approximately 10 and 11 kD in the LPS electrophoretic profile (FIG. 1, arrows). Our results suggest that two low-molecular-mass proteins present in porcine respiratory tract mucus bind *A. pleuropneumoniae* LPS.

REFERENCES

1. ABRAHAM, S. N. & E. H. BEACHEY. 1985. Host defenses against adhesion of bacteria to mucosal surfaces. *In* Advances in Host Defense Mechanisms. J. I. Gallin & A. S. Fauci, Eds.: 63–88. Raven Press. New York.
2. BEACHEY, E. H. 1981. J. Infect. Dis. **143:** 325–345.
3. RUTTER, J. M. 1985. Adv. Vet. Sci. Comp. Med. **29:** 239–279.
4. LETELLIER, A., D. DUBREUIL, G. ROY, J. M. FAIRBROTHER & M. JACQUES. 1991. Am. J. Vet. Res. **52:** 34–39.
5. NICOLET, J. 1986. *Haemophilus* infections. *In* Disease of Swine. A. D. Leman, B. Straw, R. D. Glock, W. L. Mengeling, R. H. C. Penny & E. Scoll, Eds. 6th ed.: 426–436. Iowa State University Press. Ames.
6. BÉLANGER, M., S. RIOUX, B. FOIRY & M. JACQUES. 1992. FEMS Microbiol. Lett. **97:** 119–126.

Cloning and Molecular Analysis of the *galE* Gene of *Neisseria meningitidis* and Its Role in Lipopolysaccharide Biosynthesis

MICHAEL P. JENNINGS,[a] PETER van der LEY,[b]
KATHY E. WILKS,[a] DUNCAN J. MASKELL,[c]
JAN T. POOLMAN,[b] AND E. RICHARD MOXON[a]

[a]*Molecular Infectious Diseases Group*
Institute of Molecular Medicine
John Radcliffe Hospital
Headington, Oxford OX3 9DU, United Kingdom

[b]*National Institute of Public Health and Environmental Protection*
Antonie van Leeuwenhoeklaan 9
Bilthoven, the Netherlands

Meningococcal meningitis and septicemia remain significant health problems worldwide. Vaccines are available which give a limited degree of protection against Group A and C strains, but not the Group B organisms, which are the major cause of disease in many countries. The lipopolysaccharide (LPS) of *Neisseria meningitidis* is known to be a major determinant of virulence[1] and of host defense against infection.[2] Present in the LPS are the galactose-containing structures, galα1-4galβ and lacto-*N*-neotetraose, which are also found on the surface of epithelial cells or in host secretions.[3,4] The biologic role of these structures in the pathogenesis of *N. meningitidis* infection is not known.

In this study, the *galE* gene from *Haemophilus influenzae* was used as a hybridization probe for the *galE* gene of *N. meningitidis* Group B, identifying two different homologous loci. Each of the loci was cloned, and nucleotide sequence analysis revealed that both loci contained sequences similar to *galE*. One contained a functional *galE* gene and mapped to the capsule biosynthetic locus. The second contained only a partial *galE* coding sequence which did not express a functional gene product. A *galE* mutant meningococcal strain was constructed by transformation with an inactivated *galE* gene. Analysis of the LPS from the *galE* mutant strain revealed an apparent reduction in molecular weight (Fig. 1) and a loss of reactivity with monoclonal antibodies specific for L3 and L8 immunotypes known to contain galactose. These results are consistent with the loss of galactose from the LPS and defines the galactose-

---

[c]PRESENT ADDRESS: Department of Biochemistry, Imperial College of Science, Technology and Medicine, London, SW7, 2AY, UK.

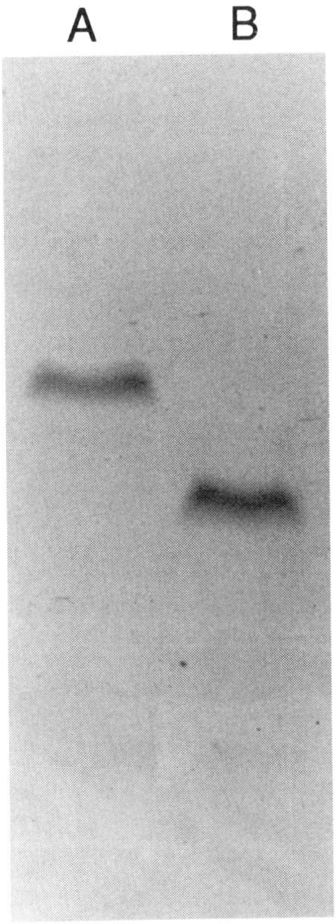

FIGURE 1. Tricine-SDS-polyacrylamide electrophoresis of LPS prepared from MC58 (**A**) and MC58*galE* (**B**). LPS was visualized by silver staining. Migration of the *galE* derivative of MC58 displayed an apparent reduction in molecular weight in comparison to the parent.

containing structures of L3 (lacto-*N*-neotetraose) and L8 (gluc-gal) as essential components of the L3 and L8 epitopes (FIG. 2).

Meningococcal LPS has potential as a vaccine component. However, the presence of structures also found on human glycolipids, such as lacto-*N*-neotetraose on L3 and galα1-4βgal on L1 LPS, may be problematic as they could potentially result in immunopathology. The absence of these structures in *galE* mutants may thus be useful in vaccine development. In addition, the loss of galactose residues may expose the more conserved parts of LPS, which are not subject to phase variation, to the immune system. Investigation of the immunogenicity of the truncated *galE* LPS will demonstrate whether antibodies cross-reacting with multiple immunotypes can be induced in this way.

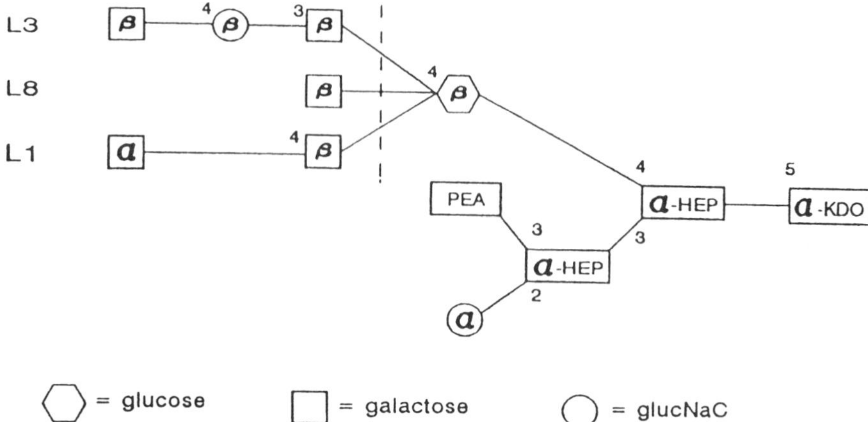

FIGURE 2. Primary structure of meningococcal oligosaccharides of immunotypes L1, L3, and L8. Differences between the three immunotypes are presented to the *left of the dotted line.* *Arabic numbers* indicate the position of the binding site. α and β indicate the anomeric configuration. KDO = 2-keto-3-deoxyoctulosonic acid; PEA = phosphoethanolamine; HEP = heptose. Reproduced, with permission, from Scholten *et al.* 1994. (Submitted to J. Med. Microbiol.)

REFERENCES

1. JONES, D. M., R. BORROW, A. J. FOX, S. GRAY, K. A. CARTWRIGHT & J. T. POOLMAN. 1992. Microb. Pathog. **13:** 219–224.
2. GRIFFISS, J. M., H. SCHNEIDER, R. E. MANDRELL, R. YAMASAKI, G. A. JARVIS, J. J. KIM, B. W. GIBSON, R. HAMADEH & M. A. APICELLA. 1988. Rev. Infect. Dis. **10:** 287–295.
3. MANDRELL, R. E., J. M. GRIFFISS & B. A. MACHER. 1988. J. Exp. Med. **168:** 107–126.
4. VIRJI, M., J. N. WEISER, A. A. LINDBERG & E. R. MOXON. 1990. Microb. Pathog. **9:** 441–450.

Analysis of the I69 Mutation of *Haemophilus influenzae*

ANDREW PRESTON,[a] DUNCAN J. MASKELL,[b] AND
E. RICHARD MOXON

Molecular Infectious Diseases Group
Institute of Molecular Medicine
John Radcliffe Hospital
Oxford OX3 9DU, UK

Haemophilus influenzae is a gram-negative bacterium that is a major cause of meningitis, cellulitis, epiglottitis, pneumonia, and lower respiratory tract infections of infants. Surface molecules such as capsular polysaccharide and lipopolysaccharide (LPS) are important contributors to the virulence of the bacterium.[1,2]

H. influenzae LPS consists of a toxic lipid A molecule linked via a single phosphorylated 2-keto-3-deoxyoctulosonic acid (KDO) residue to an oligosaccharide, which is different from, but analogous to, enterobacterial LPS core.[3] However, it lacks structures equivalent to the repeating O-antigen polysaccharides of enterobacterial LPS. I69 is a mutation of *H. influenzae* that confers an opaque colony phenotype on bacteria.[4] I69 mutant LPS is very deep rough, consisting of just lipid A and a single molecule of phosphorylated KDO which is the deepest rough LPS phenotype described for any bacterium.[5] The I69 mutation was isolated to a 9.4-kb-*Eco*RI restriction fragment (A. Johnson, unpublished data) (FIG. 1) which was sequenced on both strands.

The equivalent wild-type region was amplified by the polymerase chain reaction, cloned, and sequenced. Comparison of the mutant and wild-type DNA sequences identified the I69 mutation as a non-sense mutation of an unidentified reading frame, which we call *isn* (*I*-sixty-*n*ine) (FIG. 2). Surrounding *isn* are two periplasmic permeases,[6] dipeptide permease and histidine permease. A second unidentified reading frame maps next to *isn* and is divergently oriented with respect to *isn* (FIG. 1). The degree of homology between the *Escherichia coli* and *H. influenzae dpp* systems is high and leaves no doubt that the sequences described here are those of *H. influenzae dpp*. However, the histidine permease homologs show certain differences from the *E. coli* sequences (absence of *hisJ*, that encodes a binding protein and an unusual arrangement of genes). The significance of these differences is unknown.

The function of *isn* is unknown. There are two obvious possibilities for its function. One is that *isn* is involved in a transport function as it is positioned between two

---

[a]To whom correspondence should be addressed.

[b]PRESENT ADDRESS: Department of Biochemistry, Imperial College of Science, Technology and Medicine, London SW7 2AY, UK.

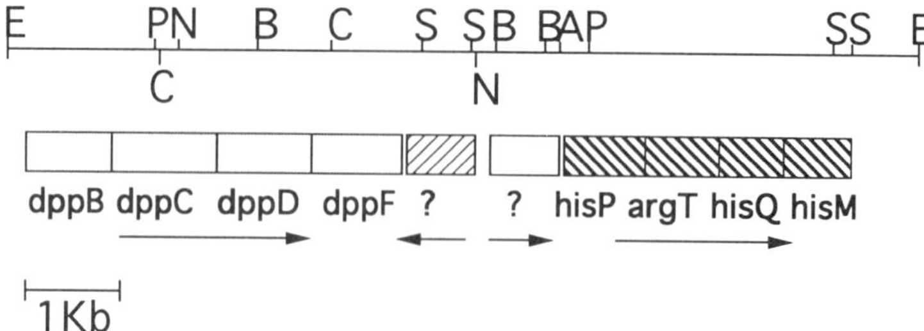

FIGURE 1. Restriction enzyme map of the 9.4-kb chromosomal locus on which the I69 mutation was isolated. E = *Eco*RI; P = *Pvu*I; C = *Cla*I; N = *Nru*I; B = *Nsi*I; S = *Sna*BI. Also shown are open reading frames (ORFs) identified from the nucleotide sequence of the 9.4-kb locus. DppB-F are ORFs that are highly homologous to the Dpp proteins of *E. coli*. The HisP, Q, and M and ArgT are ORFs that are homologous to the His proteins of the histidine permease of *E. coli* and *Salmonella typhimurium*. ? = ORFs that show no homology to proteins held in the Swissprot, translated Genbank, or translated EMBL databases. *Arrows* represent the direction of transcription of the ORFs.

```
Wild            M    Y    L    D    Q    I ....
Type    CAATCAATGTATTTAGATCAAATC..

                M    Y    *
I69     CAATCAATGTATTAGATCAAATC....
```

FIGURE 2. 5′ nucleotide sequence of *isn* and the deduced translation product from both wild-type and I69 mutants of *H. influenzae*. The mutant DNA sequence contains a single base pair deletion that causes premature termination of the reading frame. The deleted base pair is represented by the underlined T-nucleotide of the wild-type DNA sequence.

transport loci, and the second is that it is involved, in addition of heptose, to the lipid A-KDO molecule.

Current work is aimed at elucidating the function of *isn*.

REFERENCES

1. Moxon, E. R. & K. A. Vaughn. 1981. J. Infect. Dis. **143:** 517–524.
2. Zwahlen, A., L. G. Rubin & E. R. Moxon. 1986. Microb. Pathog. **1:** 465–473.
3. Moxon, E. R. & D. J. Maskell. 1992. *Haemophilus influenzae* lipopolysaccharide: The biology of a virulence factor. *In* Molecular Biology of Bacterial Infection: Current Status and Future Perspectives. C. E. Hormaeche, C. W. Penn & C. J. Smyth, Eds.: 75–96. Cambridge University Press. Cambridge.
4. Zawahlen, A., L. G. Rubin, C. J. Connelly, T. J. Inzana & E. R. Moxon. 1985. J. Infect. Dis. **152:** 485–492.
5. Helander, I. M., B. Lindner, H. Brade, K. Altmann, A. A. Lindberg, E. T. Rietschel & U. Zahringer. 1988. Eur. J. Biochem. **177:** 483–492.
6. Ames, G. F., C. S. Mimura, S. R. Holbrook & V. Shyamala. 1992. Adv. Enzymol. Relat. Areas Mol. Biol. **65:** 1–47.

Use of Tissue Culture Invasion Assays to Compare Strains of *Neisseria meningitidis*

KRISTIN A. BIRKNESS,[a] VELMA G. GEORGE,[a]
DAVID S. STEPHENS,[b] EFRAIN RIBOT,[a] AND
FREDERICK D. QUINN[a]

[a]*Centers for Disease Control and Prevention*
Atlanta, Georgia 30333

[b]*Emory University School of Medicine*
Atlanta, Georgia 30322

Meningococcal disease continues to be a serious world health problem, causing recent epidemics in South America and the Middle East and remaining a principal cause of morbidity and mortality in young children in developing countries where the disease is endemic.[1] Pharyngeal carriage of *Neisseria meningitidis* is common, but the mechanism by which the organism penetrates the mucosal surface and enters the bloodstream is largely unknown. This bacterium is an exclusively human pathogen which limits the relevance of animal models in the study of its pathogenesis. Human buccal epithelial cells have been used by many researchers to study attachment and invasion of meningococci; these cells are readily available, but vary greatly in age, size, and viability, and, in addition, are not the cells normally colonized by pathogenic Neisseria. Stephens[2] and coworkers have developed a nasopharyngeal organ culture system that permits study of the interaction between bacteria and the intact mucosal surface as it would occur in a natural infection. These tissues, however, are difficult to obtain, extremely variable from donor to donor, require the initial use of high concentrations of antibiotics, and have limited viability.

An artificial organ system based on layering epithelial and endothelial monolayers is an alternative approach to examining the process of attachment and invasion that must occur as the bacterium makes its way from the mucosal surface through the epithelial cells and into the vascular system. As a first step toward developing such a model we looked at a variety of cell lines to observe meningococcal attachment and invasion in single monolayers. Using a modification of the assay described by Shaw and Falkow[3] we focused our study on HeclB cells, an endometrial carcinoma cell line frequently used with gonococci, and HMEC-1 cells, a human microvascular endothelial cell line. We examined a variety of meningococcal strains including epidemic and sporadic case and carrier isolates from seven countries, strains with and without pili or capsule, and other spontaneous and transposon-induced mutants.

Attachment to host cells ranged from 1–1,000 bacteria/tissue culture cell. However, invasion was variable (FIGS. 1 and 2). Of 24 serogroup A strains tested in HMEC-1 cells, 5 did not invade; 18 invaded at a range of 1 bacterium/10^2–10^4 tissue culture cells; and 1 strain consistently invaded at >1 bacterium/tissue culture cell.

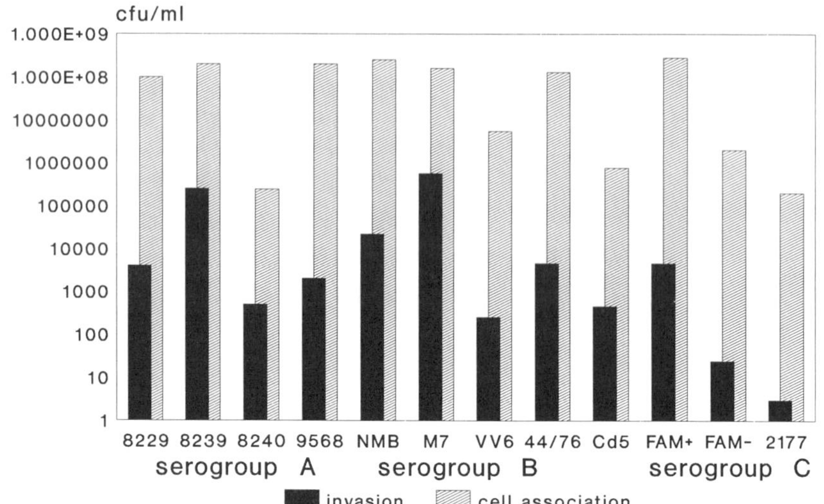

FIGURE 1. Human endometrial carcinoma cells (HeclB). Cell association and cell invasion of HeclB cells by representative strains of *Ne. meningitidis.* M7 and VVV6 are Tn916 transposon-induced mutants of strain NMB. FAM18[+] and FAM18[-] are piliated and nonpiliated, respectively.

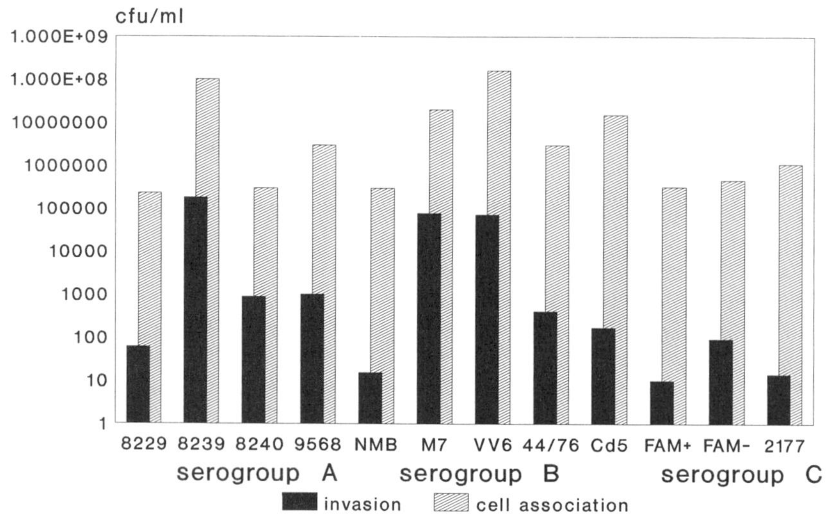

FIGURE 2. Human microvascular endothelial cells (HMEC-1). Cell association and cell invasion of HMEC-1 cells by representative strains of *Ne. meningitidis.* M7 and VVV6 are Tn916 transposon-induced mutants of strain NMB. FAM18[+] and FAM18[-] are piliated and nonpiliated, respectively.

Of 6 group B strains, 4 strains invaded HMEC-1 cells at a range of 1 bacterium/ 10^2-10^4 tissue culture cells; 2 mutant strains invaded at a range of ≥ 1 bacterium/ tissue culture cell. Group C strains were not as invasive; of 7 tested, all invaded at a range of 1 bacterium/ $\geq 10^2$ tissue culture cells. Invasion of HeclB cells was less variable, but in general greater than HMEC-1 invasion (FIGS. 1 and 2); most strains showed a range of 1 internalized bacterium/10^2-10^4 tissue culture cells. The A strain that invaded HMEC-1 cells in high numbers and 1 of the 2 mutant B strains also invaded HeclB cells at >1 bacterium/tissue culture cell. Although we see considerable variation in both attachment and invasion in each of these cell lines, these differences do not appear to be serogroup-specific, carrier- or case-specific, or epidemic or sporadic case-specific. Our preliminary findings suggest that tissue culture monolayers may be an appropriate model for the study of factors involved in meningococcal invasion.

REFERENCES

1. APICELLA, M. A. 1991. *Neisseria meningitidis:* Pathogenesis and immune response. *In* Infections of the Central Nervous System. H. P. Lambert, Ed.: 75-83. B. C. Decker Inc. Philadelphia.
2. STEPHENS, D. S. 1989. Gonococcal and meningococcal pathogenesis as defined by human cell, cell culture, and organ culture assays. Clin. Microbiol. Rev. **2** (suppl.): S104-S111.
3. SHAW, J. H. & S. FALKOW. 1988. Model for invasion of human tissue culture cells by *Neisseria gonorrhoeae.* Infect. Immun. **56:** 1625-1632.

A Tissue Culture Model for Studying the Pathogenesis of Brazilian Purpuric Fever

FREDERICK D. QUINN, ROBBIN S. WEYANT,
MICAH J. WORLEY, VELMA G. GEORGE,
ELIZABETH H. WHITE, EDWIN A. ADES,
EARL G. LONG, AND ERIC A. UTT

Centers for Disease Control and Prevention
Atlanta, Georgia 30333

Brazilian purpuric fever (BPF) is a frequently fatal infectious disease of young children.[1] This illness is preceded by purulent conjunctivitis, which resolves, but is followed 10 to 14 days later by an acute onset of fever associated with systemic toxicity, petechiae, purpura, and vascular collapse. Initially, all confirmed BPF cases were caused by a single HAE clone.[2] However, recent cases in Valparaiso, Brazil, and Australia were caused by HAE which are not the original BPF clone.[3] Common virulence factors shared by clone and non-clone BPF case strains have not been identified.

Using an immortalized human microvascular endothelial cell line, HMEC-1,[4] we developed an *in vitro* assay which identifies all known BPF-causing HAE strains. A unique cytotoxic effect was observed in which tissue culture cells detached and aggregated in large floating masses after 48 hours of incubation (FIG. 1). The cytotoxic phenotype was observed in all HAE strains isolated from patients with BPF *versus* only 14% of non-BPF HAE control strains. Viable count studies indicate that the cytotoxic phenotype is generated during bacterial replication in association with tissue culture (FIG. 2). Analysis of infected monolayers by electron microscopy and confocal microscopy suggests that BPF-causing HAE strains invade individual cells and likely multiply intracellularly, whereas non-BPF-causing HAE strains attach but do not intracellularly replicate. The cytotoxic phenotype is not the product of endotoxin release inasmuch as gamma irradiation-killed whole bacteria, viable bacteria separated from the monolayer by a small-pore membrane, bacterial cell fractions, or bacteria treated with chloramphenicol did not produce the cytotoxic phenotype. The ability of the bacterium to invade, replicate, and produce the phenotype appears to be primarily parasite-directed because phagocytosis, pinocytosis, and protein synthesis inhibitors including cyclohexamide, cytochalasin D, and methylamine had no effect on the ability of the bacteria to invade and cause a cytotoxic response.

We have succeeded in developing an *in vitro* tissue culture virulence model that apparently is capable of identifying BPF-causing strains of HAE by their ability to attach, invade, perhaps intracellularly replicate, and ultimately cause a cytotoxic phenotype. This system represents a convenient *in vitro* approach to the identification of potential BPF virulence factors.

260

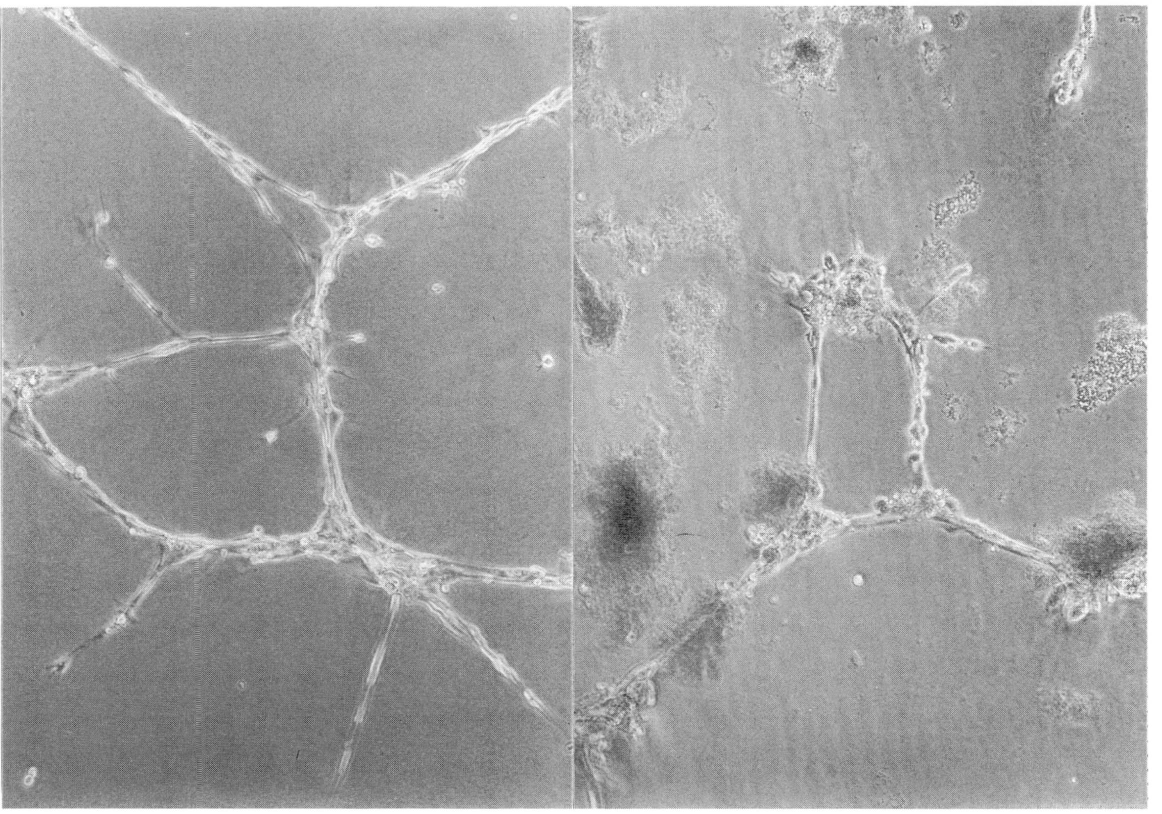

FIGURE 1. Human microvascular endothelial cell line (HMEC-1) tubules infected with BPF case strain 3031 (**A**) and non-BPF–associated strain 1947 (**B**). Inoculum = 1,000 HAE cells per well.

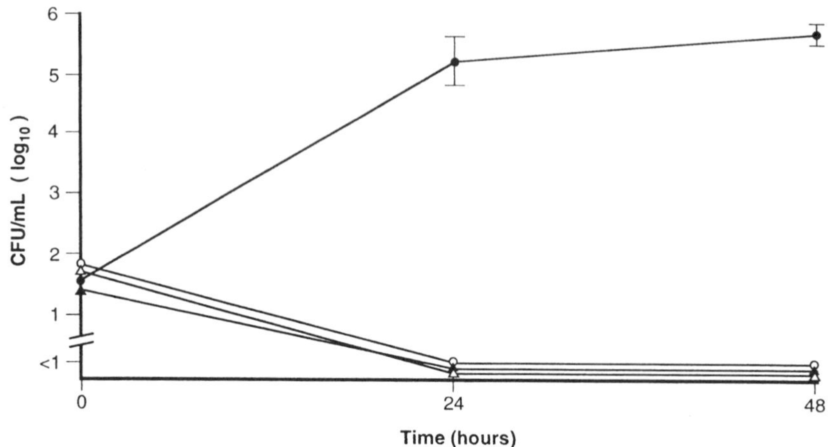

FIGURE 2. Growth of BPF case strain 3031 (BPF clone) and case-associated strain 1947 (non-BPF clone) in HMEC-1 tissue culture. *Closed circle* = case strain 3031 in tissue culture medium with HMEC-1 cells; *open triangle* = case-associated strain 1947 in tissue culture medium with HMEC-1 cells; *open circle* = case strain 3031 grown in tissue culture medium alone; *closed triangle* = case-associated strain 1947 grown in tissue culture medium alone.

REFERENCES

1. BRAZILIAN PURPURIC FEVER STUDY GROUP. 1987. Brazilian purpuric fever: Epidemic purpura fulminans associated with antecedent purulent conjunctivitis. Lancet **2:** 757-761.
2. BRAZILIAN PURPURIC FEVER STUDY GROUP. 1987. *Haemophilus influenzae* biogroup aegyptius bacteraemia in Brazilian purpuric fever. Lancet **2:** 761-763.
3. MCINTYRE, P. G., G. WHEATON, J. ERLICH & D. HANSMAN. 1987. Brasilian purpuric fever in central Australia. Lancet **2:** 112.
4. ADES, E. W., F. CANDAL, R. A. SWERLICK *et al.* 1992. HMEC-1: Establishment of an immortalized human microvascular endothelial cell line. J. Invest. Dermatol. **99:** 683-690.

Methods for the Identification of Virulence Genes Expressed in *Mycobacterium tuberculosis* Strain H37Rv

LYNNE C. KIKUTA-OSHIMA, C. HAROLD KING,
THOMAS M. SHINNICK, AND FREDERICK D. QUINN

National Center for Infectious Diseases
Centers for Disease Control and Prevention
Atlanta, Georgia 30333

Dramatic increases in infections due to *Mycobacterium tuberculosis* over the last few years have prompted renewed efforts to characterize virulence factors and other aspects of the pathogenesis of this disease. The study of microbial virulence was greatly facilitated in recent years through the use of molecular genetics.[1-3] Previous methods for the identification of such genes involved the development of a shuttle vector system for gene transfer, mutagenesis methods, genetic library development, and subsequent screening of library clones. These methods are generally time-consuming and may be particularly difficult when working with newly discovered pathogens.

RNA subtractive hybridization (RSH) is useful for the detection of constitutively expressed virulence factors whether or not an observable phenotype is present. This subtractive hybridization method requires RNA to be extracted rapidly after the lysis of a large volume of mid-log phase bacteria; therefore, a safe and novel lysis method using large scale nitrogen decompression and phenol-chloroform extraction was developed. cDNA was made to the extracted RNA from strain H37Rv and hybridized to a large excess of RNA from strain H37Ra on a hydroxylapatite column. Residual cDNA subtraction products were made double-stranded, polymerase chain reaction-amplified, and subsequently used as colony and Southern blot probes (FIG. 1). Approximately 8.8 kb of DNA were identified in Southern blots which contain genes expressed in the virulent H37Rv strain that are not expressed in the avirulent H37Ra (FIG. 2). These genes have been isolated and are currently being sequenced from an H37Rv *Pst*I genomic library.

In addition, we began a series of infections of H37Rv in the J774 mouse macrophage cell line to identify bacterial genes that are induced during macrophage infection. This cell line displays many relevant properties of macrophages such as phagocytosis, antigen presentation, activation, and free radical production as well as allowing *M. tuberculosis* to invade and multiply.[4,5] During the days and weeks following invasion, bacteria will be harvested, RNA isolated, and electron microscopy and the RSH protocol will be followed as just described. Bacterial genes induced during the infectious process can be temporally identified using this procedure.

These three techniques may simplify identification of the factors necessary for the pathogenesis of tuberculosis.

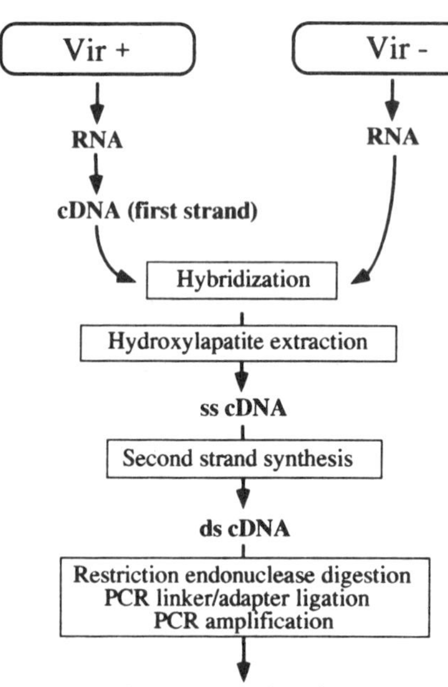

FIGURE 1. Schematic outline for RNA subtractive hybridization (RSH).

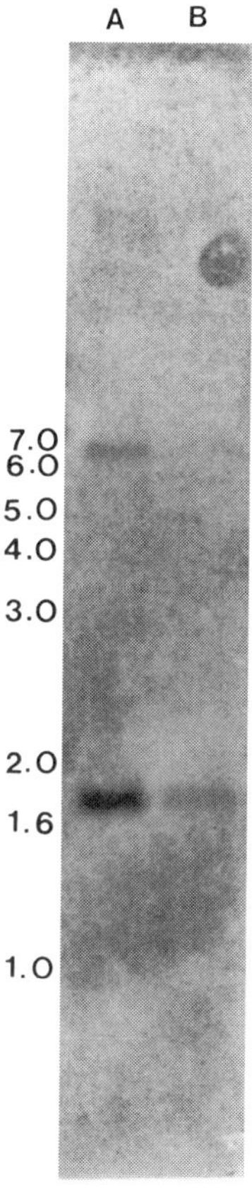

FIGURE 2. Digoxigenin-labeled Southern hybridization of an RNA subtractive hybridization polymerase chain reaction product probed against *Sau*3A1 chromosomal restriction digestions: (**A**) *M. tuberculosis* H37Rv (virulent) strain genomic DNA; (**B**) *M. tuberculosis* H37Ra (less virulent) strain genomic DNA. Each lane contains 0.35 to 0.50 μg of restricted DNA.

REFERENCES

1. MILLER, V. L., J. B. BLISKA & S. FALKOW. 1990. J. Bacteriol. **172:** 1062–1069.
2. MILLER, V. L. & S. FALKOW. 1988. Infect. Immun. **56:** 1242–1248.
3. PORTNOY, D., P. S. JACKS & D. HINRICHS. 1988. J. Exp. Med. **167:** 1459–1471.
4. RASTOGI, N., M. POTAR & H. L. DAVID. 1987. Curr. Microbiol. **16:** 79–92.
5. SYNDERMAN, R., M. C. PIKE, D. G. FISCHER & H. S. KOREN. 1977. J. Immun. **119:** 2060–2066.

Use of the Chick Embryo for the Determination of the Relative Virulence of *Neisseria meningitidis* Strains

LEO PINE,[a] EDWIN P. EWING, Jr.,[a]
KRISTIN A. BIRKNESS,[a] ELIZABETH H. WHITE,[a]
DAVID S. STEPHENS,[b] AND FREDERICK D. QUINN[a]

[a]*Centers for Disease Control and Prevention
Atlanta, Georgia 30333*

[b]*Emory University
Atlanta, Georgia 30322*

Buddingh and Polk[1–3] reported that infection of the chick embryo by *Neisseria meningitidis* produced disease similar to that observed in human infection. We attempted

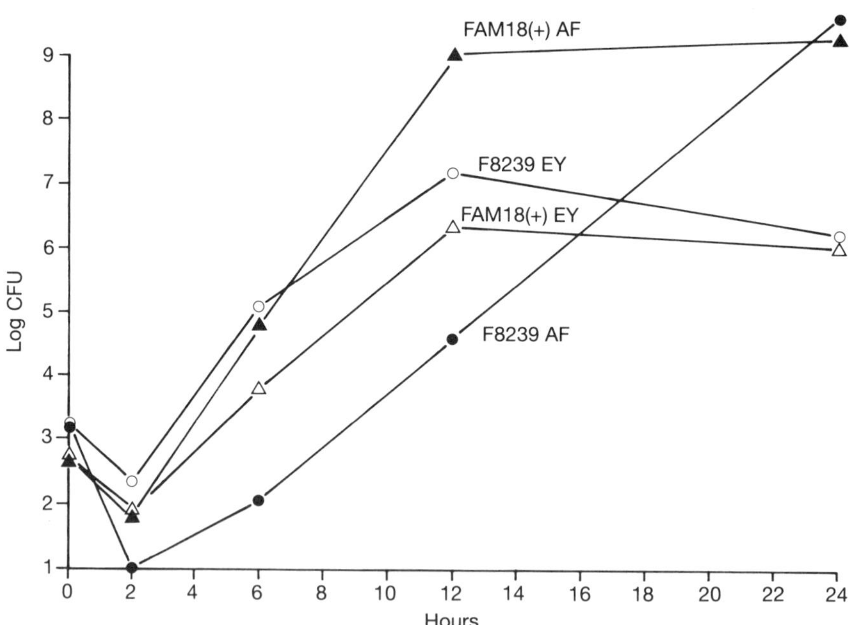

FIGURE 1. Growth of FAM18(+) and F8239 in 9-day-old eggs inoculated via the egg yolk. Colony-forming units (CFU) were determined in the egg yolk and allantoic fluid; the averages of the CFU of three eggs are given for each time point.

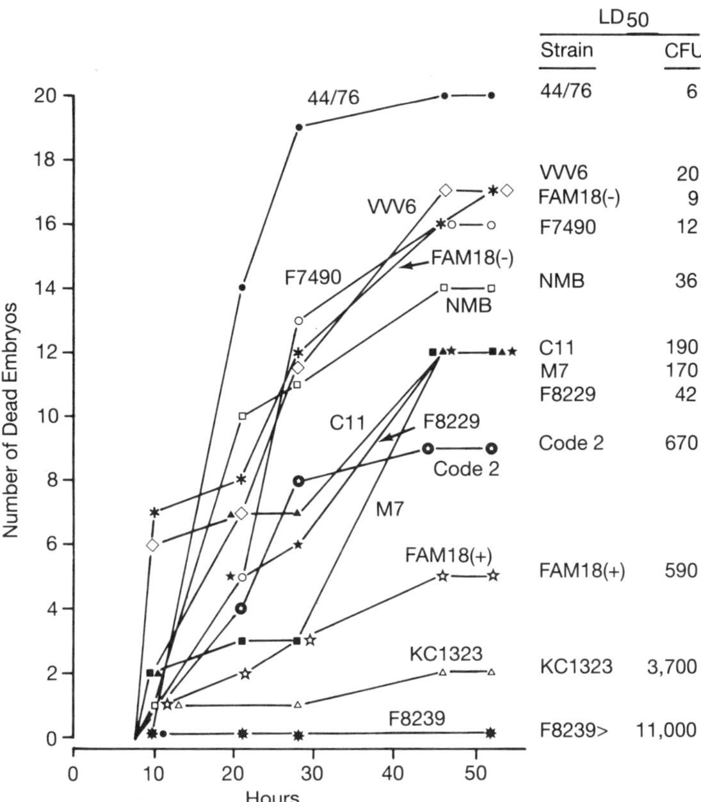

FIGURE 2. Death of 13-day-old eggs inoculated via egg yolk at 10^{-4}, 10^{-5}, 10^{-6}, and 10^{-7} dilutions of approximately 5×10^8 CFU/ml. Five eggs were inoculated per dilution; each point represents the sum of the total dead embryos of the four dilutions.

to determine if the chick embryo model can delineate relative virulence among laboratory and epidemic strains, between transposon-constructed mutants and their wild-type strain, and among strains known to differ in their infection of selected tissue culture monolayers. Parameters considered were: routes of infection such as the chorioallantoic membrane (CAM), allantoic fluid (AF), and egg yolk (EY); age of the embryo; commercial source of the egg; and effect on the LD_{50} of the antibiotic diet fed to the hens from which the eggs were obtained. Pathology was determined with stained sections using light and electron microscopic observations. Experimental results were obtained by calculation of LD_{50} values, determination of killing curves with time, and determination of colony-forming units (CFU) in AF and EY during the infection period.

The following 12 strains of *Neisseria* were compared. Strains F7490, 44/76, and C11 are used for vaccine production and represent serogroups A, B, and C, respectively. Strain KC1323 is the type strain of *Neisseria lactamica.* Strain NMB is a case strain of serogroup B, M7 is a polysaccharide-deficient transposon mutant of NMB, and strain VVV6 is a transposon mutant of NMB infecting at lower efficiency in tissue culture monolayers with complement-inactivated human serum. Strains F8229 and F8239 represent serogroup A, clonal group III-1, and are case and carrier strains, respectively. Strains FAM18(+) and FAM18(−) are pili-positive and pili-negative strains, respectively, of serogroup C. Code 2 is a serogroup B strain isolated from a case of meningitis and maintained without laboratory passage after isolation.

Meningococci were observed, by light and electron microscopy, within the cells and blood vessels of various organs depending on the site of inoculation. Bacteria infecting eggs from hens currently fed aureomycin gave higher LD_{50} values than did those obtained with eggs taken 10 days after the antibiotic was withdrawn. Bacitracin in the chicken feed did not affect the LD_{50} values. In a comparison of the routes of inoculation, LD_{50} values determined in 9-day-old eggs infected via the CAM were 10^2 to 10^4, via the AF they were 10^1 to 10^3, and via the EY they were 10^1 to 10^2. In 9-day-old eggs, the rates of growth determined in AF, but not in EY, differentiated the more virulent FAM18(+) from the "avirulent" F8239 (Fig. 1). The use of 13-day-old eggs infected via the EY demonstrated differences among the 12 strains as assessed by LD_{50} values and death curves (Fig. 2). The avirulent strains, *N. lactamica* and strain F8239, had LD_{50} values of 10^3 to 10^4, whereas the most virulent strains had values of 6–36 CFU. Thirteen-day-old eggs infected via the CAM gave similar death curves, but with higher LD_{50} values, as compared to those obtained with eggs inoculated via the EY.

REFERENCES

1. BUDDINGH, G. J. & A. POLK. 1937. Meningococcus infection of the chick embryo. Science **86:** 20–21.
2. BUDDINGH, G. J. & A. D. POLK. 1939. Experimental meningococcus infection of the chick embryo. J. Exp. Med. **70:** 485–498.
3. BUDDINGH, G. J. & A. D. POLK. 1939. The pathogenesis of meningococcus meningitis in the chick embryo. J. Exp. Med. **70:** 499–510.

mRNA Subtractive Hybridization for the Isolation and Identification of Tissue Culture-Induced Determinants from *Haemophilus influenzae* Biogroup Aegyptius, the Causative Agent of Brazilian Purpuric Fever

ERIC A. UTT AND FREDERICK D. QUINN

Centers for Disease Control and Prevention
Atlanta, Georgia 30333

Brazilian purpuric fever (BPF) is an acute, fulminant, pediatric disease that is usually preceded by purulent conjunctivitis and characterized by a rapidly progressive fever,

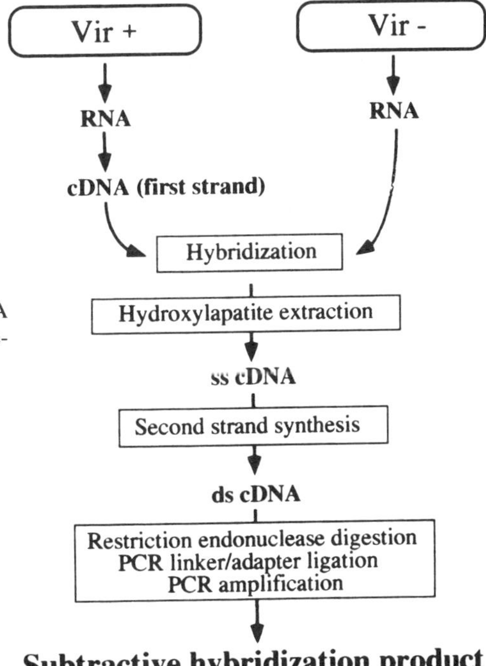

FIGURE 1. Schematic outline for mRNA subtractive hybridization. (See text for details.)

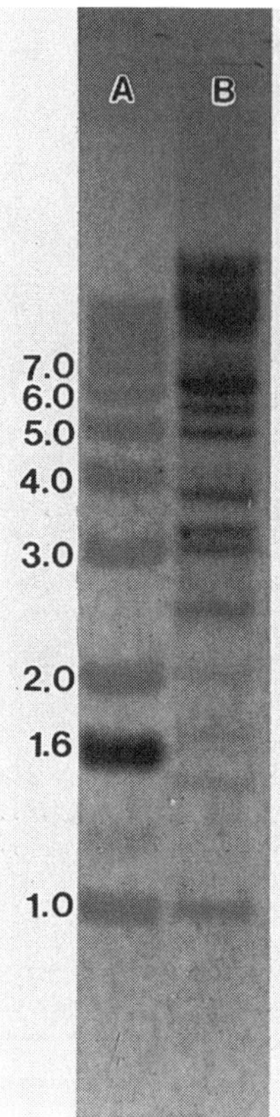

FIGURE 2. Detection of gene expression differences between tissue culture-propagated and broth-propagated HAE. The subtraction product was enzymatically labeled with digoxigenin using the Genius DIG DNA detection kit (Boehringer Mannheim) and used as a probe in a Southern hybridization. Hybridization proceeded at 65°C. *Lane A:* Molecular size markers (1-kb ladder); *lane B: Eco*RI-restricted genomic DNA from HAE F3031.

purpura, vascular collapse, and death.[1] *Haemophilus influenzae* biogroup aegyptius (HAE) is the etiologic agent of BPF.[2]

A newly developed method, mRNA subtractive hybridization,[3] has identified genetic determinants that are involved in the attachment and/or invasion of the bacteria to human microvascular endothelial (HMEC-1) tissue culture cells.[4] The mRNA from HAE that had attached to and invaded the HMEC-1 tissue culture monolayer was reverse transcribed and subtractively hybridized to mRNA from agar-grown HAE (Fig. 1). All eukaryotic mRNA was removed using an oligo-dT cellulose column prior to hybridization. The remaining cDNA in the oligo-dT column eluate, which did not hybridize, represents differences in gene expression between HAE propagated in the HMEC-1 tissue culture and that on chocolate agar plates. The cDNA was isolated from the column eluate by precipitation, and a complementary strand was synthesized to yield the double-stranded subtractive hybridization product. The ds cDNA was amplified using the polymerase chain reaction, and the product was labeled with digoxigenin.

A total of 30 kilobase pairs of chromosomal DNA from the BPF-causing HAE clone, which represents genes that are differentially expressed in the tissue culture

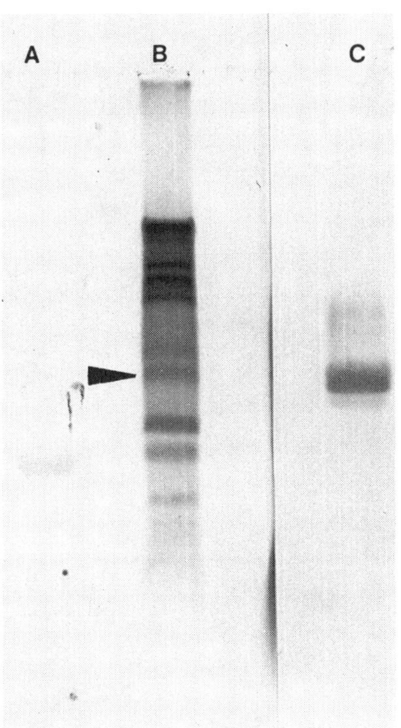

FIGURE 3. The γgt11-cloned DNA insert was subcloned into pUC 18 and electroporated into *E. coli* DH5α (pEU 1001). The DNA insert in pEU 1001 was confirmed to be a 3.2-kb HAE DNA fragment in a Southern hybridization analysis using the DIG-labeled subtraction product as a probe. *Lane A: Eco*RI-restricted *E. coli* DH5α genomic DNA; *lane B: Eco*RI-restricted HAE F3031 genomic DNA; *lane C: Eco*RI-restricted pEU 1001.

virulence model, were identified in a Southern hybridization using the subtractive hybridization product to probe an HAE chromosomal digest (FIG. 2). In control experiments in which the mRNA from tissue culture-propagated HAE or agar-propagated HAE was subtracted against self-derived mRNAs, no subtractive hybridization products were observed. The labeled subtractive hybridization products were probed against a γgt11 genomic library of HAE, using plaque hybridizations to identify the relevant gene fragments. The positive plaques were amplified, ligated into the *Eco*RI site of pUC18, and electroporated into *Escherichia coli* DH5α. A 3.2-kb HAE DNA insert was confirmed in a Southern hybridization analysis as having homology to the subtraction product and corresponded to a 3.2-kb *Eco*RI fragment from the HAE chromosome (FIG. 3).

The hypothesis that this fragment harbors a gene or genes that is/are differentially expressed in the HMEC-1 tissue culture model was explored in an mRNA time course experiment. Approximately 1×10^7 HAE cells were inoculated into HMEC-1 tissue culture in T-150 flasks containing 100 ml of tissue culture and medium. mRNA samples were removed at different times postinoculation. Northern hybridization analysis indicated that a single mRNA transcript was expressed within 10 minutes postinfection (FIG. 4). This message was not expressed in control experiments in the absence of the HMEC-1 tissue culture cells. The corresponding gene on the cloned 3.2-kb fragment is currently being sequenced.

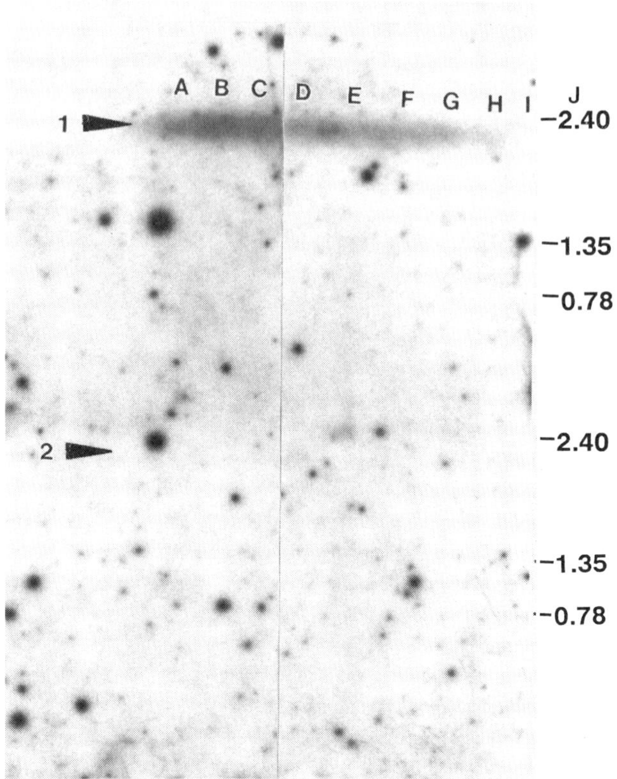

FIGURE 4. Northern hybridization analysis of differential gene induction with and without the presence of the HMEC-1 tissue culture cells. Briefly, 0.5 ml of an 0.5 OD_{600} broth culture of HAE (F 3031) was added to T-150 tissue culture bottles with and without the HMEC-1 monolayer propagated in 50 ml of EMB basal medium. At the time points indicated the total 50 ml was removed and placed in an ice-water bath for 20 minutes. The mRNA from each fraction was isolated using the guanidine isothiocyanate–phenol/chloroform method. A total of 12 μg total RNA for each time point was loaded onto a 1.2% formaldehyde gel and electrophoresed at a constant voltage of 150 V. The resolved RNAs were transferred onto a nylon membrane using the Posi-blot system (Stratagene, Inc.) following the manufacturer's instructions. The membrane was probed under high stringency using the isolated 3.2-kb cloned fragment from pEU1001 that had been end-labeled with [32]P. Lane assignments: *A*, 6 hours; *B*, 3 hours; *C*, 2 hours; *D*, 1 hour; *E*, 30 minutes; *F*, 20 minutes; *G*, 15 minutes; *H*, 10 minutes; *I*, 0 minutes; *J*, molecular size markers in kilobase. *Panel 1* is total RNA from bacteria in the presence of the HMEC-1 cells. *Panel 2* is total RNA from bacteria incubated in the absence of the HMEC-1 cells.

REFERENCES

1. CENTERS FOR DISEASE CONTROL. 1985. Morbid. Mortal. Weekly Rep. **34:** 217–219.
2. CENTERS FOR DISEASE CONTROL. 1986. Morbid. Mortal. Weekly Rep. **35:** 553–554.
3. UTT, E. A., J. P. BROUSAL, L. C. K. OSHIMA & F. D. QUINN. 1993. Can. J. Microbiol., in press.
4. WEYANT, R. S., F. D. QUINN, E. A. UTT, M. J. WORLEY, V. G. GEORGE, F. J. CANDEL & E. W. ADES. 1994. J. Infect. Dis. **169:** 430–433.

Fluorescent Labeling of *Listeria* and *Salmonella*

Analysis of Bacteria-Host Cell Interactions by Flow Microfluorimetry

V. K. BUNNING AND R. B. RAYBOURNE

Food and Drug Administration
Immunobiology (HFS326)
8301 Muirkirk Road
Laurel, Maryland 20708

The interaction between pathogenic bacteria and host cells is central to the induction of immunity. Flow microfluorimetry (FMF) is a potential method for studying this relation on a cellular level, particularly if nontoxic fluorophores are used to label bacteria. The site-specific pathology of autoimmune arthritogenic sequelae to gram-negative enteric infection impelled us to develop this approach.[1] We proposed to validate an FMF assay by duplicating and extending previous work with cell lines[2,3] and showing utility in appropriate rodent models.

Certain pathogens such as *Listeria monocytogenes* and *Salmonella typhimurium* appear to survive and grow in host macrophages.[2,3] We labeled these bacteria with the lipophilic fluorophore PKH-2,[4] and the interaction with J774 cells *in vitro* was

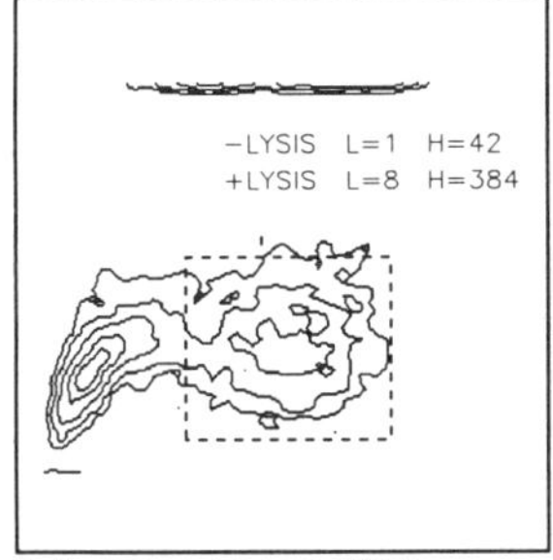

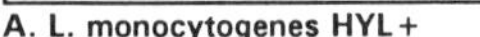

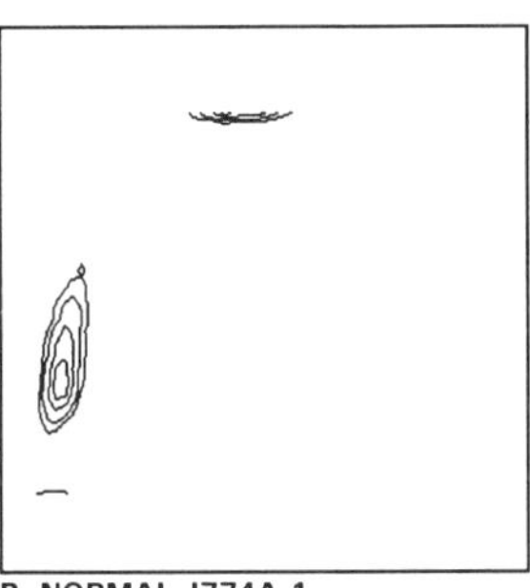

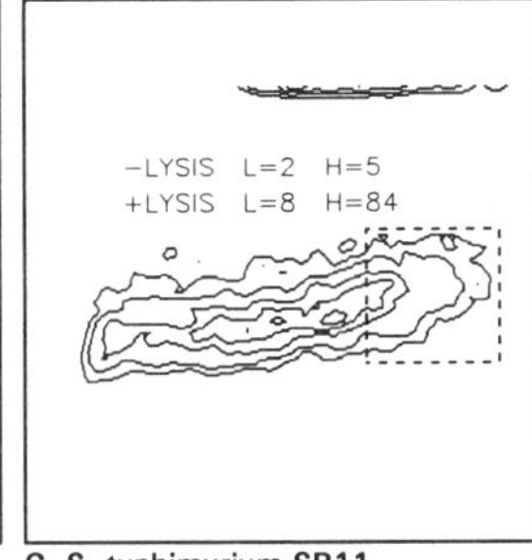

FIGURE 1. Comparison of *L. monocytogenes* (**A**) and *S. typhimurium* (**C**) infection of J774 cells. Autofluorescence of uninfected J774 cells is shown in **B**. The X-axis represents logarithmically amplified green (PKH-2 excitation) fluorescence (LGFL) and the Y-axis represents logarithmically amplified red (propidium iodide-stained dead cells) fluorescence (LRFL). Each histogram represents 5,000 macrophages. Positive (+) lysis indicates that osmotic and mechanical disruption was used to release intracellular bacteria from macrophages; negative (−) lysis, vice versa. H and L refer to high and low LGFL intensity infected macrophage populations. The *dashed box* outlines the bitmap used for sorting the H population.

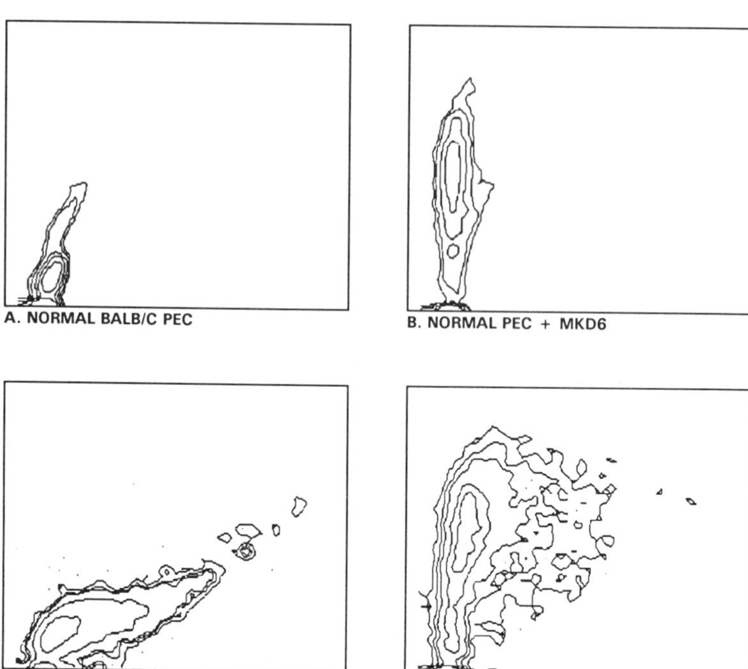

FIGURE 2. Simultaneous detection using two-color flow microfluorimetry (X-axis, LGFL; Y-axis, LRFL) of (1) PKH-2 labeled *Listeria,* intraperitoneally injected into BALB/c mice, within peritoneal exudate cells (PEC) recovered 24 hours later (**C**) and (2) class II major histocompatibility antigen (MHC) (**B,C**). For the latter, PEC were treated with biotinylated monoclonal antibody (moAb) MKD6 (previous blocking of Fc with moAb 24G2), and class II MHC antigen was visualized with an R-phycoerythrin conjugate (red fluorescence). Virtually all of the bacterially infected cells were Ia-positive (**D**). Autofluorescence of normal BALB/c PEC are shown in **A**.

examined. Fluorescence intensity (FI) of labeled bacteria was consistent: *S. typhimurium* cells appeared about 14 times brighter with a broader fluorescence intensity range than did *L. monocytogenes* cells. Stable dye binding was shown by a proportional decrease in fluorescence intensity with growth rate. Labeled and unlabeled bacteria were identical in terms of viability, growth, and intracellular survival, but recovery per macrophage was greater for *Listeria* than for *Salmonella* (FIG. 1).

The fate of labeled *Listeria* during phagocytosis (1-hour incubation; 10-minute intervals) and after extracellular washing with the addition of gentamicin (T = 0) was examined over 24 hours. *Listeria* recovery was directly proportional to the fluorescence intensity of viable infected J774 cells sorted by logarithmic or linear signals. Propidium iodide staining showed that bacterially induced cell death increased over time, paralleling intracellular growth. The addition of uninfected J774 cells, which were selectively sorted by natural fluorescence, indicated that *Listeria* spread from cell to cell; this mechanism optimized intracellular growth yields. Interval analysis of phagocytosis indicated that *Listeria* were rapidly killed, that the percentage of surviving *Listeria* was lower in heavily infected macrophages, and that J774 cells were heterogeneous for bacterial intracellular survival. Overall, our FMF/sorting method defined distinct phases of *Listeria* uptake, killing, adaptation, intracellular growth, cell spreading, and ultimate cell lysis. The ability to selectively sort *Listeria*-infected cells at these phases and to simultaneously analyze bacteria and host cells provide a strong technical advantage for elucidating pathogenesis.

With *Salmonella,* macrophage (J774 or BALB/c bone marrow) viability was stable over a lengthy incubation, surviving bacteria were an infrequent event, and no intracellular growth was detected. Lengthy enrichments of 100 to 1,000 viable infected J774 cells were required to detect intracellular *Salmonella* survivors. These data indicated a very low level carrier state for *S. typhimurium* within J774 cells. Contrastingly, *Salmonella* invaded and replicated in the epithelial-like cell line CACO-2. Labeled bacteria had to be grown statically to the late exponential phase to achieve adequate invasion, which confirmed previous results.[5] These data also indicated that PKH-2 labeling of the bacteria did not affect the ability to invade and grow in epithelial-like cells, as previously demonstrated by others.[6]

Initial *in vivo* studies showed an efficient ability to detect and sort cells infected with labeled *Listeria* from perfused spleens and peritoneal exudates 24 hours after intravenous and intraperitoneal injections, respectively, of BALB/c mice. For the latter (FIG. 2), viable bacteria were recovered and two-color FMF was used to simultaneously detect class II MHC antigens, which are important in the presentation of bacterial antigens to the immune system.[7]

REFERENCES

1. RAYBOURNE, R. B., V. K. BUNNING & K. M. WILLIAMS. 1988. J. Immunol. **140:** 3489-3495.
2. PORTNOY, D. A., P. S. JACKS & D. J. HINRICHS. 1988. J. Exp. Med. **167:** 1459-1471.
3. BUCHMEIER, N. A. & F. HEFFRON. 1989. Infect. Immun. **57:** 1-7.
4. HORAN, P. K. & S. E. SLEZAK. 1989. Nature **340:** 167-168.
5. LEE, C. A. & S. FALKOW. 1990. Proc. Natl. Acad. Sci, USA **87:** 4304-4308.
6. GAHRING, L. C., F. HEFFRON, B. B. FINLAY & S. FALKOW. 1990. Infect. Immun. **58:** 443-448.
7. BANCROFT, G. J., R. D. SCHREIBER & E. R. UNANUE. 1991. Immunol. Rev. **124:** 5-24.

The Monocytic Cell Line U-937, Physiologically Differentiated by Retinoic Acid and Vitamin D$_3$, Is a Model for Intracellular Behavior of *Brucella* spp.[a]

EMMANUELLE CARON, JEAN-PIERRE LIAUTARD,
AND STEPHAN KÖHLER

Institut National de la Santé et de la Recherche Médicale U-65
Université Montpellier II
C.P. 100
34095 Montpellier, France

In the study of interactions between pathogens and macrophages, monocytic cell lines have the advantage of showing defined states of activation and lacking genetic variation, thus yielding reproducible results. The human cell line U-937, differentiated by phorbol esters (PMA), was used to study survival of *Salmonella typhimurium* and *Legionella pneumophila* in macrophages.[1,2] We favored the physiologically active differentiation agents retinoic acid (RA) and vitamin D$_3$ (VD) that, unlike PMA, do not interfere with eukaryotic signal transduction.[3]

We established a model for the intracellular behavior of bacteria using RA/VD-differentiated U-937. Infections were performed as previously described,[4] with the following modifications: bacteria were added at a ratio of 20 bacteria/U-937 cell for 30 minutes; extracellular bacteria were killed using medium with gentamicin at 10–50 μg/ml for at least 1 hour (intracellular survival = 100%); macrophages were lysed in 0.2% triton X-100.

A nonpathogenic *Escherichia coli* K12 strain was eliminated over a period of 3 days by both RA/VD- and PMA-differentiated U-937. However, whereas the RA/VD differentiation pathway did not alter cell viability even 6 days after infection, most PMA-differentiated cells died 2 days postinfection (not shown). Over a 24-hour period, the animal pathogen *Listeria ivanovii* was killed, whereas the human pathogen *Listeria monocytogenes* survived and multiplied in U-937 differentiated by PMA or RA/VD. Overall conditions for survival of *Listeria* were less favorable in the latter case (FIG. 1). Infection of U-937, differentiated by RA/VD, with the human pathogen *Brucella suis* S1 led to 100-fold intracellular multiplication in 3 days after an initial killing phase of 7 hours, as previously observed in murine macrophages.[5] Opsonization of this strain with specific human anti-*Brucella* antiserum before infec-

[a]This work was supported by a grant from the Caisse Nationale d'Assurance Maladie and by a long-term EMBO fellowship to S.K.

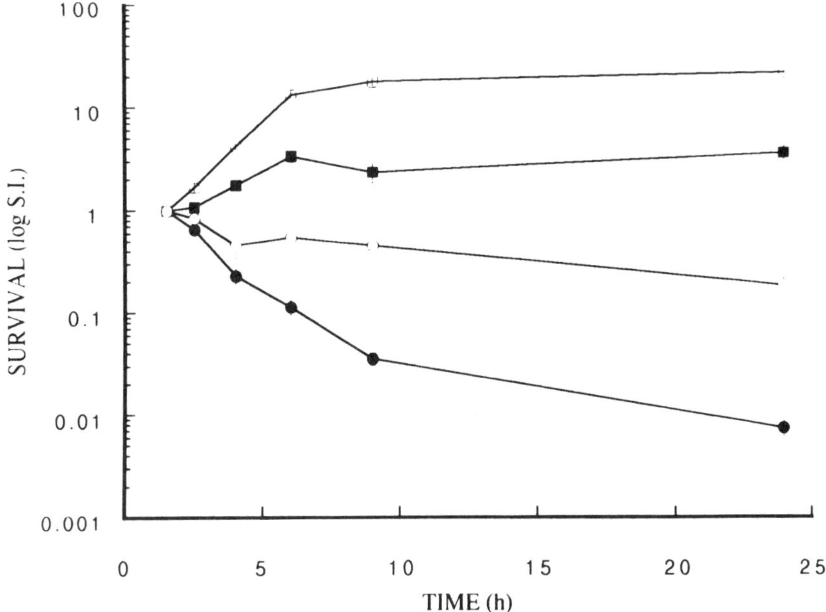

FIGURE 1. Intracellular behavior of *Listeria monocytogenes* Sv1/2a (SLCC 5764) in U-937 cells differentiated by PMA (□) or RA/VD (■) and of *L. ivanovii* (ATCC 19119) in U-937 cells differentiated by PMA (○) or RA/VD (●). S.I. = survival index = $\dfrac{\text{viable intracellular bacteria (\%)}}{100\%}$.

tion resulted in enhanced intracellular killing and very slow recovery (FIG. 2). The animal pathogen *B. canis* and strain *B. suis* S4 did not multiply within the phagocytic cells after an initial killing of 50-60% (FIG. 2).

Adhesion and phagocytosis of nonopsonized, smooth strains of *B. suis* were very low (0.3-0.4%) compared to rough strains *B. canis* and *E. coli* K12 (4-5%). IgG opsonization leveled adhesion and ingestion rates for *B. suis* and *E. coli*. It remains to be determined by which receptor(s) *Brucella* adheres to the macrophage and why phagocytosis is extremely low.

Using bacteria belonging to two different classes of intracellular pathogens, we were able to validate the use of U-937 differentiated by RA/VD as a model for the study of facultatively intracellular bacteria. *L. monocytogenes* represents the group of bacteria that is able to escape from the phagocytic vacuole into the cytoplasm, and *B. suis* is an example of pathogens remaining within the phagocytic vacuole throughout the infection. We showed that the type of differentiation seemed to influence macrophage activation and hence bacterial multiplication or killing.

This first model for the intracellular behavior of *Brucella* in a human monocytic cell line will be a helpful tool in the characterization of *Brucella* virulence factors.

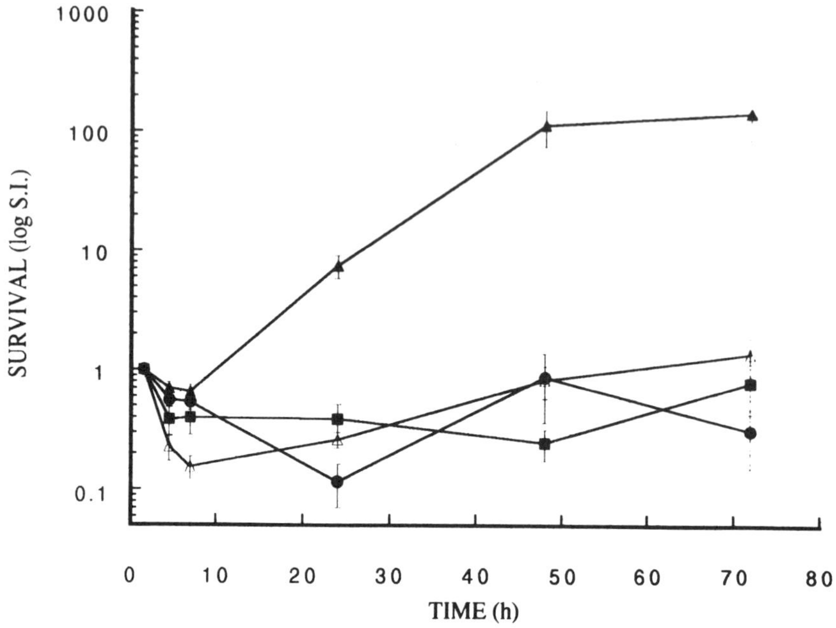

FIGURE 2. Intracellular behavior of *Brucella* strains after phagocytosis by U-937 differentiated by RA/VD: *B. canis* (●); *B. suis* S4 ATCC (■); nonopsonized *B. suis* S1 (▲); *B. suis* S1 opsonized with anti-*Brucella* IgG (△).

REFERENCES

1. ABSHIRE, K. Z. & F. C. NEIDHARDT. 1993. J. Bacteriol. **175:** 3734–3743.
2. KWAIK, Y. A., B. I. EISENSTEIN & N. C. ENGLEBERG. 1993. Infect. Immun. **61:** 1320–1329.
3. TAIMI, M., M.-T. CHÂTEAU, S. CABANE & J. MARTI. 1991. Leuk. Res. **15:** 1145–1152.
4. KUHN, M., S. KATHARIOU & W. GOEBEL. 1988. Infect. Immun. **56:** 79–82.
5. JIANG, X. & C. L. BALDWIN. 1993. Infect. Immun. **61:** 124–134.

Identification of an Adhesin-Like Gene of *Mycoplasma pirum* Isolated from AIDS Patients

T. N. THAM,[a] S. FERRIS,[a] E. BAHRAOUI,[b]
S. CANARELLI,[b] L. MONTAGNIER,[a] AND
A. BLANCHARD [a,c]

[a]*Institut Pasteur*
Departement du SIDA et des Rétrovirus
Paris, France

[b]*CNRS URA 1455*
Faculté Médecine Nord
13015 Marseilles, France

The goal of the present study is to isolate and determine the sequence of the adhesin gene of *Mycoplasma pirum*. Mycoplasmas have been suggested as cofactors in the development of AIDS.[1] The mycoplasmal species that have been implicated include *M. fermentans*, *M. penetrans*, and *M. pirum*. The latter has been sporadically isolated from contaminated cell cultures; its natural host was unknown until its recent isolation from mononuclear cells purified from the blood of HIV-infected individuals.[1,2] *M. pirum* is phylogenetically related to mycoplasmas such as *M. genitalium* and *M. pneumoniae*. The major cytoadhesins of the latter two mycoplasmas were identified and shown to be clustered at the tip of the cell as an organized structure for adherence.[3]

Synthetic oligonucleotides derived from conserved regions of adhesin genes of *M. pneumoniae* and *M. genitalium* were used as probes to localize the adhesin gene of *M. pirum*. Five *Eco*RI products of the *M. pirum* genome hybridized with one of the oligonucleotides which was homologous to the 3'-end of the adhesin genes. After cloning and sequencing, the amino acid sequence deduced from one of the five fragments presented highest scores of homology in databases with *M. pneumoniae* and *M. genitalium* adhesins. With TGA used as a Trp codon in mycoplasmas, including *M. pirum*,[4] a 5' open reading frame (ORF) of 967 bp was located on this DNA fragment, and the 3' end of the ORF (3048 bp) was found on a 10 kbp partially overlapping *Hind*III fragment. The entire gene for the P1-like adhesin of *M. pirum* shows a G+C content of only 28% which is in accordance with a G+C content of 25.5% for the entire genome of this mycoplasma.[5] The 127-kD polypeptide deduced from the complete sequence has a similarity of 46.1% and 46.9% with the adhesins of *M. genitalium* and *M. pneumoniae*, respectively (FIG. 1). The highest degree of homology was found at the COOH-terminus which was proline-rich for all three

[c] Address for correspondence: Institut Pasteur, Departement du SIDA et des rétrovirus, Oncologie Virale, 28, rue du Dr. Roux, 75724 Paris Cédex 15, France.

```
        1                                                          60
pneum   MHQtKKtaLsKstWiLiLTAtaSLatglTVVGhFtstttL...krQ.....qFSYtrPD
genit   MHQpKKr.LaKksWaF.LTAaltLg.viTgVGgY.....fLfnqnkOrssVSnFaY.qPk
pirum   M...KKikF...nYkYlL...iSLvst.TIVsa...............aaISlYStfnkD
conse   Mhq-KK--L-k--W---Lta--sL----T-Vg--------l-----q----s-Fsy--pd

        61                                                         120
pneum   eValrHtnAINprLTPWTYrNtSFSSLplTGENPGaWaLVR....DN.sakgITagSGsq
genit   OlSvkHqqAVdetLTPWTWnNnnFSSLkITGENPGsFgLVR.sQNDNLNissVTKNSsdd
pirum   QIS...npiINqnv.......kSFSnpsIvGnkvGk...IRhwQNnNFNgveI.KNgG..
conse   q-s--h--aIn--ltpwt--n-sFSsl-itGenpG---lVR--qndN-n---Itknsg--

        121                                                        180
pneum   qttY.dptrtEaaLTasttFAlRRYDlaGRALYDLDFsKL.NPqTptRDqtGQitFnPFg
genit   nlkYlna..vEkyLdgqQnFAiRRYDnnGRALYDinLaKMeNPsTVqRglnGepiFdPFk
pirum   ...Fv.......vLTstQs.At.RiDafGniLWEFD......PekIasE.dsQ..YanLa
conse   ---Y------e--Lt--q-fA-rRyD--GraLYD-d--k--nP-t--r---gq--F-pF-

        181                                                        240
pneum   GFGLsGaAPqqWNEVKnKVPVEVaQD.PsNPyrFaVLLVPrsvvyYeqLqrgl...gLpq
genit   GFGLtGnAPtdWNEIKgKVPVEVvQs.PhsPNlYFVLLVPKvaleYhnLnnqvvkesLev
pirum   G...............K.KV.VEItQDegdNsNiLYlLLIPK..................
conse   Gfgl-g-ap--wne-K-KVpVEV-Qd-p-npn---vLLVPk----y--l--------l--

        241                                                        300
pneum   qrTeSgqNTstTgaMfglK...VKnAeaDtaKsnEKLqg.aEaTGSSttSGsgqSTQRgg
genit   kaTqSsfN..pTqrL..qKdsPVK....DssKqgEKL...sEtTaSSmsSGmatST.RA.
pirum   .......NT............PdKqAsiD.pKd...LyaynElTGSS......kSkQqA.
conse   --t-s--Nt--t------k--pvK-a--D--K--ekL----E-TgSS--sg---Stqra-

        301                                                        360
pneum   ssgdtkvKALKIEVkkkSdSEdngqlQLeKNDLAnaPiKrseeSGqsVqLkAD.DFgtAl
genit   .......KALKVEVergSqSDs.....LlKNDFAkkPlKhknsSGe.VkLeAEkEFteA.
pirum   ...........tV...........vQiieN..................VnL.....Yqgs.
conse   -------kalk-eV---s-s------ql-kNd-a--p-k----sg--V-L-a---F--a-

        361                                                        420
pneum   sssgsggnsnpgsptpWrPwLaTEQI..hKdLpkwsAsILiLYDAPYarNrTAidrVDHl
genit   ...............WkPlLTTDQIareKGM...gAtVvsFYDAPYseNhTAfglVDHI
pirum   ...............tWtPsFT...I...KGL.......M..................HI
conse   ----------------W-P-Ltt-qI---KgL----a-----ydapy--n-ta---vdHi

        421                                                        480
pneum   DPKaMtaNYPPSWrTPKWNHHGlWDWkARdvLLQTTGFFNPRRHPEWFDgGQtVADNekt
genit   DPKKMVENYPPSWKTPKWNHHGiWDYnARnlLLQTTGFFNPRRHPEWFDeGQakADNtsp
pirum   DPKKMVDNYPnqWKssqss................sT.FFtkedHPsWY.....VAnNse.
conse   DPKkMv-NYPpsWktpkwnhhg-wd--ar--llqtTgFFnprrHPeWFd-gq-vAdN---

        481                                                        540
pneum   GFdV.dnsEntKqGFqKeadSdKSAPIALPFEAYFANIGNLtwfGqalLVFGGNGHVTKs
genit   GFKV.gDtDhkKdGFkK..NS..SsPIALPFEAYFANIGNMvAiGnsVFIFGGNGHaTKm
pirum   ..KVhnDaDqntnqY....NglKSAnmvLPWkqYitNlGNMfAkngiVLIFGGNGsIyn.
conse   gfkV--d-D--k-gF-k--ns-kSapiaLPFeaYfaNiGNM-a-g--vLIFGGNGh-tk-

        541                                                        600
pneum   ahTaPLSIGVFRV....rYnatgtsa.tVTGWPYAlLFsGMVNkQTDGLKDLPFnn...N
genit   ftTnPLSIGVFRI....kYtdNfsks.sVTGWPYAvLFgGLINpQTnGLKDLPLGT...N
pirum   .dpeaLSIGmWkldflkpYsgNidnnqnygGiPYAvLLryL...ryDpsKpL.LGTsapN
conse   --t-pLSIGvFr------Y--n------vtGwPYA-LF-gL-n-qtdglKdLpLgt---N

        601                                                        660
pneum   RWFE.............YVPRMAVaGaKFVGreLVLAGTiTMGDTATVPRLLYDeLEsnL
genit   RWFE.............YVPRMAVsGVKWVGnqLVLAGTlTMGDTATVPRLkYDqLEkhL
pirum   RRWnqsyapigqtdnftYVPRLAVgGVq......InAsT....DeAT...yLY..Laagi
conse   RWFe------------YVPRMAV-Gvk-vg--lVlAgT-tmgDtATVprllYd-Le--l

        661                                                        720
pneum   NLVAQG.QGLLREDLQlFTPYGWANRPDlPIGAWsssssSShn.aPyYFhNNFFwQDrpi
genit   NLVAQG.QGLLREDLQiFTPYGWANRPDiPVGAWlQDemgSkF.GPhYFlNNFDiQDnvn
pirum   t.VgQakesqaRE..vIsnsntstNk....VvtkiQDkrSlqLtGantitNtkE....ta
conse   nlVaQg-qgllREdlqiftpygwaNrpd-pVgaw-qd--ss---gp-yf-NnfD-qd---

        721                                                        780
pneum   qNvVD.AFIkpWedKNgkDdaKyIYPYRYSGMWAWQVYNWSNKLTdqPLSAdF.VNENaY
genit   ndtVE.ALIssY..KNt.DklKhVYPYRYSGLYAWQlFNWSNKLTnTPLSANF.VNENsY
pirum   aNsIDpALl..................Fgt..AFnIdsliN.LptTkLneNLtIfqNvF
conse   -n-VD-ALi-----kn--d--k--ypyrYsg--AWq--nwsNkLt-tpLsanF-VneN-Y

        781                                                        840
pneum   QPNSLF..AAILNpELLaALpDKVkYGKENEFAaNEyERFNQkLtvAPtqqTKWshFspt
genit   aPNSLF..AAILNeDLLtgLsDKIFYGKENEFAeNEaDRFNQlLslnPnpnTKWarYlnv
pirum   QyeSyFdvgAtMs..vssAvgtyyYFdKkNh...............AssstTi......
conse   qpnSlF--aAiLn--ll-al-dk--YqKeNefa-ne--rfnq-l--ap---TKW------
```

FIGURE 1. Alignment of the adhesin amino acid sequences from *M. pneumoniae, M. genitalium, and M. pirum.* The polypeptides were aligned using the PILEUP program provided by the GCG package, with a value of 1 as a gap weight. By using the PRETTY program, a consensus polypeptide (conse) was created. Positions occupied by the same or similar (conservative change) amino acids in all three sequences are indicated by *uppercase letters* in the consensus sequence.

```
      841                                                        900
pneum lsRFsTGfNLvgSvLDQvLDYvPWIGNGYrY.gNNhrgVddItaPqTSAgSSsgistnTs
genit VqRFTTGpNLdsStFDQfLDFLPWIGNGkpF.sNs.......psPsTSAsSS......Tp
pirum IntYTTasN....gWnn....LgRtafpWsYkpNN..dIgsIfqPkTndnnn........
conse --rFtTg-Nl--s--dq-ld-lpWigng--Y--Nn------i--P-Tsa-ss------t-

      901                                                        960
pneum gsrsfLPTFSNIgVGLKanVqatLggsqTmitggspRRtLdqaNL..qlWTGAGWRndka
genit .....LPTFSNINVGvKsMItqhLNkenT.......RWvFi.pNFSpdiWTGAGYR....
pirum ......aTYS.yNlsL..LIenaiN.............YyystLS...F...GY.....
conse -----lpTFSninvglk--I---ln---t-------r------nLs---WtgaGYr----

      961                                                        1020
pneum sSgQSdeNhTKftsatgMDQqgqSgtSag.NPdSlkqDN.IskSGdSlttqdGnAidqqe
genit ..vQS.aNq.K..ngIpfEQvkPSnnStpfdPnS..dDNkVtpSGgS...........sK
pirum .SlkclgglTK....IeM....PSke....NP.....ENtI..........yGyAmqvgK
conse -s-qs--n-tK----i-m-q--pS--s---nP-s---DN-I--sg-s------g-a----k

      1021                                                       1080
pneum aTnYtNLPpnltPTaDWpNALsFTNKNNaQRaQLFLRgLL..GsIPVLVNrSGsDSN.KF
genit pTtYpaLPnsisPTSDWiNALtFTNKNNpQRnQLLLRSLL..GtIPVLINkSG.DSNdqF
pirum sivYlN.....ePkSD..................LRSiayhGpssIsIgeSnlvgsaKY
conse -t-Y-nlp----PtsDw-nal-ftnknn-qr-ql-LRsll--G-ipVlIn-Sg-dsn-kF

      1081                                                       1140
pneum .qatDQKWsYTDlhsdqtklNLP.aYGEV.NGLlNpALVeTYfgntraGgsGsNTtSs.P
genit nkdsEQKWdkTEtNeg....NLP.gFGEV.NGLyNaALlhTY......GffGtNTnSTdP
pirum ...gDmdYpYvkiNnsnigy.vPsdYsnItNniiNtg.VaiYv....tGikdfN..dTiP
conse ----DqkW-yt--n------nlP--YgeV-Ngl-N-alv-tY------G--g-Nt-st-P

      1141                                                       1200
pneum gIG..FKIpEqn.nDSkaTLITpGLaWTpQ.DV..GNLVV.sgTtvsFQLGGWLV....T
genit kIG..FK.aDSs.ssSSSTLVgsGLnWTsQ.DV..GNLVViNdTsFgFQLGGWFI....T
pirum tIasqFeIgnSpyeDnSSTtkTnG...TlQptIpwndFVglNsTnFnseisslWlnnnqT
conse -Ig--Fki--s---dssstl-t-Gl-wT-Q-dV--gnLVv-n-T-f-fqlggw------T

      1201                                                       1260
pneum FTDFVkPRaGYLGlqLtgLDaSDaTqrAlIWApRPWaaFrGSW..vnRlGrveSvWD...
genit FTDFIrPRtGYLGITLsSLq..DqT...iIWADqPWtsFkGSY..lDsdGtpkSlWDpta
pirum kTn....nnehFiVT.kSpEiSEyygnA.IWtERfYynY.GSsnnaDWkGskrawFEvkd
conse fTdf--pr-gyLg-tl-sl--sD-t--a-IWa-rpW--F-GS----d--G---s-WD---

      1261                                                       1320
pneum LKgvwadqaqSdSqgSTTtaTrnaLpehPnAlaFQVsvveasaYkPNtssg.QTQsTNss
genit LKSL......pNS..STTydTnptLs..P...SFQl.......YQPNkvkayQT..TN..
pirum snSL......SNS..STTvgwqvgLdsnltAdSYyV........QkNne...QpQgd...
conse lksl------snS--STT--t---L---p-a-sFqv-------yqpN-----Qtq-tn--

      1321                                                       1380
pneum pYlhLVkPkkvT.QsdkLDddLKnLLdpnq..Vr.tKLrQsFGTdhStQp..qpqsLktT
genit tYnkLIePvDaTsaatNMtsLLK.LLtTkn..Ik.aKLgk..GTa.SsQgnnnggqvsqT
pirum .FdvLlrtrDdT.QknN.DiFFgqinnTrepgIsycKLkQnYG...Sy........FyeT
conse -Y--L--p-d-T-q--n-d--lk-ll-t----I---KL-q--Gt--S-q---------T

      1381                                                       1440
pneum tpvfgTssGNLSsvLsgggagggssGSGQsgvdlspvEkvsgWLVgqlpstsDgntsStN
genit IntItT.tGNiSegLkee.......tSiQa.......EtlkkFF........D....Skq
pirum IseI....drLS.1L............GnGQ.............FV.............N
conse i--i-t--gnlS--L----------gsgQ--------e-----Fv-------d----s-N

      1441                                                       1500
pneum NLapntNtgNdVVGVGrlsESNaAKMnddVdGIVrTPLaeLLDGeGqTaDtgpqsVkF.K
genit N.....NkSe..IGIG...DStFtKMdgkltGVVSTPLvNLinGqGaTsDsdtekIsF.K
pirum NL......SNqIlt.......nNLAnLlvqVn..lSTvtgNpLDsks.T.......IrivK
conse Nl----n-sn---g-g----sn-akM---v-g-vsTpl-nlldg-g-T-d------I-f-K

      1501                                                       1560
pneum spdQIDFNRLFThPVTD..LFDPvTMLVYDQYIPLFIdIPasVn..pkmVRLKVlSFdtn
genit pgNQIDFNRLFTlPVTE..LFDPnTMFVYDQYVPLLVnlPSgfD..qaSIRLKViSYsve
pirum ..NQf.LNevF..qVTknpiiEgsT....ptYgPviI.VaSnVDfvsqSatFtaySWn..
conse --nQidFNrlFt-pVT---lfDp-Tm-vydqY-Pl-I--ps-vd----s-rLkv-S----

      1561                                                       1620
pneum eQSLGlRLEfFKpDqdTQpnnnvqvnpnngdFlPlLtASSqGPQTlFsPFNQWpDYVLPL
genit nQtLGvRLE.FK.DPqTQ...........qFIPVLNASStGPQTVFqPFNQWADYVLPL
pirum ..SLtknyDvm...PrTnssk..........InViNnS......IFagFsamADWILPv
conse -qsLg-rlE-fk-dp-Tq-----------fipvlnaSs-gpqt-F-pFnqwaDYVLPl

      1621                                                       1680
pneum aITVPIVVIVLCVTLGLaIGIPMIIKNK(qALIUAGFuLSNqIlVDVLTKAVGSVFKEIINRIG
genit IVTVPIVVIILSVTLGLtIGIPMHrNKKALqAGFDLSNkKVDVLTKAVGSVFKEIINRTG
pirum VIaIPIVlVaLiIgLGcsIGIPMaKhKKAiKvGFELqhdKVgtLTsAVGgVFKkIIdnTn
conse -ItVPIVvI-LsVtLGl-IGIPMhknKkAlkaGF-Lsn-KVdvLTkAVGSVFKeIInrTg

      1681                                                       1737
pneum ISqA....PKrLKQtsAaKPgaPrP...........PvPPkpgAPKPPVqppkkpa
genit ISNA....PKkLKQAtptKP.TPkt.............P.......PKPPVKq.....
pirum .SNnvkskPqmLK.AaAkKPnTvpParsqltndsvsrPtPP.ssAPKPPIK......
conse iSna----Pk-LKqa-a-KP-tp-p-----------P-pp---aPKPPVk-----
```

The consensus sequence is in *lowercase letters* when the same amino acid is found in two sequences of the adhesins; other positions are shown in *dashes*. In the adhesin sequences, amino acids identical to the consensus are in *uppercase letters*. Gaps are shown by *dots*. Amino acid sequences are: *M. pneumoniae* P1 adhesin (pneum), *M. genitalium* MgPa adhesin (genit), and *M. pirum* P1-like adhesin (pirum). Signal sequences are *underlined*.

adhesins. When analyzed by the method of Kyte and Doolittle,[6] the NH_2-terminal regions of the three adhesins presented a similar hydropathy profile, suggesting by analogy with the adhesins of *M. genitalium* and *M. pneumoniae* the presence of a sequence signal for the *M. pirum* adhesin. Moreover, in contrast to the absence of cysteine residue in *M. pneumoniae* and *M. genitalium* adhesins, three cysteine residues were found in the *M. pirum* adhesin. This would potentially contribute to the establishment of at least one disulfide bridge, leading to a more stable structure of the protein. To characterize the expression of the product of the cloned P1-like gene, antisera were produced against a peptide modeling the COOH-terminus of this adhesin-like, and they were found to specifically recognize a 126-kD polypeptide from the *M. pirum* cell lysate and also from its membrane fraction.

The results just described indicate that we have identified the gene for the *M. pirum* adhesin, which will potentially allow the production of antigenic and serologic tools for the study of the putative pathogenic potential of *M. pirum*.

REFERENCES

1. MONTAGNIER, L. & A. BLANCHARD. 1993. Mycoplasmas as cofactors in infection due to the human immunodeficiency virus infection. Clin. Infect. Dis. **17:** S309–S315.
2. GRAU, O., R. KOVACIC, R. GRIFFAIS & L. MONTAGNIER. 1993. Development of a selective and sensitive polymerase chain reaction assay for the detection of *Mycoplasma pirum*. FEMS Microbiol. Lett. **106:** 327–334.
3. RAZIN, S. & E. JACOBS. 1992. Mycoplasma adhesion. J. Gen. Microbiol. **138:** 407–422.
4. THAM, T. N., S. FERRIS, R. KOVACIC, L. MONTAGNIER & A. BLANCHARD. 1993. Identification of *Mycoplasma pirum* genes involved in the salvage pathways for nucleosides. J. Bacteriol. **175:** 5281–5285.
5. DEL GIUDICE, R. A., J. G. TULLY, D. L. ROSE & R. M. COLE. 1985. *Mycoplasma pirum* sp. nov., a terminal structured mollicute from cell culture. Int. J. Syst. Bacteriol. **35:** 285–291.
6. KYTE, J. & R. F. DOOLITTLE. 1982. A simple method for displaying the hydropathic character of a protein. J. Mol. Biol. **157:** 105–132.

A Leukotoxin Nonproducing Mutant of *Pasteurella haemolytica*

Phagocytosis and Killing by Bovine Polymorphonucleocytes

A. P. RICKETTS, J. A. GORDON,[a] M. B. HARRIGAN, AND S. FROSHAUER

*Pfizer Inc
Central Research Division
Groton, Connecticut 06340*

Pasteurella haemolytica causes an economically important, stress-related pneumonia in cattle (shipping fever). This gram-negative bacterium secretes a well-characterized leukotoxin that has been proposed to function as an important virulence factor that specifically lyses ruminant leukocytes. To explore the role of this and other bacterial and host factors during pathogenesis, we compared the interaction of *P. haemolytica* with bovine polymorphonucleocytes (PMNs) *in vitro* in the presence and absence of leukotoxin. A leukotoxin nonproducing mutant (lkt⁻) of *P. haemolytica* has been isolated,[1,2] and this strain does not cause lysis or release of the cytosolic enzyme lactate dehydrogenase from bovine PMNs. Therefore, using the mutant, we were able to develop an *in vitro* model of the interaction of the actively growing *P. haemolytica* with viable host defense cells. In initial experiments we were surprised to find that the growth rate of *P. haemolytica* measured by counting bacterial colonies was not reduced in the presence of PMNs despite phagocytic uptake of 50% of the added bacteria.[3] In contrast, *Staphylococcus aureus* or *Escherichia coli* were efficiently taken up and killed by the PMNs.[3] We here report an alternative approach to measuring the association between internalization and killing of *P. haemolytica* by PMNs.

RESULTS AND DISCUSSION

We incubated PMNs with bacteria radiolabeled with protein or DNA precursors and measured release of trichloroacetic acid (TCA) soluble radioactivity into the supernatant. We found that the optimal bacteria : PMN ratio for release of radioactivity

[a] PRESENT ADDRESS: Advanced Biosciences Laboratory, Frederick Cancer Research and Development Center, Frederick, MD 21702.

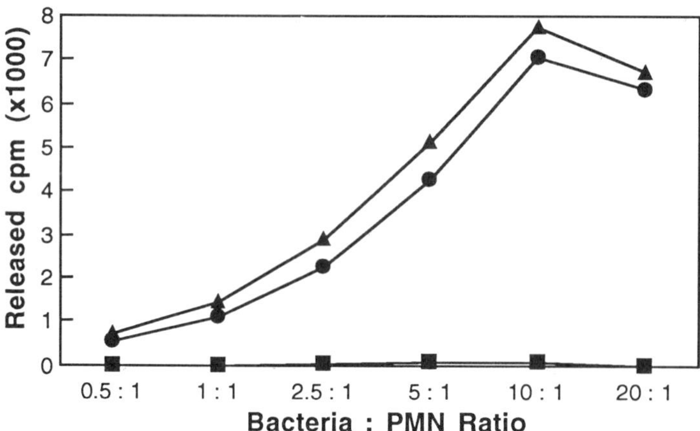

FIGURE 1. Optimal ratio of bacteria to polymorphonucleocytes (PMNs). PMNs were collected from udders of dairy cows 18 hours after instillation of 120 ml of a 0.5% solution of glycogen in physiologic saline. Mid-log lkt⁻ *P. haemolytica* in BHI broth were incubated for 30 minutes with 20 μCi/ml [³H]thymidine in M63 glucose media, and then opsonized with bovine serum (10% immune + 10% fresh whole adult). Bacteria ($1.25 \times 10^6 - 5 \times 10^7$ cfu per well) and PMNs (2.5×10^6 per well) in RPMI-1640 media were mixed in 24-well microtiter plates, centrifuged at 1,800 rpm for 5 minutes, and incubated at 5% CO_2 and 37 °C. Values are TCA soluble radioactivity in the supernatant in the presence of PMNs minus that in their absence. Results are from a representative single experiment taken at time 0 (■), 30 minutes (●), and 60 minutes (▲).

was 10:1 (FIG. 1). The time course for release of label is shown in FIGURE 2. The amount of radiolabeled lkt⁻ *P. haemolytica* added to incubations was 1.1×10^6 TCA precipitable counts per minute (cpm)/well with [³⁵S]methionine and 1.4×10^5 cpm/ well with [³H]thymidine. After 1 hour, 13% of added ³⁵S was recovered as TCA soluble radioactivity in the supernatant and 1.5% of added ³H. When radiolabeled wild-type *P. haemolytica* were used, PMNs were rapidly lysed, and substantially less radioactivity was released from the bacteria (FIG. 2). Evidence that release of radioactivity reflects phagocytic degradation comes from several modifications to the assay that we employed that block phagocytosis, judged microscopically in cytospin preparations. These manipulations all blocked release of radioactivity. Results shown in FIGURE 2 are for substitution of 20% heat-inactivated fetal calf serum as opsonin which eliminates antibody and complement; incubation of bacteria and PMNs at 0 °C instead of 37 °C to prevent cell motility; pretreatment of PMNs with cytochalasin B which inhibits actin filament formation; and omission of a centrifugation step that we normally use to promote the association of bacteria and PMNs.

Our benchmark method for scoring bacterial killing is bacterial colony counting, where incubation mixtures are treated with 0.5 mg/ml saponin to solubilize PMNs (without affecting bacterial growth) followed by spreading lysates on BHI agar plates and incubating overnight at 37 °C. We found that only 50% of added lkt⁻ *P.*

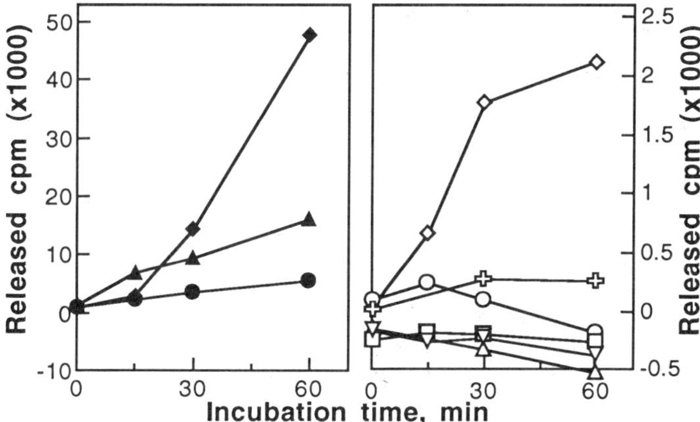

FIGURE 2. Requirement for phagocytosis. Lkt⁻ *P. haemolytica* labeled as previously described with [³H]thymidine (*open symbols*) or labeled with [³⁵S]methionine in MEM media without methionine (*filled symbols*) were incubated at a bacteria : PMN ratio of 10 : 1. Results are for standard assay conditions (◆, ◇) and several modifications that prevented phagocytosis: opsonization with heat-inactivated fetal calf serum (□), incubating at 0 °C (▽), omitting centrifugation (⊕), 15-minute pretreatment of PMNs with 10 μg/ml cytochalasin B (●, ○), and use of wild-type *P. haemolytica* (▲,△). Results are representative single experiments or the average of from two to four replicate experiments.

haemolytica are internalized in our system, and the background of extracellular bacteria reduces assay sensitivity when using colony counts. In fact, we do not detect any reduction of colony counts caused by bovine PMNs. However, release of radioactivity from labeled bacteria is detectable under the same conditions. We found that only a small percentage of added radioactivity was released on incubation with PMNs, and this may indicate that a small number of added *P. haemolytica* are killed, likely below the detection limit for colony counting. The method described is a sensitive and reproducible indicator for phagocytosis-dependent effects on *P. haemolytica* and appears internally consistent. However, we obtained paradoxical results when comparing different species of bacteria. *Staphylococcus aureus,* which is effectively killed based on colony counts, gave results by radiometric scoring that were not substantially different from *P. haemolytica.* Further work is required to resolve this anomaly.

REFERENCES

1. PETRAS, S. F., S. A. FROSHAUER, E. F. ILLYES, G. M. WEINSTOCK & C. P. REESE. 1992. 73rd Annual CRWAD Meeting, Abstr. 94.
2. CHIDAMBARAM M., B. SHARMA, G. M. WEINSTOCK, C. P. REESE, S. F. PETRAS & S. FROSHAUER. In preparation.
3. FROSHAUER, S., M. B. HARRIGAN & A. P. RICKETTS. In preparation.

Escherichia coli That Express *Neisseria gonorrhoeae* Opacity-Associated Proteins Attach to and Invade Human Fallopian Tube Epithelium

G. GORBY,[a] D. SIMON,[b] AND R. F. REST [b]

[a]*VA Medical Center*
Creighton University
University of Nebraska
Omaha, Nebraska 68105-1873

[b]*Hahnemann University School of Medicine*
Philadelphia, Pennsylvania 19102-1192

Gonococcal opacity-associated proteins (Opa) mediate adherence/invasion of *Neisseria gonorrhoeae* and *Escherichia coli* in human epithelial cell lines in culture.[1–3] Their role in invasion of normal fallopian tube epithelium has not been fully elucidated.[4,5] Studies in the human fallopian tube organ culture model indicate that differences among Opa proteins can influence the amount of attachment and damage to the mucosa[4] and suggest a subsequent effect on invasion.[5] Understanding the role of Opas in attachment and invasion is complicated by the phase variation of gonococcal antigens and the intergonococcal adherence of Opas with gonococcal lipooligosaccharides.

To see if Opas alone can mediate attachment with subsequent invasion, *E. coli* DH5α bearing plasmid pGEM-3Z carrying Opa P (GC strain F62SF), Opa A (GC strain FA1090), or Opa B (also FA1090)[2,3] was tested for the ability to attach to and invade epithelial cells in the human fallopian tube organ culture model.[5] The Opa B-producing strain which lost the ability to produce Opa on serial passage despite retaining ampicillin resistance was used as a negative control. Opa production was detected by immunoblotting (FIG. 1) with monoclonal 4B12/CII (kindly provided by Milan Blake, PhD). Fallopian tube explants were infected with 2×10^5 cfu/ml *E. coli,* harvested at 24 and 48 hours postinfection and prepared for light microscopy.[5] Tissue sections were stained with rabbit anti-*E. coli* polyclonal antisera followed by goat-anti-rabbit FITC-conjugated antisera, rhodamine phalloidin (stains F-actin), and Hoechst 33342 (stains DNA). Registered image stacks of each fluorochrome were obtained at 0.4-μ intervals and subjected to digital confocal microscopy.[6] Cell-associated bacteria were quantified via computerized image analysis[5] by measuring FITC-stained bacteria inside or touching cytoplasmic regions defined by rhodamine-stained actin. Intracellular bacteria were measured by including bacteria inside but not touching the region of interest boundary. The difference between these measurements represented extracellular adherent bacteria.

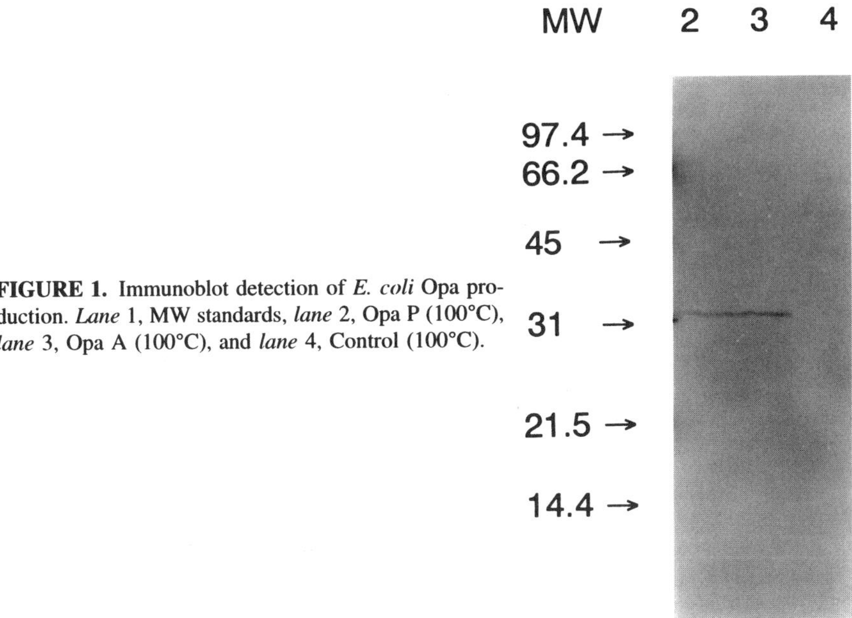

FIGURE 1. Immunoblot detection of *E. coli* Opa production. *Lane* 1, MW standards, *lane* 2, Opa P (100°C), *lane* 3, Opa A (100°C), and *lane* 4, Control (100°C).

Opa A producers were more adherent (0.9 μ^2/cell) than Opa P producers (0.017 μ^2/ cell) or the nonproducer (0.015 μ^2/cell) at 24 hours ($p < 0.001$). Opa P did not differ significantly from the control ($p > 0.05$). There was no invasion at 24 hours, but qualitative evaluation at 48 hours revealed more invasive bacteria in the Opa A group compared to the Opa P or nonproducer group (FIG. 2). By 48 hours Opa P clearly attached and modestly invaded, but the control did not. Quantitative evaluation by computerized image analysis is underway to confirm this impression. Although the amount of *E. coli* invasion appeared similar to that of GC previously investigated,[5] the morphology of invasion differed somewhat. In the fallopian tube model, GC are usually seen traversing the epithelium as multiorganism clumps in vacuoles or are seen clumped in submucosal regions. By contrast, *E. coli* that produced Opa proteins were seen as single rods traversing the epithelium and were more loosely associated in the submucosal region, perhaps due to a lack of adherence between bacteria. Attachment to and invasion of fallopian tube epithelium by some wild-type strains of *E. coli* has previously been reported.[7] Thus, Opas may complement an underlying ability of *E. coli* DH5α to trigger invasion by allowing close attachment, or Opas may single-handedly mediate both attachment and invasion.

We conclude that GC Opas are sufficient to allow adherence to and invasion of human fallopian tube epithelium by a previously nonadherent strain of *E. coli*. This ability to mediate adherence with subsequent invasion appears to differ between the two Opas tested, but both invade.

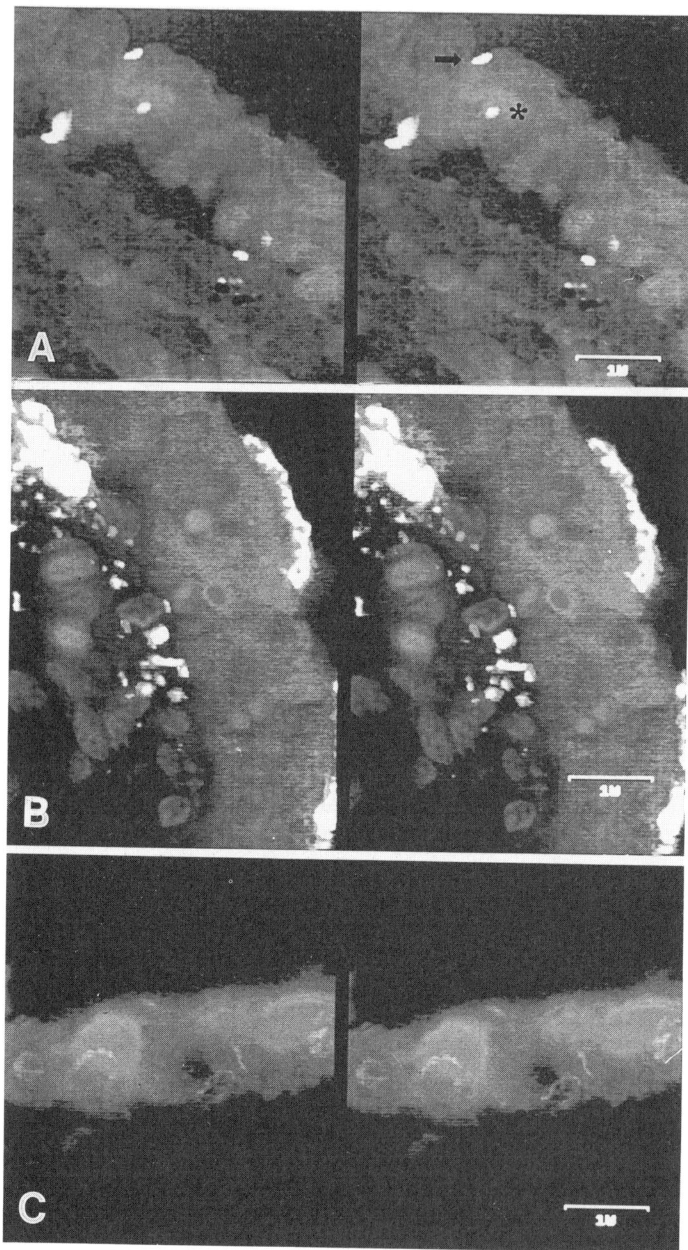

FIGURE 2.

FIGURE 2. Stereo pair three-dimensional gray-scale reconstruction of Opa-producing *E. coli* interactions with human fallopian tube epithelium 48 hours postinfection. Rhodamine-stained actin and Hoechst-stained nuclei were rendered with low contrast to outline cellular regions, whereas cell-associated bacteria were rendered with high contrast to allow them to be differentiated from cellular components. (**A**) Opa P variant depicting modest attachment and submucosal invasion of the epithelium. Bacteria undergoing early internalization (*arrow*) and transcytosis (*asterisk*) can be seen. (**B**) Opa A variant showing marked apical attachment and submucosal invasion. (**C**) Nonproducer showing lack of epithelial cell association. No attached bacteria are visible in this image, a typical finding in this experimental group. Bar = 10 μ.

REFERENCES

1. MAKINO, S., J. P. M. VAN PUTTEN & T. F. MEYER. 1991. EMBO J. **10:** 1307–1315.
2. SIMON, D. & R. F. REST. 1992. Proc. Natl. Acad. Sci. USA **89:** 5512–5516.
3. SIMON, D. & R. F. REST. 1992. *In* Eighth International Pathogenic Neisseria Conference. C. J. Conde-Glez, E. Calderon, S. A. Morse & C. Oropeza-Abundez, Eds. Vol. **1:** 89. National Institute of Public Health. Cuernavaca, Mexico.
4. DEKKER, N. P., C. J. LAMMEL, R. E. MANDRELL & G. F. BROOKS. 1990. Microb. Pathog. **9:** 19–31.
5. GORBY, G. L. & G. B. SCHAEFER. 1992. Microb. Pathog. **13:** 93–108.
6. HIRAOKA, Y., J. W. SEDAT & D. A. AGARD. 1987. Science **238:** 36–41.
7. MCGEE, Z. A., G. L. GORBY, P. B. WYRICK, R. HODINKA & L. H. HOFFMAN. 1988. Rev. Infect. Dis. **10** (Suppl. 2): 311–316.

Gestational Age-Dependent Distribution of *Escherichia coli* Fimbriae in Pregnant Patients with Pyelonephritis

BOGDAN NOWICKI,[a,b] MARK MARTENS,[a]
AUDREY HART,[a] AND STELLA NOWICKI [a,b]

Division of Infectious Disease
[a]*Department of Obstetrics & Gynecology*
and
[b]*Department of Microbiology*
The University of Texas Medical Branch
Galveston, Texas 77555

The etiology of pyelonephritis and other complications of pregnancy, including preterm labor and low birth weight, is often associated with *Escherichia coli* infections.[1] The general view is that obstruction of the urinary tract due to an enlarging uterus, in association with dilated ureters, glycosuria, and aminoaciduria, is the major factor increasing frequency of acute pyelonephritis in pregnant females. Therefore, the role of bacterial virulence and host factors, other than anatomic, involved in the development of gestational pyelonephritis and low birth weight/preterm labor has not been intensely explored.[2,3]

To the contrary, in the nonpregnant population, the mechanism of pyelonephritis is associated with *E. coli* virulence factors and tissue receptors.[4] The molecular basis for reaching the upper urogenital tract by *E. coli* is associated with ascending colonization due to *E. coli* fimbriae (e.g., P and Dr adhesins) anchoring cells to the high density receptor binding sites in the genitourinary tract.[4] Endogenous but highly virulent *E. coli* from the colon colonize the periurethral area and vaginal introitus. Some organisms may then reach uroepithelial receptors in the bladder and kidneys.

Few studies have tested the role of P and other fimbriae in renal infections of pregnant women. In this study, we tested the hypothesis that *E. coli* colonization factors may be important in the development of pyelonephritis during gestation by analyzing the frequency of expression of different fimbriae.

E. coli strains isolated from 60 pregnant patients of different gestational age with pyelonephritis were tested for expression of P, type 1, and Dr fimbriae. Expression of P fimbriae was tested by hemagglutination (HA) assay with 3% vol/vol pp erythrocytes and inhibition of HA by 0.5% gal-1-4gal. Expression of type 1 fimbriae was tested with guinea pig red cells and inhibition by 2% a-methylmannose. Dr fimbriae were identified by HA with Dr (a−) red cells and HA inhibition with 10 mM chloramphenicol.

We demonstrated that P fimbriae were expressed throughout the pregnancy with the highest frequency during the second trimester (65%) (TABLE 1). Expression of

TABLE 1. *E. coli* Fimbrial Types in Gestational Pyelonephritis

Trimester	No. of Strains	E. coli Fimbriae/Percentage		
		Type 1	P	Dr
I	13	10 (77)*	7 (54)	1 (8)
II	25	12 (48)	16 (64)	2 (8)
III	22	7 (32)	11 (50)	6 (27)*

type 1 fimbriae was observed among several strains, predominately during the first trimester (77%). To the contrary, Dr+ *E. coli* occur more frequently during the third trimester. As we proposed recently, type 1 fimbria can recognize receptors on human chorionic gonadotropin hormone (hCG). This is consistent with our proposal that hCG may be a host factor that increases the susceptibility of pregnant patients in the early trimesters to renal infection. The increased frequency of P fimbriae in the second and Dr in the third trimester may hypothetically be due to increased receptor density at this gestational age.

The frequency of P fimbriae positive *E. coli* in gestational pyelonephritis was almost as high as that in nonpregnant patients with pyelonephritis (70-80%). Therefore, it is likely that virulence factors of *E. coli* may be important in the pathogenesis of renal infection in the pregnant population. We observed a novel phenomenon that is the gestational age-dependent distribution of *E. coli* fimbriae in pregnant patients with pyelonephritis. Differential distribution of fimbrial types during pregnancy may result from gestational age-related tissue tropism. This, in turn, may suggest that pyelonephritis occurs more frequently during pregnancy due not only to anatomic changes, but also to the function of *E. coli* virulence factors and host ligands. Consequently, it is possible that preventive approaches may be developed to protect mother and fetus from serious gestational complications.

REFERENCES

1. ANDRIOLE, V. T. & T. F. PATTERSON. 1991. Med. Clin. North Am. **75:** 359-373.
2. STENQVIST, K., T. SANDBERG, G. LIDIN-JANSON, F. ØRSKOV, I. ØRSKOV & SVANBORG-EDÉN. 1987. J. Infect. Dis. **156:** 870-877.
3. MITTENDORF, R., M. A. WILLIAMS & E. H. KASS. 1992. Clin. Infect. Dis. **14:** 927-932.
4. NOWICKI, B., H. HOLTHOFER, T. SARANEVA, M. RHEN, VAISANEN-RHEN, & T. K. KORHONEN. 1986. Microb. Pathog. **1:** 169-180.

Host Factors in the Attachment of Gonococcal Cells to Pelvic Tissue

STELLA NOWICKI,[a,b] BOGDAN NOWICKI,[a,b]
MARK MARTENS,[a] ANIL KAUL,[a]
GUSTAVO FLORES,[a] AND DHRUV KUMAR [c]

*Departments of Obstetrics and Gynecology,[a] Microbiology,[b] and
Pathology [c]
The University of Texas Medical Branch
Galveston, Texas 77555*

Gonorrhea is an exclusively human disease. Human host factors are known to be involved in supporting gonococcal infections leading to severe complications such as pelvic inflammatory disease (PID). It was suggested by other investigators that gonococcal cell (GC) attachment is mediated by specific ligands that selectively recognize receptors on certain types of human cells. The host factors important in attachment of GC are poorly understood.[1] It is critical to note that different mechanisms are probably operating in the attachment of gonococci to different kinds of cells. The mechanism operating in the attachment of GC to the fallopian tube seems to be species specific. The importance of host factors (TNF and CMP-NANA) as well as GC factors (protein II, pili, and lipooligosaccharide) in infection of human tissues including fallopian tubes by GC was studied by many investigators.[2-6] To the contrary, many unanswered questions exist concerning the mechanism of infection of the uterine endometrium by *Neisseria gonorrhoeae*. The nature of the receptors and host factors that mediate specific interaction of GC with human endometrium is not completely understood. Recently, we described a new potential mechanism of GC attachment to human tissues in which complement C1q was a bridging molecule between GC and C1q receptors on human cells.[7,8] Glycoprotein C1q is a component of menstruum. Menstruum is known to be a predisposing host factor in developing upper genital tract infection. The fact that uterine and fallopian tube tissue is involved in PID raised the question of whether C1q is able to enhance attachment of GC to the uterus and fallopian tubes.

CONCLUSION

The attachment of GC to human uterus, but not to the fallopian tubes, was increased significantly in C1q-enriched medium *versus* C1q-deficient medium. Anti-C1q IgG inhibited attachment of GC in C1q-enriched medium to human endometrium but not to the fallopian tubes. Therefore, it is likely that the mechanisms of interaction of GC with the uterine tissue may differ from those with the fallopian tubes (previously described). These experiments supported the hypothesis that human factor C1q may increase the attachment of GC to uterine tissue and that this attachment seems to be

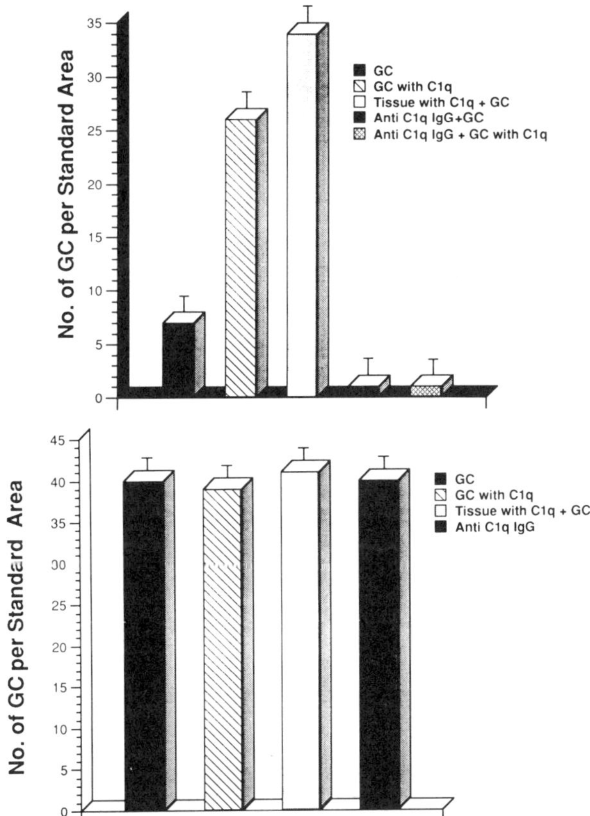

FIGURE 1. Effect of C1q on attachment of *N. gonorrhoeae* to the (**top**) endometrium and (**bottom**) fallopian tube.

tissue specific. C1q, which is thought to play a role in activation of complement cascade to killed microorganisms, plays a role in increasing GC virulence by mediating attachment to genital tissue. Overall, we suggest that C1q be considered a host-specific virulence factor of gonococcal PID (FIG. 1).

REFERENCES

1. BROOKS, G. F. 1985. *In* Gonococcal Infection. G. F. Brooks & E. A. Donegan, Eds.: 51–82. Edward Arnold Ltd. London.
2. GOTSCHLICH, E. C., M. A. APICELLA, R. E. MANDRELL, M. SHERO, M. E. WILSON, J. M. GRIFFISS, G. F. BROOKS, C. LAMMEL, J. F. BREEN & P. A. RICE. 1990. J. Infect. Dis. **162:** 506-512.
3. CORNELISSEN, C., S. A. HILL, J. M. KOOMEY, C. MARCHAL, T. F. MEYER, S. A. MORSE, S. NORMARK, A. B. SCHRYVERS, H. S. SEIFERT, P. F. SPARLING & J. SWANSON. 1991. *In* Neisseriae 1990. M. Achtman, P. Kohl, C. Marchal, B. G. Morella, A. Seiler & B. Thiesen, Eds.: 340- 341. Walter de Gryter. Berlin, New York.

4. HITCHCOCK, P. J. & T. M. BROWN. 1983. J. Bacteriol. **154:** 269–277.
5. GREGG, C. R., A. P. JOHNSON, D. TAYLOR-ROBINSON, M. A. MELLY & Z. A. MCGEE. 1981. Infect. Immunol. **34:** 1056–1058.
6. PARSONS, N. J., J. R. C. ANDRADEM, P. V. PATEL, J. A. COLE & H. SMITH. 1989. Microb. Pathog. **7:** 63–72.
7. NOWICKI, S. & M. MARTENS. 1992. American Society for Microbiology General Meeting, Abstract.
8. NOWICKI, S., M. MARTENS, A. KAUL & B. NOWICKI. 1994. *In* Pathobiology and Immunology of Neisseriae. C. Broome, J. Knapp, S. Morse, P. Rice, C. DEL RIO, P. KOHL, S. NORMARK & F. SPARLING, Eds.: 730–734. Nat'l. Institute of Public Health, Mexico. In press.

Mouse Virulence Gene A (*mviA*⁺) Is a Pleiotropic Regulator of Gene Expression in *Salmonella typhimurium*

W. EDWARD SWORDS[a] AND W. H. BENJAMIN, JR. [a,b]

Departments of Microbiology[a] and Pathology[b]
University of Alabama at Birmingham
Birmingham, Alabama 35294

Salmonella typhimurium strains of the LT2 lineage differ dramatically in their virulence for mice. Previous studies from our laboratory showed that this variation is accounted for by allelic differences in a single chromosomal gene, *mviA*.[1] Virulent LT2 strains were shown to possess one allele (*mviA*), whereas avirulent strains had a second allele (*mviA*⁺).

Complementation analysis revealed that avirulence was dominant whether on a plasmid or in the chromosome; thus, the *mviA*⁺ allele is the functional, dominant copy of the gene. Transductional crosses from other virulent *S. typhimurium* backgrounds showed that the *mviA*⁺ allele is found in all virulent backgrounds other than LT2. The model that was proposed to resolve this apparent paradox was that *mviA*⁺ constitutes an intermediate component of a genetic regulatory network. During years of passage on artificial media, strains of the LT2 lineage have undergone a mutation that renders them avirulent when they possess a functional *mviA*⁺ gene. The *mviA* allele thus represents a compensatory mutation in the LT2 background which restores virulence. In support of this model, the deduced amino acid sequence of *mviA*⁺ shows significant homology to the response regulator family of regulatory genes (Benjamin *et al.*, in preparation). These genes are usually the effector component of so-called two-component regulatory systems.[2]

Because *mviA*⁺ is apparently involved in the regulation of virulence-related genes in *S. typhimurium* strains outside the LT2 lineage, we are investigating the role of *mviA*⁺ in the virulence of these strains. We showed that the insertional inactivation of *mviA*⁺ induces a significant reduction in the size of colonies on solid media, which we have named the small colony morphology or Scm⁺ phenotype. Most virulent strains exhibit this phenotype (ATCC14028, C5, SL1344, TML, UK-1, W118-2); strains SR-11 and LT2 do not. Comparison of the growth rates of parental and Scm⁺ strains revealed that the Scm⁺ phenotype is a growth-related phenomenon. Transposon insertions (Mu*d*J, Tn*10*) which abolish the Scm⁺ phenotype were mapped to 57-60 minutes on the chromosome, a region that is known to contain virulence-related genes.[3–5] We further demonstrated that Scm⁺ *mviA* knockout mutants are avirulent, thus establishing that *mviA*⁺ is an essential virulence gene.

Using Western blots, we also showed that inactivation of *mviA*⁺ causes distinct changes in the expression of immunoreactive proteins. The most notable of these is a 55-kD protein that is prominent in all parental strains and is not expressed in Scm⁺ *mviA* knockout mutants. Of particular interest is that this protein is expressed in *mviA* (virulent) and not in *mviA⁺* (avirulent) strains of the LT2 lineage. Therefore, we established that *mviA⁺* is a component of a regulon that modulates the expression of a number of virulence-related genes. We also found considerable experimental support for the hypothesis that the LT2 lineage of *S. typhimurium* strains harbors multiple mutations related to virulence.

REFERENCES

1. BENJAMIN, W. H., JR., J. YOTHER, P. HALL & D. E. BRILES. 1991. The *Salmonella typhimurium* locus *mviA* regulates virulence in *Ity^s* but not *Ity^r* mice: Functional *mviA* results in avirulence; mutant (nonfunctional) *mviA* results in virulence. J. Exp. Med. **174:** 1073–1083.
2. STOCK, J. B., A. J. NIFKA & A. M. STOCK. 1989. Protein phosphorylation and regulation of adaptive responses in bacteria. Microbiol. Rev. **53:** 450–490.
3. GALAN, J. E., C. GINOCCHIO & P. COSTEAS. 1992. Molecular and functional characterization of the *Salmonella* invasion gene *invA:* Homology of InvA to members of a new protein family. J. Bacteriol. **174:** 4338–4349.
4. LEE, C. A., B. D. JONES & S. FALKOW. 1992. Identification of a *Salmonella typhimurium* invasion locus by selection for hyperinvasive mutants. Proc. Natl. Acad. Sci. USA **89:** 1847–1851.
5. FANG, F. C., S. J. LIBBY, N. A. BUCHMEIR, P. C. LOEWEN, J. SWITALA, J. HARWOOD & D. G. GUINEY. 1992. The alternative σ factor KatF (RpoS) regulates *Salmonella* virulence. Proc. Natl. Acad. Sci. USA **89:** 11978–11982.

Role of the 145-Kilodalton Surface Protein in Virulence of the Brazilian Purpuric Fever Clone of *Haemophilus influenzae* Biogroup Aegyptius for Infant Rats

LORRY G. RUBIN [a]

Division of Infectious Diseases
Department of Pediatrics
Schneider Children's Hospital of Long Island Jewish Medical Center
New Hyde Park, New York 11042
Long Island Campus for the Albert Einstein College of Medicine

Brazilian purpuric fever (BPF) is a fulminant, often fatal disease of young children associated with bacteremia with clonally related strains of *Haemophilus influenzae* biogroup aegyptius (*H. aegyptius*).[1,2] Symptoms and signs of sepsis develop abruptly 7-16 days after an episode of purulent conjunctivitis due to *H. influenzae* biogroup aegyptius, an organism previously associated only with conjunctivitis.[1] Case-clone *H. influenzae* biogroup aegyptius strains are more virulent for infant rats than are non-BPF case-associated strains,[3] but the basis for this enhanced virulence is poorly understood. Lipooligosaccharide (LOS) phenotype contributes to the virulence of the case clone strain for infant rats.[4]

To determine the additional attributes of the BPF case clone that contribute to virulence, we examined the role of P145, a 145-kilodalton surface protein that is a target of bactericidal and protective antibodies[5] and is subject to phase-variable expression by case clone strains. We first compared the virulence of case clone isolates from the blood of two children with BPF from Serrana, Brazil. These isolates had similar LOS phenotypes determined by SDS-urea-PAGE and reactivity with a panel of monoclonal anti-LOS antibodies, were piliated (as measured by human erythrocyte binding to colonies), and had identical outer membrane protein electrophoretic patterns except for P145 expression. Twenty-four hours after intraperitoneal inoculation, a significantly higher incidence (51% vs 26%, $p = 0.035$) and magnitude (2.9 ± 5.8 vs 0.7 ± 2.0 cfu/0.01 ml, $p = 0.024$) of bacteremia were found in rats inoculated with the P145-expressing strain. Because these strains may have unrecognized differences in phenotype in addition to P145 expression which could have contributed to the observed differences in virulence, we compared the virulence

[a] Address for correspondence: Schneider Children's Hospital, 269-01 76th Ave., New Hyde Park, NY 11040.

of animal-passaged P145-expressing case clone strain F3037 and a spontaneously occurring P145-nonexpressing phase variant of this strain. These variants had similar lipooligosaccharide phenotypes designated LOS2,[4] were nonpiliated, and had identical outer membrane protein electrophoretic patterns except for P145 expression. The geometric mean magnitude of bacteremia for P145-expressing F3037 (44 ± 4.9 cfu/0.01 ml blood) was significantly higher than that for the P145-nonexpressing variant (4.4 ± 5.1 cfu/0.01 ml blood, $p < 0.0001$). Colonies grown from blood cultures maintained the P145 phenotype of the inoculated strain. Thus, P145 expression contributes to the virulence of the BPF case clone for infant rats. These findings suggest that P145 expression by the BPF case clone may contribute to intravascular survival of bacteria.

REFERENCES

1. HARRISON, L. H., G. A. DA SILVA, M. PITTMAN, D. W. FLEMING, A. VRANJAC, C. V. BROOME & the Brazilian Purpuric Fever Study Group. 1989. Epidemiology and clinical spectrum of Brazilian purpuric fever. J. Clin. Microbiol. **27:** 599–604.
2. BRENNER, D. J., L. W. MAYER, G. M. CARLONE, L. H. HARRISON, W. BIBB, M. C. DECUNTO BRANDILEONE, F. O. SOOTNEK, K. IRINO, M. W. REEVES, J. M. SWENSON, K. A. BIRKNESS, R. S. WEYANT, S. F. BERKLEY, T. C. WOODS, A. G. STEIGERWALT, P. A. D. GRIMONT, R. M. MCKINNEY, D. W. FLEMING, L. L. GHEESLING, R. C. COOKSEY, R. J. ARKO, C. V. BROOME & the Brazilian Purpuric Fever Study Group. 1988. Biochemical, genetic, and epidemiologic characterization of *Haemophilus influenzae* biogroup aegyptius (*H. aegyptius*) strains associated with Brazilian purpuric fever. J. Clin. Microbiol. **26:** 1524–1534.
3. RUBIN, L. G., E. S. GLOSTER, G. M. CARLONE & THE BPF STUDY GROUP. 1989. An infant rat model of bacteremia with Brazilian purpuric fever isolates of *Haemophilus influenzae* biogroup aegyptius (*H. aegyptius*). J. Infect. Dis. **160:** 476–482.
4. RUBIN, L. G. & J. W. ST. GEME, III. 1993. Role of lipooligosaccharide in virulence of the Brazilian purpuric fever clone of *Haemophilus influenzae* biogroup aegyptius. Infect. Immunol. **61:** 650–655.
5. RUBIN, L. G., A. RIZVI & THE BRAZILIAN PURPURIC FEVER STUDY GROUP. 1991. Antibody to a 145-kilodalton outer membrane protein has bactericidal activity and protective activity against experimental bacteremia caused by a Brazilian purpuric fever isolate of *Haemophilus influenzae* biogroup aegyptius. Infect. Immunol. **59:** 1501–1503.

Size Variation of a Major Serotype-Specific Antigen of *Ureaplasma urealyticum*

XIAOTIAN ZHENG,[a] LEE-JENE TENG,[a,b]
JOHN I. GLASS,[a] ALAIN BLANCHARD,[c]
ZUHUA CAO,[a] MIRJAM C. KEMPF,[a]
HAROLD L. WATSON,[a] AND GAIL H. CASSELL[a]

[a]Department of Microbiology
University of Alabama at Birmingham
Schools of Medicine and Dentistry
Birmingham, Alabama 35294

[c]Institut Pasteur
Paris, France

Ureaplasma urealyticum (*Uu*) is a commensal in the lower urogenital tract in women. Recently, this organism was implicated in various human diseases including respiratory infection, chorioamnionitis, and central nervous system diseases in newborn infants.[1] Our interests lie in understanding the human immune response to this organism and precisely how it may affect the organism's success as a pathogen. We characterized a major surface-localized antigen, multiple banded (MB) antigen, that displays multiple banded patterns on immunoblot. We[2,3] showed that this antigen (1) is specific for *Uu*; (2) contains serotype-specific as well as cross-reactive epitopes; (3) has a high rate of size variation both *in vitro* and *in vivo* (FIG. 1), and (4) is one of the predominant antigens recognized during infections in humans. Monoclonal antibodies (mAb) directed to this antigen can inhibit the growth of this organism *in vitro*. In addition, by using serotype-specific reagents, including mAbs, to analyze clinical isolates from cerebrospinal fluid (CSF), 70% of the CSF isolates were identifiable as serotypes 1, 3, 6, 8, or 10 representing 5 of the 14 established serotypes.[4] These data support the hypothesis that the property of invasiveness for ureaplasmas is not likely to be limited to 1 of the 14 established serovars. The study also showed that even in isolates of the same serotype there can be size variation in the antigens expressed. Therefore, it appears that many serotypes are invasive and that perhaps antigenic variation and host factors are more important determinants of ureaplasma infections than are different serotypes. Using a serotype 3 clinical isolate, we observed that after exposure of organisms to mAb directed to the MB antigen, higher molecular weight variants of this antigen appeared. This is in contrast to previous *in vitro* subcloning experiments in which the molecular weights of variant antigens in all

[b]On leave from the School of Medical Technology, College of Medicine, National Taiwan University, Taipei, Taiwan, ROC.

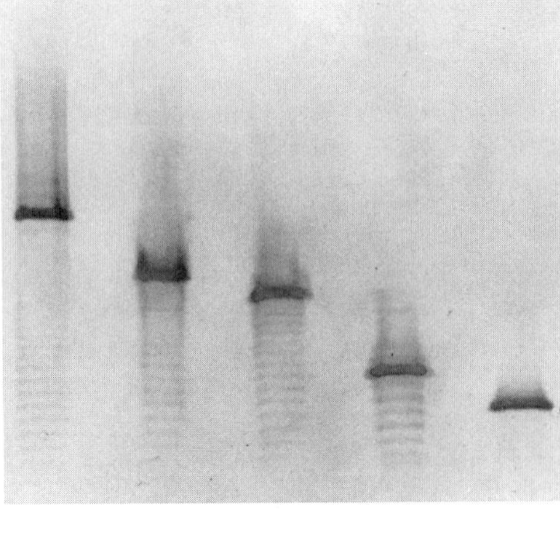

FIGURE 1. Immunoblot of five serotype 3 *U. urealyticum* strains. The blot was developed with mAb 3B1.5 which is directed to the MB antigen. *Lane 1* was loaded with protein of reference strain; *lanes 2-4* were those of subclones generated from a clinical isolate; and *lane 5* was loaded with an isolate from amniotic fluid. Molecular weight for antigen bands are 67.8, 53, 47, 39, and 36 kD from lanes 1 to 5, respectively.

cases shifted downward. Prior to the current study, the only time an upward shift in the size of this antigen was observed was in organisms recovered from experimentally infected mice. This difference in the size of antigens synthesized under *in vivo* and *in vitro* conditions could have important implications as to how the organism interacts with its host. Although the exact mechanism of this variation is to be analyzed, this capacity to respond to specific antibody may be found to play a significant role in this organism's *in vivo* survival strategy.

To further understand size variation of this antigen, the gene encoding the serotype 3 MB antigen of the reference strain was cloned and sequenced.[5] It has been shown that sequence of this antigen contains a signal peptide followed by an acylation site. Surprisingly, we found that two thirds of the gene at the COOH-terminus of the protein was composed of identical 18 nucleotide (6 amino acid) repeats. Synthetic peptide analysis indicated that the repeat sequence contained both serovar-specific and cross-reactive epitopes. Analysis of different variants with Southern blot hybridization (with a probe to the repeat region) and polymerase chain reactions suggest that although the NH_2-terminal regions are conserved among different variants, the length of the COOH-terminal repeat region varied in correspondence with the size variation at protein level. Furthermore, DNA sequence analysis showed that the copy number of the repeat was the only difference between the MB antigen genes of two *Uus* which had been isolated from different geographic locations and had different molecular weights for the antigen. Therefore, the size variation seen with this antigen is likely a result of regulation of the number of repeats in this gene. The result also showed that antigen size variants can be generated from a homogeneous population and that the organism can change this phenotypic property during the reproduction process.

Surface protein size variation resulting from changes in repetitive structures has been seen on both eukaryotic and prokaryotic pathogens including malaria, group A streptococcus, group B streptococcus, pathogenic *Neisseria,* and *Streptococcus pneumoniae.* Many of the proteins on these organisms are considered to be virulence associated. Antigen size variation has also been found in mycoplasmas. Our previous studies showed that the difference in V-1 antigen in *Mycoplasma pulmonis,* a genital and respiratory tract pathogen of rodents, is the only difference detectable between virulent and avirulent strains, and this difference is associated with differences in disease severity.

For pathogenic bacteria, genetic variation is an important method for escaping the immune response of the host or a way of adapting to the microenvironment. A repetitive structure enables recombination events to happen at a much higher frequency than do random mutations in a single gene. It has been proposed[6] that the high frequency with which intragenic recombination events occur could accelerate the evolution of a structural gene and result in the generation of new antigenic variants.

REFERENCES

1. CASSELL, G. H., K. B. WAITES, H. L. WATSON, D. T. CROUSE & R. HARASAWA. 1993. *Ureaplasma urealyticum* intrauterine infection: Role in prematurity and disease in the newborn. Clin. Microbial. Rev. **6:** 69–87.
2. WATSON, H. L., D. K. BLALOCK & G. H. CASSELL. 1990. Variable antigens of *Ureaplasma urealyticum* containing both serovar-specific and serovar-cross-reactive epitopes. Infect. Immunol. **58:** 3679–3688.
3. WATSON, H. L., X. ZHENG & G. H. CASSELL. 1993. Structural variations and phenotypic switching of mycoplasmal antigens. Clin. Infect. Dis. **17**(Suppl 1): S183–186.
4. ZHENG, X., H. L. WATSON, K. B. WAITES & G. H. CASSELL. 1992. Serotype diversity and antigen variation among invasive isolates of *Ureaplasma urealyticum* from neonates. Infect. Immunol. **60:** 3472–3474.
5. ZHENG, X., L.-J. TENG, J. I. GLASS, A. BLANCHARD, H. L. WATSON & G. H. CASSELL. 1994. Genotypic characterization of a *Ureaplasma urealyticum* serotype-specific antigen. Manuscript in preparation.
6. HOLLINGSHEAD, S. K., V. A. FISCHETTI & J. R. SCOTT. 1987. Size variation in group A streptococcal M protein is generated by homologous recombination between intragenic repeats. Mol. Gen. Genet. **207:** 196–203.

Moderate Stress Protects Female Mice against Bacterial Infection of the Bladder by Eliciting Uroepithelial Shedding

EILATA DALAL, ORA MEDALIA, ORNA HARARI,
AND MOSHE ARONSON

Department of Histology and Cell Biology
Tel Aviv University
Sackler School of Medicine
Ramat Aviv, Tel Aviv 69978, Israel

We previously showed[1] that shedding of viable uroepithelial cells, elicited by invading microorganisms, constitutes an antimicrobial defense mechanism, because the adhering bacteria are washed out together with the cells. We demonstrated that most of the shed cells are viable and that the active agent that induces shedding is the bacterial endotoxin. Our results also indicated that the uroepithelium is preprogrammed to respond by rapid shedding when required, as the process already begins within 1 hour after administration of lipopolysaccharide to the bladder.

The present studies were initiated to determine if perturbation of circadian rhythms will affect the course of experimental vesical infection. The spontaneous clearance of bacteria, which usually requires 2-3 weeks, was expected to be prolonged under these conditions. However, female mice exposed to 4 days of constant illumination, in order to develop a state of "free running," failed altogether to become infected (10-20% *vs* 70% in the controls, $p < 0.0001$). We subsequently showed that constant illumination is accompanied by increased epithelial shedding.

A causal connection with stress was suspected when accidental exposure of mice to high temperatures (37°C for 24 hours) also resulted in extensive shedding. The state of augmented shedding lasted at least 2 weeks after termination of exposure to either light or heat (TABLE 1).

We also showed that exposure both to heat and to constant illumination is accompanied by thymic involution and elevation of blood corticosterone levels. In addition, shedding was elicited by intraperitoneal administration of hydrocortisone together with norepinephrine or by injection of corticosterone into the bladder. Constant illumination as well as heat facilitated migration of polymorphonuclear cells into the bladder following chemotactic stimuli.

Male mice subjected to identical stress-generating conditions did not display considerable epithelial shedding and were not protected from intravesical infection.

Finally, we showed (manuscript in preparation) that the excessive epithelial shedding induced in our stressed animals terminated after benzodiazepam administration for several days.

TABLE 1. Extent and Duration of Shedding following Stress in Female Mice[a]

| | Days after Stress Termination | | |
Mode of Stress	1	7	14
Controls	0.927 ± 0.59	—	—
Constant illumination[b]	2.58 ± 0.86 ($p = 0.0008$)	2.666 ± 0.84 ($p = 0.0014$)	2.333 ± 0.623 ($p = 0.0032$)
Heat exposure[c]	2.66 ± 0.64 ($p = 0.0001$)	2.447 ± 1.5 ($p = 0.0001$)	2.1666 ± 0.89 ($p = 0.0024$)

[a] p values relate to difference from the controls.
[b] Results of three experiments in groups of six mice.
[c] Results of six experiments in groups of six mice.
Extent of shedding was graded according to the following scale (representing number of cells following collection and cytospinning): 1 = control values (100–400); 2 = 2–3,000; 3 = 4–7,000; 4 = 10,000 and over.

REFERENCE

1. ARONSON, M., O. MEDALIA, D. AMICHAY & O. NATIV. 1988. Endotoxin-induced shedding of viable uroepithelial cells is an antimicrobial defence mechanism. Infect. Immun. **56:** 1615–1616.

Role of Tryptophan in Gamma Interferon-Mediated Chlamydial Persistence

W. L. BEATTY,[a] T. A. BELANGER,[a] A. A. DESAI,[a]
R. P. MORRISON,[b] AND G. I. BYRNE [a]

[a]Department of Medical Microbiology and Immunology
University of Wisconsin
Madison, Wisconsin 53706

[b]Laboratory of Intracellular Parasites
Rocky Mountain Laboratories
Hamilton, Montana 59340

Chlamydia trachomatis is an important human obligate intracellular pathogen responsible for a significant proportion of ocular and sexually transmitted diseases. Repeated infection promotes chronic inflammation which contributes to scarring associated with blindness and infertility. Chlamydial persistence also is thought to augment the disease process by providing prolonged antigenic stimulation, leading to immunopathologic sequelae.

Gamma interferon (IFN-γ) is an immune effector molecule responsible for inhibiting intracellular chlamydial growth and the generation of persistent chlamydial development. IFN-γ inhibits chlamydial growth by induction of indoleamine 2,3-dioxygenase (IDO), a nonconstitutive enzyme associated with tryptophan degradation.[1] IFN-γ-mediated activation of host cells to restrict intracellular chlamydial development requires relatively large amounts of the cytokine. Induction of persistence occurs at greatly reduced amounts of IFN-γ, and persistence is characterized by the presence of morphologically and biochemically unique forms of chlamydiae.[2] These enlarged, aberrant chlamydial forms are noninfectious and exhibit altered expression in key chlamydial proteins, such as decreased levels of structural constituents (the major outer membrane protein [MOMP], 60-kD outer membrane protein, and lipopolysaccharide) and continued synthesis of hsp60, a stress protein associated with local immunopathologic changes.[2]

Studies were performed to determine if the mechanism for induction of chlamydial persistence in the presence of subinhibitory levels of IFN-γ was similar to that reported to inhibit chlamydial growth. First, levels of IDO activity were measured and the amount of both extracellular and intracellular tryptophan catabolism was determined to evaluate tryptophan availability for chlamydial growth. Then, induction of persistence was measured in an IDO-deficient mutant host cell and compared with its normal parental line. Finally, induction of persistence was investigated in host cells incubated in tryptophan-deficient medium supplemented with specified amounts of exogenous tryptophan.

TABLE 1. Effects of IFN-γ and Tryptophan Deprivation on Chlamydial-Infected Host Cells

Host Cells	Treatment	Support *C. trachomatis* Growth	IDO Activity	Chlamydial Development	MOMP-Deficient
HeLa	Untreated	+	−	Normal	−
HeLa	IFN-γ-treated	+	+	Aberrant	+
HeLa	Tryptophan-depleted	+	−	Aberrant	+
Me180	Untreated	+	−	Normal	−
Me180	IFN-γ-treated	+	+	Aberrant	+
IDO mutants	Untreated	+	−	Normal	−
IDO mutants	IFN-γ-treated	+	−	Normal	−

Persistence-inducing levels of IFN-γ were assessed for IDO activity by HPLC analysis of exogenous tryptophan and its catabolites. Levels of IDO activity, as reflected by the accumulation of extracellular tryptophan catabolites, revealed only 5% specific catabolism in culture supernatants of persistently infected cells, well below the activity required for chlamydial growth inhibition.[1] However, analysis of intracellular acid-soluble pools revealed a much greater level of cytoplasmic tryptophan catabolism (60%), indicating that although tryptophan was plentiful in the growth medium, the availability of this essential amino acid was limited in intracellular pools.

A mutant cell line (ME180-IR3B6A) responsive to IFN-γ but deficient in IDO activity has been shown to lack the capacity to restrict intracellular chlamydial growth in the presence of IFN-γ.[3] These IDO-deficient mutant cells were tested for their capacity to induce chlamydial persistence in the presence of IFN-γ. Dose-dependent IFN-γ-induced persistence occurred in the parental ME180 cells. The mutant cells supported *C. trachomatis* growth; however, normal chlamydial development was observed at concentrations of IFN-γ that induced aberrant growth in the parental line.

To more directly address the role of IFN-γ-mediated nutrient deprivation in the generation of persistence, infected HeLa cells were incubated in growth medium supplemented with incremental levels of tryptophan. Chlamydial growth during tryptophan deprivation resulted in the development of enlarged, atypical noninfectious forms with altered levels of chlamydial proteins, consistent with the findings described for IFN-γ- induced persistence (TABLE 1).

These studies confirm that essential nutrient deprivation by IDO-mediated tryptophan catabolism is responsible for IFN-γ-induced *C. trachomatis* persistence. Results suggest that *in vivo* IFN-γ-mediated activation of chlamydial host cells may contribute to chronic infection and tissue damage associated with ocular disease and infertility.

REFERENCES

1. BYRNE, G. I., L. K. LEHMANN & G. J. LANDRY. 1986. Induction of tryptophan catabolism is the mechanism of gamma interferon-mediated inhibition of intracellular *Chlamydia psittaci* replication in T24 cells. Infect. Immunol. **53:** 347–351.

2. BEATTY, W. L., G. I. BYRNE & R. P. MORRISON. 1993. Morphologic and antigenic characterization of interferon γ-mediated persistent *Chlamydia trachomatis* infection *in vitro*. Proc. Natl. Acad. Sci. USA **90:** 3998–4002.

3. THOMAS, S. M., L. F. GARRITY, C. R. BRANDT, C. S. SCHOBERT, G.-S. FENG, M. W. TAYLOR, J. M. CARLIN & G. I. BYRNE. 1993. IFN-γ-mediated antimicrobial response. Indoleamine 2,3-dioxygenase-deficient mutant host cells no longer inhibit intracellular *Chlamydia* spp. or *Toxoplasma* growth. J. Immunol. **150:** 5529–5534.

Normal MØ Cell-Associated TNF$_\alpha$ Is Resistant to PGE$_2$ as Well as TGF$_\beta$ Downregulation[a]

C. L. MILLER-GRAZIANO, K. KODYS, AND
K. JHAVER

Department of Surgery
University of Massachusetts Medical Center
Worcester, Massachusetts 01655

Eighty percent of patients with severe thermal or mechanical trauma who die more than 2 days postinjury succumb not as a direct result of their injuries, but from organ failure (kidney, lung, and heart) due to cytokine and septic shock.[1] These immunoaberrant trauma patients experience both depressed T-lymphocyte function with subsequent increased septic episodes and elevated monocyte (MØ) tumor necrosis factor alpha (TNF$_\alpha$) of both cell-associated and secreted types.[1,2] Normal human MØ TNF$_\alpha$ production is downregulated by both prostaglandin E$_2$ (PGE$_2$) and TGF$_\beta$ at the mRNA level.[3,4] However, trauma patients with depressed T-cell proliferation responses (immunoaberrant) because of excessive MØ PGE$_2$ production also experience excessive TNF$_\alpha$ production concomitant to increased MØ TGF$_\beta$ production.[5,6] This report compares the sensitivity of paired trauma patients' and normal control subjects' MØ TNF$_\alpha$ production to the addition of exogenous PGE$_2$ or TGF$_\beta$. Because trauma patients' MØ produce large excesses of biologically active cell-associated TNF$_\alpha$ (cell TNF$_\alpha$), both cell-associated and secreted TNF$_\alpha$ were assessed.

Patients with severe mechanical (injury severity score >35) or thermal trauma (>30% 3° burn) and normal controls were selected for this study. Mitogen responses were assessed. Patients with depressed responses were classified as immunoaberrant and selected for further study of the monocyte (MØ) functions. Trauma patients' and normal subjects' MØ were separated by selective microexudate adherence of the Ficoll-Hypaque density isolated mononuclear cells.[2] In some experiments, normal MØ were cross-link stimulated through their 72-kD FcγRI by rosetting the T-cell-depleted mononuclear cells with anti- Rh-coated erythrocytes, followed by density isolation of the rosetted cells, then further purification by adherence to microexudate-coated plates.[2] MØ equaled 95% of the final population by CD14 staining. The isolated MØ population, FcγRI-stimulated and FcγRI-nonstimulated MØ (3 × 10^6 MØ in 3 ml of medium), was further induced with 20 µg/ ml of muramyl dipeptide (MDP) or a combination of 3 hours' priming with either 10 U or 100 U IFNγ/ml plus 20 µg/ml MDP. Then 10^{-7} M PGE$_2$ or 2.4 ng/ml TGF$_\beta$ was added with the IFN-γ primer. Appropriate ethanol controls were included in the PGE$_2$ experiments. Using

[a]This work was supported by Public Health Service grant GM36214-09 and Department of Defense grant DAMD17-92-C-2033.

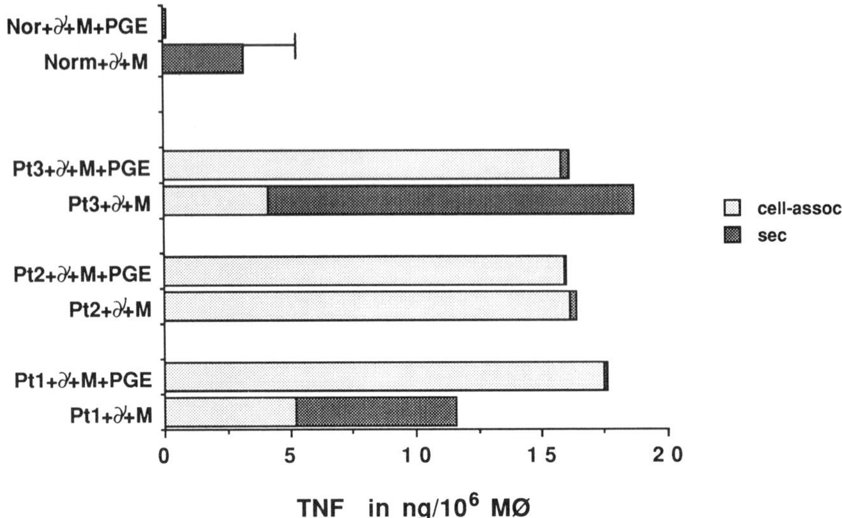

FIGURE 1. PGE_2 addition downregulates both patients' and normals' Secreted TNF_α. 10^6/ml trauma patient (Pt) or normal (Nor) MØ cultured with 10 U IFN-γ plus 20 μg/ml MDP (γ + M) in the presence or absence of 10^{-7} M exogenously added PGE_2. TNF_α was measured in LM bioassay as described. Cell-associated TNF_α (cell-assoc) was measured in MØ membrane sonicates, whereas secreted TNF_α (sec) was measured in MØ supernatants. Normal TNF_α values represent the medium and range for paired normals.

the LM bioassay, secreted TNF_α was measured in the MØ supernatants, and cell-associated TNF_α activity was determined in the sonicated MØ lysates after repeated freezing-thawing.[2] Both secreted and cell-associated MØ TNF_α activity was totally neutralized by anti-TNF_α antibody. PGE_2 was measured by ELISA in the MØ supernatants.[2] MØ supernatants were assayed for TGF_β using the mink lung bioassay against a recombinant human TGF_β standard, as described.[2]

Patients' MØ producing PGE_2 levels of >30 ng/10^6 MØ and TGF_β levels of 50-200 pM 10^6 MØ were concomitantly producing elevated total TNF_α levels (secreted and cell-associated) of 30 to 130 ng/10^6 MØ/ml. These data implied that ongoing patients' MØ TNF_α production is resistant to downregulation by both PGE_2 and TGF_β. However, new induction of MØ TNF_α might still be sensitive to PGE_2 or TGF_β downregulation. The exogenous addition of 10^{-7} M/ml PGE_2 to patients' or normal subjects' MØ stimulated with a suboptimal IFN-γ prime (10 U/ml) plus MDP resulted in suppression of new TNF_α production by both normal and immunocompetent trauma patients' MØ, while having no significant effect on total MØ TNF_α levels induced in immunoaberrant patients, but significantly altering the ratio of secreted to cell-associated TNF_α in the aberrant trauma patients' MØ (FIG. 1). Exogenous TGF_β (2.4 ng/ml) added to the same suboptimal stimulation system had no inhibitory effect on patients' MØ secreted or cell-associated TNF_α, whereas induction of normal MØ-secreted TNF_α was significantly inhibited (TABLE 1). Because of the differential inhibitory effect of PGE_2 on patients' secreted *versus* cell-associated TNF_α, we investi-

TABLE 1. TGF$_\beta$ Increases MØ TNFα Levels in IFN-γ + MDP-Stimulated Trauma Patients' MØ While Decreasing TNF$_\alpha$ in Controls' MØ[a])

	TNF Bioactivity			
	Secreted/Cell-Associated (ng/10^6 MØ)			
	Nor	Pt	Nor	Pt
10 IFN-$_\gamma$ + MDP	15.8/1.6	23.1/4.5	4.0/0	10.2/24.7
10 IFN-$_\gamma$ + MDP + TGF$_\beta$	4.9/2.1	32.4/3.5	3.1/0	11.4/27.4
10 IFN-$_\gamma$ + MDP	9.5/5.7	38.1/7.3	11.4/2.6	8.7/24.3
10 IFN-$_\gamma$ + MDP + TGF$_\beta$	5.9/4.7	38.2/7.8	6.9/3.2	12.2/29.6
10 IFN-$_\gamma$ + MDP	15.1/0	38.1/10.3	2.1/0	10.5/0.3
10 IFN-$_\gamma$ + MDP + TGF$_\beta$	12.4/0	105.8/16.2	1.6/0	17.1/0.3

[a] TNF$_\alpha$ activity in LM bioassay of 3×10^6 normal control (Nor) or trauma patients' (Pt) MØ stimulated by 10 U/ml IFN-$_\gamma$ + 20 μg/ml MDP in the presence or absence of 2.4 ng/ml TGF$_\beta$. Secreted TNF$_\alpha$ was assayed in MØ supernatants and cell-associated TNF$_\alpha$ in MØ lysates.

gated the effect of the exogenous addition of either PGE$_2$ or TGF$_\beta$ in a system in which normal MØ were induced to produce cell-associated as well as secreted TNF$_\alpha$. Cross-linking the normal MØ FcγRI receptor induces significant MØ cell-associated as well as secreted TNF$_\alpha$.[2,5] In this system, normal MØ cell-associated TNF$_\alpha$ induced by FcγRI cross-linking was resistant to PGE$_2$ downregulation and TGF$_\beta$ inhibition. However, secreted TNF$_\alpha$ was still inhibited by the addition of either TGF$_\beta$ or PGE$_2$.

These data suggest that although immunoaberrant patients' MØ are concomitantly producing high levels of TNF$_\alpha$, TGF$_\beta$, and PGE$_2$, new induction of secreted TNF$_\alpha$ is still sensitive to PGE$_2$ inhibition, whereas cell-associated TNF$_\alpha$ induced before the addition of PGE$_2$ is resistant to inhibition in both patients and normal subjects. In contrast, TGF$_\beta$ inhibits induction of normal subjects' MØ-secreted TNF$_\alpha$ but not patients' secreted TNF$_\alpha$. The posttrauma induction of high levels of PGE$_2$ resistance to cell-associated TNF$_\alpha$, along with the altered sensitivity of TNF$_\alpha$ to TGF$_\beta$ inhibition can contribute to excessive TNF$_\alpha$ production by trauma patients' MØ.

REFERENCES

1. WAAGE, A. & A. O. AASEN. 1992. Immunol. Rev. **127:** 221–230.
2. MILLER-GRAZIANO, C. L., G. SZABO, K. KODYS & K. GRIFFEY. 1990. J. Trauma **30:** S86–S97.
3. CHANTRY, D., M. TURNER, E. ABNEY & M. FELDMANN. 1989. J. Immunol. **142:** 4295–4300.
4. SPENGLER, R. N., M. L. SPENGLER, R. M. STRIETER, D. G. REMICK, J. W. LARRICK & S. L. KUNKEL. 1989. J. Immunol. **142:** 4346–4350.
5. MILLER-GRAZIANO, C. L., G. SZABO & K. KODYS. 1993. *In* Host Defense Dysfunction in Trauma, Shock, and Sepsis. E. Faist, Ed.: 637–650. Springer-Verlag. Berlin, Germany.
6. GRBIC, J. T., J. A. MANNICK, D. B. GOUGH & M. L. RODRICK. 1991. Ann. Surg. **214:** 253–263.

Enhanced Susceptibility of Young Rats with Alloxan-Induced Diabetes Mellitus to Enterohemorrhagic *Escherichia coli*

F. V. DIMA, D. LAKY, AND S. V. DIMA

Cantacuzino and Victor Babes Institutes
Bucharest, Romania

Enterohemorrhagic *Escherichia coli* strains have been associated with hemorrhagic colitis and hemolytic uremic syndrome as well as with sporadic cases of gastrointestinal illness in the United States, Canada, England, and Japan.[1] By contrast to the situation regarding enteropathogenic and enterohemorrhagic *E. coli* strains in human and animal models,[2] relatively little information is available on infection with enterohemorrhagic *E. coli* 0157 : H7 in humans and animals with diabetes mellitus.

In this study we investigated the colonizing ability as well as the association of *E. coli* 0157 : H7 with epithelial cells of the intestinal tract in alloxan-induced diabetes mellitus in young rats and controls.

Diabetic and nondiabetic rats infected with *E. coli* 0157 : H7 were evaluated using three experimental parameters: (1) colonization of the intestinal tract; (2) location of bacteria on enterocyte cells by two methods: (a) plate count of bacteria localized on epithelial cells and (b) association of (^{3}H) thymidine-labeled bacteria on enterocyte cells; and (3) histopathologic observations.

The severity of experimental bacterial infection in these experiments with *E. coli* 0157 : H7 in young rats with diabetes mellitus was characterized by: (1) higher susceptibility to oral infection with *E. coli* 0157 : H7 in diabetic than in nondiabetic rats; (2) *E. coli*-colonizing values in the range of 10^6-10^7 CFU/g of feces; (3) maximum colonization values in the distal ileum, cecum, and proximal colon; (4) colonization values 100-1,000 times lower in the controls than in the test lot; (5) association of (^{3}H)-TdR-*E. coli* 0157 : H7 cells with enterocyte and colonocyte cells in 27.2% of diabetic rats by contrast with only 8.34% of control rats; and (6) the finding that the main histopathologic changes, namely, enterohemorrhagic colitis (FIG. 1) and corticotubular necrosis in kidneys (FIG. 2), were presumably induced by Shiga-like toxins.

In the pathogenic factors specific to enterohemorrhagic *E. coli* 0157 : H7 strains (verocytotoxins, Shiga-like toxins, and plasmid 60 MDa),[1,3,4] we emphasized the

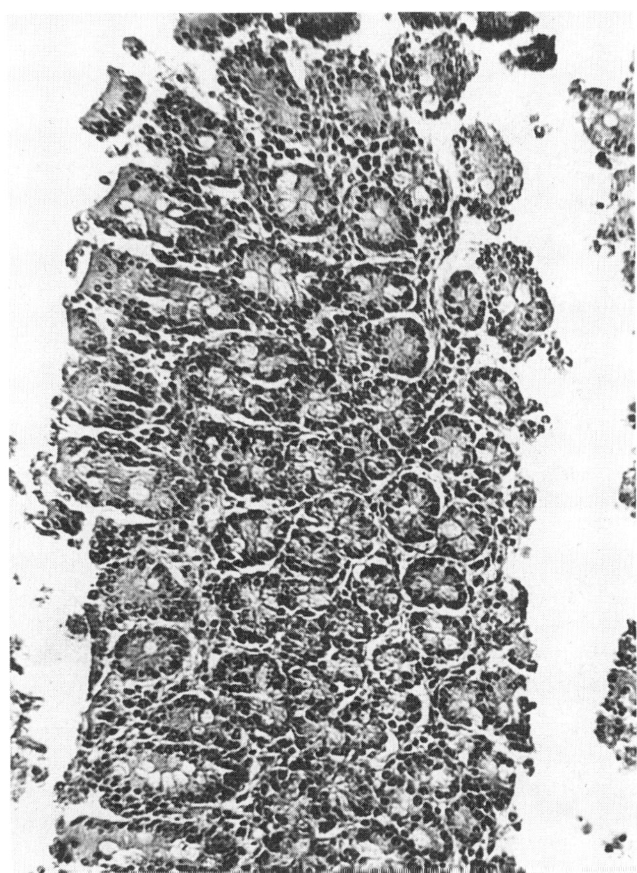

FIGURE 1. Proximal colon. Note the ulcerations of the colonic mucosa and the cell exfoliations in the lumen and leukocytes. Hematoxylin-eosin stain; magnification × 194.

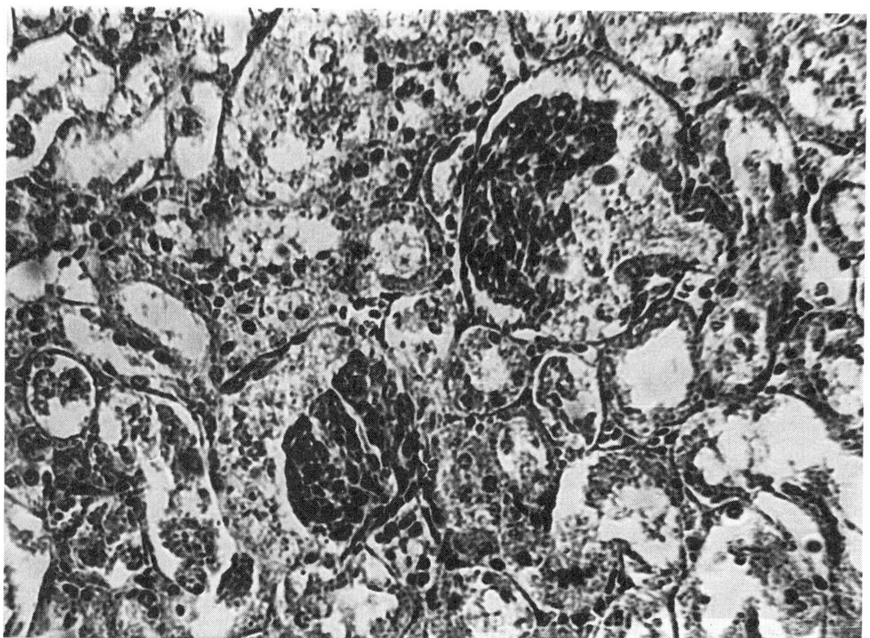

FIGURE 2. Kidneys with severe glomerular lesions. Note the disaggregation of some portions and granular content in the capsular cavity and the severe tubular ulcerative lesions and desquamations. Hematoxylin-eosin stain; magnification × 388.

metabolic and immunologic status of animals with diabetes mellitus,[5] which is responsible for the severe evolution of bacterial infection with *E. coli* 0157 : H7.

Summing up, these results demonstrate that young diabetic rats were more susceptible to enterohemorrhagic *E. coli* 0157 : H7 than were normal rats.

REFERENCES

1. YAMADA, S., S. MATSUSHITA, A. KAI, A. TSUJI, S. KANEMITSU, N. YAMASHITA, E. ANZAI & Y. KUDOH. 1993. Microbiol. Immunol. **37:** 111–118.
2. RICHARDSON, E. S., A. R. ROTMAN, R. C. JAY, C. R. SMITH, L. E. BECKER, M. PETRIC, N. F. OLIVIERI & M. A. KARMALI. 1992. Infect. Immun. **60:** 4154–4167.
3. KARMALI, A. M. 1990. Clin. Microbiol. Rev. **2:** 15–38.
4. TESH, L. V. & A. D. O'BRIEN. 1992. Microbiol. Path. **12:** 245–254.
5. FOREHAND, R. J. & R. B. JOHNSTON. 1985. Clin. Immunol. Allergy **5:** 351–369.

Resistance to Mycobacterial Infection and Cytokine Production in Mouse Macrophages

REIKO M. NAKAMURA[a] AND FUMIO AMANO[b]

Department of Bacteriology[a] and Chemistry[b]
National Institute of Health
1-23-1 Toyama, Shinjuku-ku, Tokyo, Japan

Host resistance to mycobacterial infection is regulated in two ways, immunity and natural resistance. In both cases the effector cells for killing bacteria are macrophages. Immune T cells release gamma interferon (IFN-γ) by antigenic stimuli and activate macrophages to become bactericidal. Naturally resistant macrophages, however, are bacteriostatic without immunologic activation. The natural resistance gene, *Bcg*, controls the resistance to mycobacteria in mice.[1] A *Bcg*-congenic mouse strain C.D2 was developed by introducing *Bcg*^{r} gene into the *Bcg*^{s} background of BALB/c mouse. Cytokine profiles were determined in the macrophages of BALB/c and C.D2 mice infected with *Mycobacterium avium* Mino to detect the influence of *Bcg* gene on cytokine production by macrophages. It was found that interleukin-1 (IL-1) is produced equally by *M. avium*-infected macrophages of *Bcg*^{s} and *Bcg*^{r} mice. More tumor necrosis factor-alpha (TNF$_\alpha$) was produced in *Bcg*^{s} than in *Bcg*^{r} macrophages at the mycobacterial infection. Tumor necrosis factor production correlated with O_2^- production and granuloma formation. Interleukin-6 (IL-6) production was higher in *Bcg*^{r} than in *Bcg*^{s}. Interestingly, IL-10 production was much higher in *Bcg*^{s} macrophages than in *Bcg*^{r} macrophages with mycobacterial stimuli. This IL-10 may inhibit IFN-γ activity in the *Bcg*^{s} mouse and consequently suppress macrophages in mycobacterial killing.

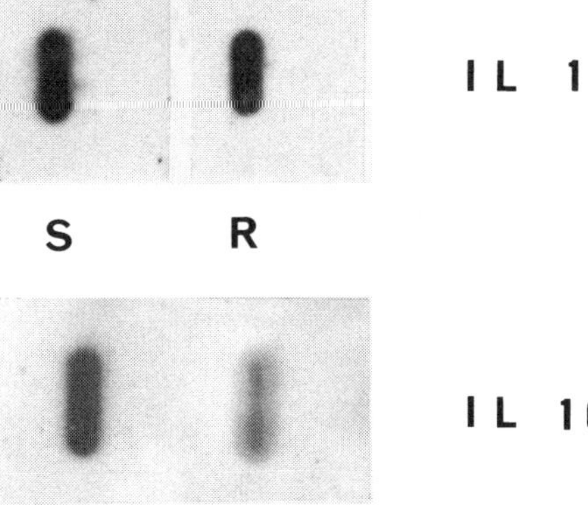

FIGURE 1. Northern hybridization with IL-1 and IL-10 cDNA. RNA was extracted from the spleen of BALB/c (S) or C.D2 (R) mouse infected with *Mycobacterium avium* Mino 24 hours before. A total of 25 μg RNA was applied.

TABLE 1. Phenotypes of *Bcg* Gene[a]

Characteristics	*Bcg*[s]	*Bcg*[r]
Growth of *M. avium* Mino *in vivo*	+++	−
Growth of *M. bovis* BCG *in vivo*	++	−
AcM.1 expression on macrophages	−	+
O_2^- production by macrophages	++	±
Granuloma formation	++	−
TNF$_\alpha$ production by macrophages	++	+
IL-6 production by macrophages	+	++
IL-10 production by macrophages	++	+
Nitric oxide production by macrophages at mycobacterial infection	+	++

[a] *Bcg* gene expression in various characteristics related to macrophages was compared in *Bcg*[s] and *Bcg*[r] mice infected with *M. avium* Mino.

The *Bcg*[s] background macrophage cell line JA-4 and its lipopolysaccharide-resistant mutant LPS1916[2] were examined for their resistance to mycobacterial infection and cytokine production. JA-4 produces more TNF$_\alpha$ by lipopolysaccharide stimulation and shows more susceptibility to mycobacteria. LPS1916 does not produce TNF$_\alpha$ by lipopolysaccharide stimulation, but it does with mycobacterial infection. Whether or not TNF$_\alpha$ increases the susceptibility of macrophages to mycobacteria is under investigation.

The question remains, what is the killer molecule of mycobacteria in a macrophage. *Bcg*[s] macrophages produce much O_2^- as well as JA-4 cells, but both are susceptible to mycobacteria. JA-4 produces nitric oxide and the production is enhanced by IFN-γ as well as *Bcg*[r] macrophages. However, these macrophages show different resistance to mycobacterial infection, suggesting that neither O_2^- nor nitric oxide is the effector killer molecule of mycobacteria.

REFERENCES

1. SKAMENE, E., P. GROS, A. FORGET, *et al.* 1982. Nature **297:** 506.
2. AMANO, F. & Y. AKAMATSU. 1991. Infect. Immun. **59:** 2166.

Salicylate Enhances Opsonization of *Klebsiella pneumoniae* with Anticapsular Antibodies

P. DOMENICO,[a] R. J. SALO,[b] A. S. CROSS,[c] AND
B. A. CUNHA[a]

[a]*Winthrop-University Hospital
Mineola, New York 11501*

[b]*Nassau County Medical Center
East Meadow, New York*

[c]*Walter Reed Army Institute of Research
Washington, DC 20307–5100*

Encapsulated gram-negative bacteria are among the leading causes of morbidity and mortality in the hospital environment. *Klebsiella pneumoniae* virulence is predicated on the production of capsular polysaccharide (CPS). The capsule envelopes bacteria and shields them from host defenses.[1] Encapsulated *K. pneumoniae* also produce large quantities of cell-free CPS, which is aggregated with toxic lipopolysaccharide and contributes to pathogenicity.[2] Circulating, cell-free CPS may also tie up and neutralize antibodies that would otherwise attach to and opsonize bacteria.[3]

Recently, salicylate was used to reduce CPS expression in *K. pneumoniae*. Decapsulation of bacteria with salicylate enhanced their phagocytic uptake, but only in the presence of whole-cell antiserum.[4] The present report evaluates the opsonic and protective potential of CPS-specific antisera against a number of *K. pneumoniae* serotypes after decapsulation.

K. pneumoniae serotypes O1:K1, O1:K2, and O1:K66 were decapsulated with salicylate and subjected to phagocytosis by human neutrophils (PMN). Rabbit antisera raised against encapsulated whole cells, and human hyperimmune globulin (hIgG, Nosocuman®) raised against 24 capsular serotypes were used to enhance the uptake and clearing of bacteria. Salicylate (2.5 mM) treatment significantly enhanced phagocytosis of all bacteria in the presence of homologous, but not heterologous, whole-cell antisera, as illustrated in FIGURE 1. Diluted rabbit antisera at 1:40 no longer opsonized fully encapsulated O1:K2, but it still promoted multiple uptake of decapsulated bacteria in >90% of polymorphonuclear cells ($p < 0.001$). Opsonization with hIgG was also significantly enhanced after salicylate treatment. As little as 0.25 mM salicylate significantly increased opsonophagocytosis of O1:K2 in the presence of hIgG.

K-specific antibodies may be rendered nonfunctional either by attachment to cell-free CPS or by being masked underneath the capsule surface. Extensive washing of fully-encapsulated bacteria to remove cell-free and loosely attached capsular material did not influence anti-K phagocytosis. However, decapsulated bacteria were no longer phagocytized by anti-K antisera after the addition of minute quantities of purified

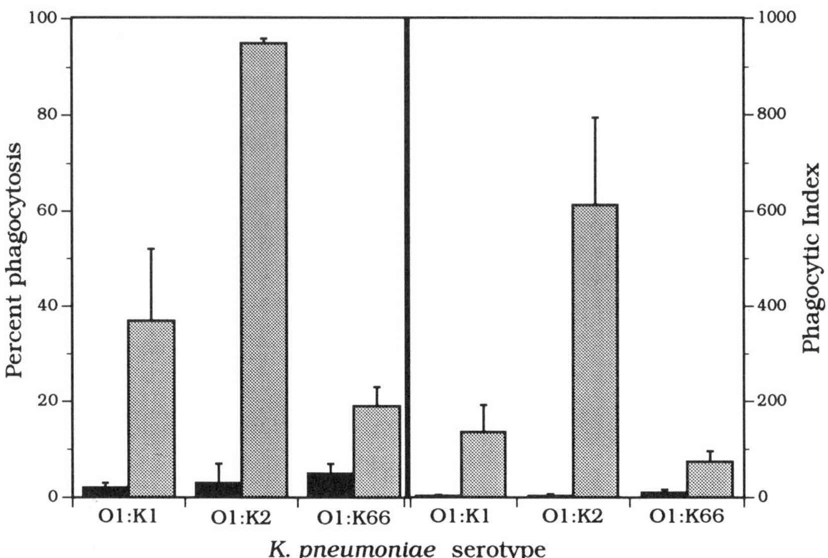

FIGURE 1. Effect of salicylate and homologous, K-specific antiserum on opsonophagocytosis. *K. pneumoniae* serotypes O1:K1, O1:K2, and O1:K66 were cultured overnight with (*gray bars*) and without (*black bars*) 2.5 mM salicylate and incubated with human polymorphonuclear cells in 10% fresh normal serum and 10% K-specific antiserum for 30 minutes at 37°C. Phagocytic index is expressed as the number of bacteria per active phagocyte × 100 phagocytes counted.

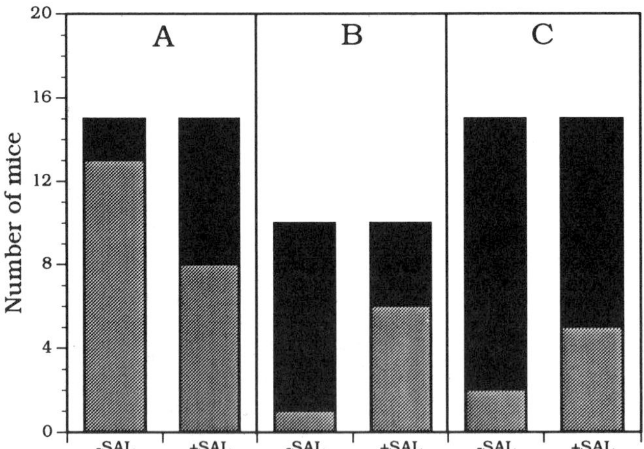

FIGURE 2. Mouse protection studies with Nosocuman and salicylate. Mice were administered 50 μg (**A**), 10 μg (**B**), or no (**C**) K-specific hIgG 1 hour before challenge with 25 LD_{50} units of *K. pneumoniae* O1:K2. Half the mice received salicylate at 114 mg/kg at the time of challenge. Death (*black bars*) and survival (*gray bars*) were monitored over a 5-day period.

CPS. Thus, K-specific antibodies can be neutralized by soluble CPS. Immunofluorescence was used to visualize antibody binding to bacteria. Fluorescein-tagged, K-specific antibodies reacted with CPS throughout the capsule, indicating that much of the IgG may be buried underneath the capsule surface.

The effects of salicylate (114 mg/kg) on immunotherapy gave encouraging, but conflicting results, as shown in FIGURE 2. Mice challenged intraperitoneally with 25 LD_{50} of O1:K2 and treated with 10 μg hIgG were provided 50% greater protection when also receiving salicylate, yet animals treated with 50 μg hIgG were 33.4% more likely to die with salicylate treatment. In conclusion, K-specific opsonins are more efficient against bacteria decapsulated by salicylate, apparently through a variety of mechanisms, but the medical importance of this finding is inconclusive.

REFERENCES

1. SIMOONS-SMIT, A. M., J. J. VERWEIJ-VAN VUGHT & D. M. MACLAREN. 1986. J. Med. Microbiol. **21:** 133–137.
2. STRAUS, D. C. 1987. Infect. Immun. **55:** 44–48.
3. POLLACK, M. 1976. Infect. Immun. **13:** 1543–1548.
4. DOMENICO, P., R. J. SALO, D. C. STRAUS, J. C. HUTSON & B. A. CUNHA. 1992. Infection **20:** 66–72.

Immunohistochemical Detection of Cytokines in Tissues of *Aotus* Monkeys Infected with Hepatitis A Virus

Y. E. POLOTSKY, R. A. VASSELL, L. N. BINN, AND
L. V. S. ASHER

Walter Reed Army Institute of Research
Washington, DC 20307–5100

The major pathologic alterations in human hepatitis A virus (HAV) infection are lymphocytic portal inflammation in the liver with piecemeal parenchymal necrosis. Because HAV is not cytotoxic, a cell-mediated immune response has been suggested as causing the hepatic injury.[1,2] In other viral infections cytotoxic lymphocytes are known to damage target cells.[3] We studied the immunohistopathology of experimental HAV hepatitis to gain insight into the role of cell-mediated immunity.

Aotus trivirgatus monkeys were infected by oral inoculation and developed hepatitis that was confirmed virologically, immunologically, and histopathologically.[4] Animals were subjected to necropsy 4 hours to 9 weeks postinoculation. Frozen and paraffin sections were stained to identify immunotypes of inflammatory cells and to detect cells producing cytokines. Paraffin sections 3-4 μm thick were deparaffinized and digested with 0.05% protease VIII. Frozen sections 4-6 μm thick were fixed in cold acetone. We then applied primary monoclonal and polyclonal antibodies to 17 human cell-differentiation (CD) antigens (Dako, Becton Dickinson) and 14 cytokines (Genzyme, Endogen). Primary antibody binding was revealed by secondary antispecies antibodies from either peroxidase-labeled avidin-biotin complex (Vectastain ABC, Vector), peroxidase-antiperoxidase (PAP, Dako), alkaline phosphatase-antialkaline phosphatase (APAAP, Dako) kits, or fluorescein-isothiocyanate labels (Kirkegaard and Perry, Cappel).

Mononuclear inflammatory infiltrates, consisting mostly of lymphocytes, gradually developed in portal areas starting 3 weeks after infection and increasing with time. Lymphocytes were a mixture of CD3$^+$ T cells, scattered uniformly, and CD20$^+$ B cells with HLA-DR antigen on their surfaces, which expanded locally around bile ducts. The majority of CD3$^+$ cells were CD4$^+$ helper cells, whereas a few CD8$^+$ cytotoxic cells (FIG. 1) were located close to those hepatocytes that developed dystrophic lesions. A few Kupffer cells and monocytes in lobular sinusoids and single macrophages in portal infiltrates were positive for MAC 387 antigen. No pathologic changes were seen in the spleens.

Occasional solitary interleukin-1 beta (IL-1β^+), tumor necrosis factor-alpha (TNFα)$^+$, and IL-2$^+$ cells were found in portal areas at 3 weeks and later, but they were very few and did not increase in number as the infection progressed. At 4 weeks, large IL-6$^+$ and IL-4$^+$ lymphocytes were seen in the liver around portal veins

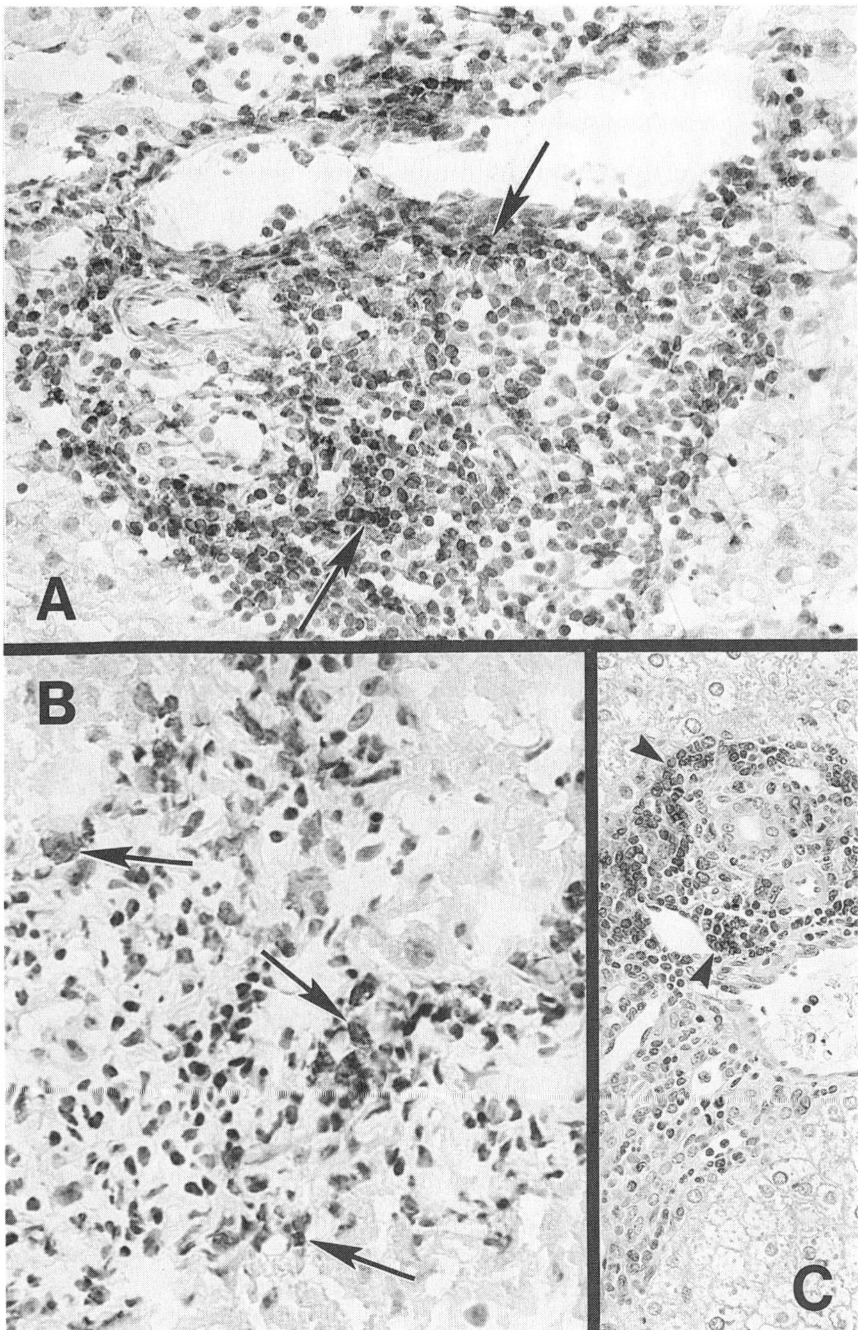

FIGURE 1. Immunotypes of lymphocytes in inflammatory portal infiltrates. Frozen sections. Immunoperoxidase ABC. (**A**) Most of the infiltrate consists of CD4$^+$ T helper lymphocytes (*arrows*) (5 weeks × 200 magnification). (**B**) A few peripheral CD8$^+$ lymphocytes (*arrows*) (6 weeks × 300 magnification). (**C**) Clusters of CD20$^+$ B lymphocytes (*arrowheads*) (5 weeks × 150 magnification).

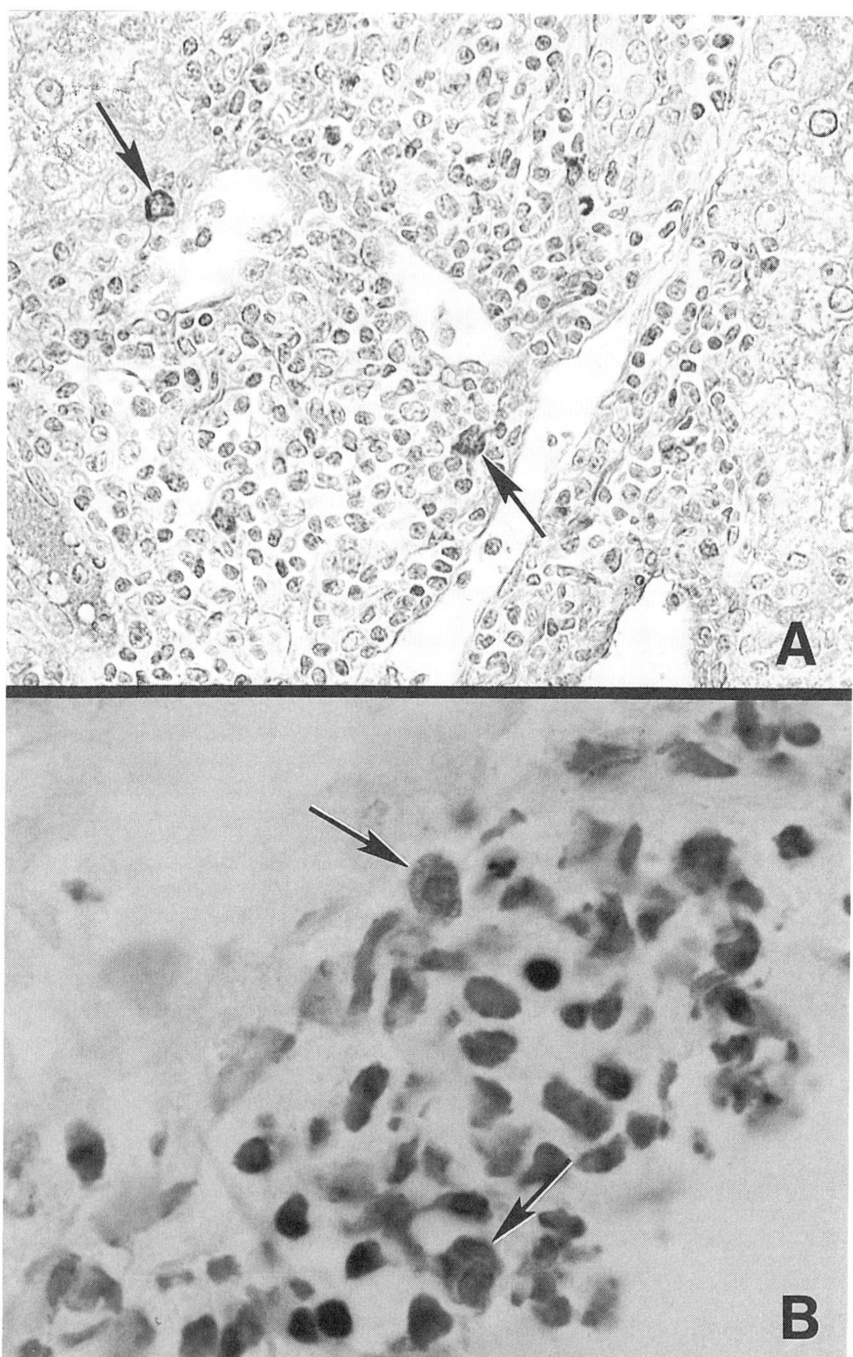

FIGURE 2. A few large cytokine-producing lymphocytes in portal inflammatory infiltrates. Immunoperoxidase ABC. (**A**) IL-6 (*arrows*). (5-week paraffin section; magnification × 300.) (**B**) IL-4 (*arrows*). (6-week frozen section; magnification × 900.)

and in the spleen around arterioles and in the red pulp. Their appearance coincided with activation and proliferation of B cells. The number of T lymphocytes producing IL-6 and IL-4 increased as portal inflammation progressed (FIG. 2).

Our findings suggest that cytokines IL-6 and IL-4, derived from T-helper subset 2 cells,[5] stimulate B cells, resulting in their local expansion and probably the production of antibodies to HAV. IL-6 and IL-4 might also stimulate cytotoxic activity of CD8[+] cells found adjacent to dystrophic and disintegrating hepatocytes.

SUMMARY

Cytokines IL-1-beta, IL-2, and TNF_α were detected in occasional cells within portal inflammatory infiltrates beginning 3 weeks after oral inoculation of monkeys with HAV. The number of cells secreting those cytokines did not increase, and they were not of importance in the pathogenesis. Production of cytokines IL-6 and IL-4 by T lymphocytes infiltrating portal areas started 4 weeks after inoculation, stimulating local expansion of B cells, probably secreting antibodies to HAV. IL-6 and IL-4 may also stimulate cytotoxic activity of a few CD8[+] lymphocytes.

REFERENCES

1. HOLLINGER, F. B. & J. TICEHURST. 1990. *In* Virology. B. N. Fields, D. M. Knipe, R. M. CHANOCK, M. S. HIRSCH, J. L. MELNICK, T. P. MONATH & B. ROIZMAN, Eds. 2nd Ed.: 631–667. Raven Press. New York.
2. FLEISCHER, B., S. FLEISCHER, K. MAIER, K. H. WIEDMANN, M. SACHER, H. THALER & A. VALLBRACHT. 1990. Immunology **69:** 14–19.
3. DOHERTY, P. C. 1993. Semin. Virol. **4:** 117–122.
4. ASHER, L. V. S., L. N. BINN, T. MENSING, R. H. MARCHWICKI, D. YOUNG, R. A. VASSELL & D. DYKSTRA. 1994. Pathogenesis of Hepatitis A virus in owl monkeys following oral inoculation. In preparation.
5. KIYONO, H., J. BIENENSTOCK, J. R. McGHEE & P. B. ERNST. 1992. Reg. Immunol. **4:** 54–62.

Inflammatory Cytokine Response to Experimental Human Infection with *Neisseria gonorrhoeae*

KYLE H. RAMSEY,[a] HERMAN SCHNEIDER,
ROBERT A. KUSCHNER, ANDREW F. TROFA,
ALAN S. CROSS, AND CAROLYN D. DEAL

Division of Communicable Disease and Immunology
Walter Reed Army Institute of Research
Washington, DC 20307-5100

The specificity of *Neisseria gonorrhoeae* for the human and the subsequent lack of an animal model has led to the use of a human male intraurethral challenge model to study pathogenesis.[1] In the present study, we describe urine and plasma levels of four inflammatory cytokines: interleukin-1 beta (IL-1β); interleukin-6 (IL-6); interleukin-8 (IL-8); and tumor necrosis factor-alpha (TNF$_\alpha$) in male volunteers inoculated intraurethrally with *N. gonorrhoeae* strain MS11mk.

Seventeen volunteers were inoculated and urine specimens were collected at 2 hours following inoculation and 12-hour intervals thereafter. Ten volunteers developed urethritis with viable *N. gonorrhoeae* in urine sediments (symptomatic volunteers). Seven volunteers displayed no symptoms with positive cultures in four of seven in the 2-hour urine specimens only followed by repeated sterile urine (asymptomatic volunteers). Volunteers were treated with one oral 500-mg dose of ciprofloxacin following development of dysuria and discharge containing gram-negative diplococci in polymorphonuclear leukocytes (PMNs). Urine was sterile 12 hours after treatment. Leukocytes were observed in urine sediment gram stains within the first 2–38 hours following inoculation (mean = 20 hours). The mean time to onset of symptoms was 86 hours (3.6 days, range 62–146 hours). In all symptomatic volunteers, viable bacteria were being shed for at least 48 hours before the onset of symptoms and often longer.

Of the 10 symptomatic volunteers, each had elevated urine levels of IL-8, IL-6, TNF$_\alpha$, and IL-1β at the onset of symptoms (Fig. 1). Preinoculation urine had undetectable levels of each cytokine. Following treatment there was a rapid return to baseline or near baseline levels. Of particular interest was the rapid manner in which IL-8, IL-6, and TNF$_\alpha$ were detected in the urine (within 2–14 hours) in 8 of 10, 6 of 10, and 4 of 10 symptomatic volunteers, respectively. A similar initial increase in IL-8 and IL-6 levels was observed in 4 of 7 asymptomatic challenge volunteers. By comparison, these returned to baseline levels within 24 hours, whereas the quantity

---

[a] PRESENT ADDRESS: Department of Microbiology, Midwestern University, 555 31st Street, Downers Grove, IL 60515.

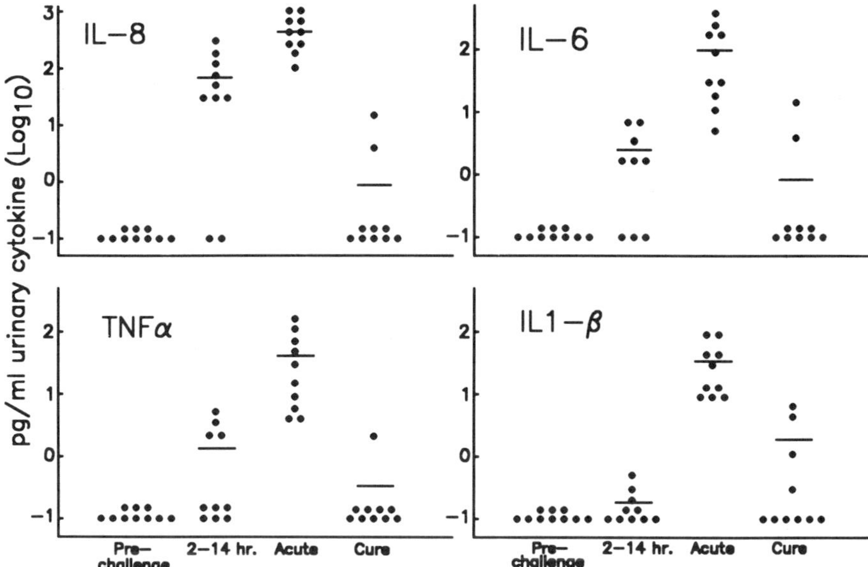

FIGURE 1. Urine cytokine levels of symptomatic volunteers. Urine was sedimented by centrifugation immediately after collection of the sample. Sediments were used for culture of the organism and for Gram stain. Supernatants were aliquoted and frozen at −70°C until assayed. Cytokines were measured in urine supernatants by commercially available antigen capture ELISA kits (R&D Systems, Minneapolis, Minnesota). Prechallenge sample was collected 1 hour before inoculation; 2–14 hour, sample was collected either 2 or 14 hours after inoculation; acute, sample was collected at the onset of symptoms and just prior to antibiotic therapy; cure, sample was collected within 24–48 hours following antibiotic therapy. *Bars* represent the mean of 10 symptomatic volunteers. Actual quantities for acute samples were as follows: IL-8, mean = 489 pg/ml, range = 149–902; IL-6, mean = 104 pg/ml, range = 5–285; TNF$_\alpha$, mean = 43 pg/ml, range = 4–141; and IL-1β, mean = 35 pg/ml, range = 8.3– 94.1.

in symptomatic volunteers continued to increase. Whether this early response is due to mild tissue damage incurred as a result of the inoculation procedure or is a true response to the bacterial inoculation was not determined. Because of the rapid nature of their appearance, it is likely that IL-8, IL-6, and TNF$_\alpha$ were produced locally, particularly during the early stages of the response to the gonococcus. Other investigators have found that IL-6 and IL-8 are produced locally in a rapid fashion in response to urinary tract infection with gram-negative bacteria.[2,3] By contrast to our study, no elevated TNF$_\alpha$ or IL-1β levels were found. However, TNF$_\alpha$ induction may be common to gonococcal infections. McGee *et al.*[4] found that *N. gonorrhoeae* induced increased TNF$_\alpha$ in explanted genital tract tissue culture supernatants as early as 3 hours postinfection. Hence, in their model, *N. gonorrhoeae* induced local and rapid production of the cytokine. In the present study, urinary IL-1β remained near baseline in all symptomatic volunteers until just before the onset of symptoms and it was not elevated at any time in asymptomatic volunteers. This pattern of IL-1β production correlated

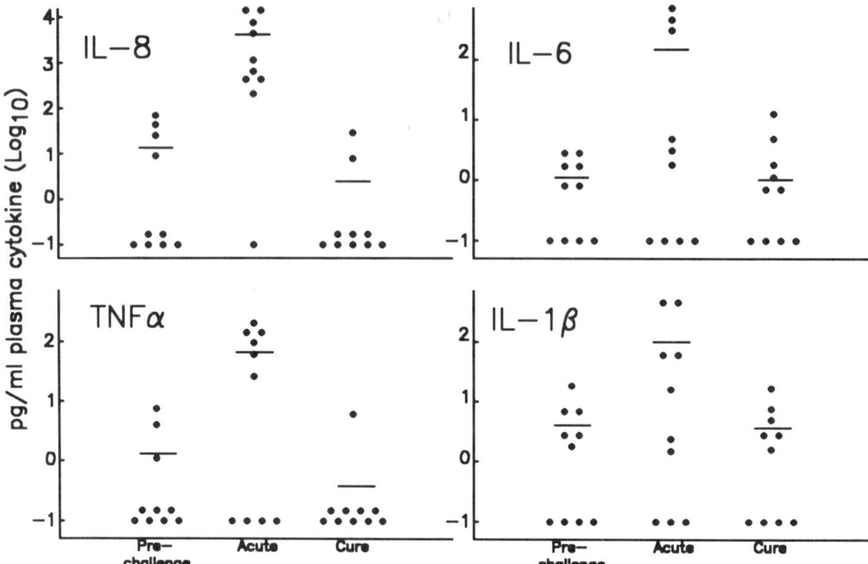

FIGURE 2. Plasma cytokine levels of symptomatic volunteers. Blood was collected in heparinized Vaccutainer tubes (Becton-Dickinson, Indianapolis, Indiana). Cells were sedimented by centrifugation and plasma was aliquoted and stored at –70°C. Actual quantities for acute samples were as follows: IL-8, mean = 4,706 pg/ml, range = 182-14,647; TNF_α, mean = 112 pg/ml, range = 32-203; IL-1β mean = 205 pg/ml, range 1-465; and IL-6, mean = 188, range = 2-547.

with an increased presence of leukocytes in urine sediment gram stains. Hence, IL-1β may have been derived from inflammatory cells recruited to the site of infection.

Blood samples were collected before inoculation, at the onset of symptoms, and 24- 48 hours after treatment. Several volunteers had detectable levels of each cytokine in the plasma before inoculation (FIG. 2). Nonetheless, 9 of 10, 6 of 10, 5 of 10, and 5 of 10 volunteers responded with elevated IL-8, TNF_α, IL-1β, and IL-6, respectively, at the onset of symptoms. As with urine, cytokine returned to baseline or near baseline levels in the plasma soon after treatment. Elevated plasma cytokine levels were not found in asymptomatic challenge volunteers.

Considering its propensity to attract and activate PMNs, it is not surprising to find that urinary IL-8 is a prominent cytokine in a disease noted for its inflammatory exudate. However, despite the localized nature of the infection, IL-8 and other cytokines were elevated systemically. This is especially noteworthy in light of the relatively short lag time between inoculation, onset of symptoms, and treatment. Other investigators studying urinary tract infection, found no concomitant increase in serum levels of IL-6 or IL-8.[2,3]

REFERENCES

1. SCHNEIDER, H., J. M. GRIFFIS, J. W. BOSLEGO, P. J. HITCHCOCK, K. M. ZAHOS & M. A. APICELLA. 1991. Expression of paragloboside-like lipooligosaccharides may be a necessary component of gonococcal pathogenesis in men. J. Exp. Med. **174:** 1601–1605.
2. HEDGES, S., P. ANDERSON, G. LIDIN-JANSON, P. DEMAN & C. SVANBORG. 1991. IL-6 response to deliberate colonization of the human urinary tract with Gram-negative bacteria. Infect. Immun. **60:** 421–427.
3. KO, Y.-C., N. MUKAIDA, S. ISHIYAMA, A. TOKUE, T. KAWAI, K. MATSUSHIMA & T. KASAHARA. 1993. Elevated IL-8 levels in the urine of patients with urinary tract infections. Infect. Immun. **61:** 1307–1314.
4. MCGEE, Z. A., C. M. CLEMENS, R. L. JENSEN, J. J. KLEIN, L. R. BAILEY & G. L. GORBY. 1992. Local induction of TNFα as a molecular mechanism of mucosal damage by gonococci. Microb. Pathog. **12:** 333–341.

Selective Translocation of Annexins III, IV, and V during Intracellular Redistribution of *Chlamydia trachomatis* Serovar L2 in HeLa and McCoy Cells

MEYTHAM MAJEED,[a] JOEL D. ERNST,[b]
KARL-ERIC MAGNUSSON,[c] ERIK KIHLSTRÖM,[d]
AND OLLE STENDAHL[c]

Departments of Clinical Microbiology[a] and Medical Microbiology[c]
University of Linköping
S-581 85 Linköping, Sweden

[b]Department of Medicine
Division of Infectious Diseases
and Rosalind Russell Arthritis Research Laboratory
San Francisco General Hospital
San Francisco, California 94143-0868

[d]Department of Clinical Microbiology
Örebro Medical Center Hospital
Örebro, Sweden

Chlamydia trachomatis is an obligate intracellular microorganism with a unique biphasic developmental cycle, alternating between the infectious, metabolically inactive, elementary body (EB) which penetrates susceptible host cells and reorganizes into the reproductive, reticulate body (RB).[1]

Elementary body-containing vesicles fuse with each other early in the infectious process, giving rise to one inclusion per infected cell.[2] However, these vesicles avoid fusion with host cell lysosomes.[3] Indeed, viable EBs are not required for inhibition of endosome-lysosome formation, because EB envelopes can avoid this formation.[4]

We recently showed that *C. trachomatis* infecting eukaryotic cells redistributes intracellularly and that clathrin and F-actin are involved.[5] This process and the subsequent formation of chlamydial inclusions require normal homeostasis of intracellular Ca^{2+}.[6]

Members of the Ca^{2+}-binding annexin family have been implicated in mediating calcium-regulated membrane traffic during endo- and exocytosis.[7] We therefore studied the intracellular distribution of certain annexins following invasion of HeLa and McCoy cells by *C. trachomatis*.

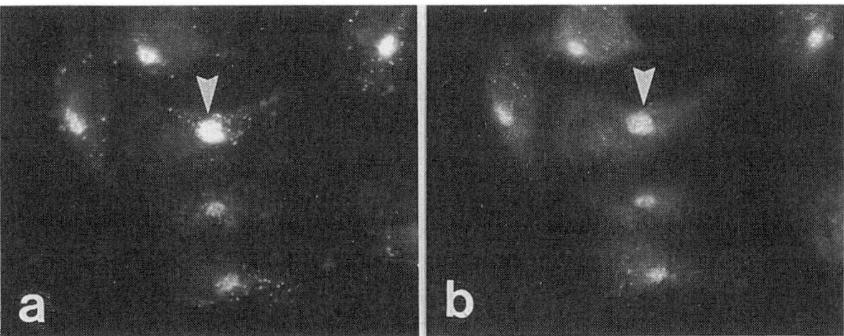

FIGURE 1. *C. trachomatis*-infected HeLa cells incubated for 3 hours at 37°C. Infected cells were fixed and double stained with a monoclonal antibody to major outer membrane protein (**a**) and with a polyclonal antiannexin III antibody (**b**). Aggregations of elementary bodies and annexin III are indicated by *arrowheads*.

MATERIALS AND METHODS

Microorganisms. C. trachomatis serovar L2 was propagated in McCoy cells, purified by centrifugation, titrated by inclusion formation, and stored at −70°C until used.

Infectious Procedure. HeLa and McCoy cells were infected with 70 μl of *C. trachomatis* at a multiplicity of infection of about 300 EBs per cell in Ca^{2+}-free buffer and incubated for 2 hours at 4°C. Then the cells were washed and incubated for different times at 37°C in either CA^{2+}-containing or Ca^{2+}-free medium in the presence of the calcium chelator 1,2-bis-5-methyl-amino-phenoxylethane-N,N,n′-tetra-acetoxymethyl acetate (MAPT/AM, Calbiochem-Behring Corp. AG, La Jolla, California). In some cell preparations chloramphenicol was added 12 hours postinfection. The cells were fixed and stained for chlamydiae with anti-*C. trachomatis* monoclonal antibody reacting with the major outer membrane protein (MOMP) (Washington Research Foundation, Seattle, Washington) and for annexins with polyclonal antiannexin antibodies. Fluorescent preparations were examined in a fluorescence microscope or a confocal scanning laser microscope.

RESULTS

Immunofluorescence staining showed that annexin III, IV, and V translocated within the cytoplasm to the area where chlamydiae aggregate (FIG. 1), whereas annexin I and VI were not affected. These results were supported by confocal microscopy which revealed an intimate association between chlamydial inclusions and annexin III. Depletion of intracellular Ca^{2+} did not prevent the association of annexin III with individual EB-containing endosomes, but it did prevent formation of chlamydial aggregates and translocation of annexin. Furthermore, chloramphenicol-treated cells also showed association between chlamydial aggregates and annexin III, indicating that the annexins are of host cell origin.

CONCLUSION

These data suggest that certain cytosolic annexins may be involved in the Ca^{2+}-dependent aggregation and fusion of chlamydia-containing vesicles. The fact that these Ca^{2+}-binding proteins differ in their ability to associate with chlamydia-containing vesicles and inclusions implies that the factors that regulate the interaction of annexin I and annexin III with endosomes are different and suggests a selective regulatory mechanism for endosome aggregation and avoided lysosome fusion during chlamydia infection.

REFERENCES

1. MOULDER, J. W. 1985. Microbiol. Rev. **49:** 298-337.
2. RIDDERHOF, J. C. & R. C. BARNES. 1989. Infect. Immun. **57:** 3189-3193.
3. FRIIS, R. R. 1972. J. Bacteriol. **110:** 706-721.
4. EISSENBERG, L. G., P. B. WYRICK, C. H. DAVIS & J. W. RUMPP. 1983. Infect. Immun. **40:** 741-751.
5. MAJEED, M. & E. KIHLSTRÖM. 1991. Infect. Immun. **59:** 4465-4472.
6. MAJEED, M., M. GUSTAFSSON, E. KIHLSTRÖM & O. STENDAHL. 1993. Infect. Immun. **4:** 1406-1414.
7. ERNST, J. D., E. HOYE, R. A. BLACKWOOD & D. JAYE. 1990. J. Clin. Invest. **85:** 1065-1071.

Role of Nitric Oxide in Hepatic Injury following Acute Endotoxemia

M. RODRIGUEZ-DEL VALLE,[a] S. M. HWANG,[b]
D. E. HECK,[c] J. D. LASKIN,[c] AND D. L. LASKIN[a]

[a]Rutgers University
Department of Pharmacology and Toxicology
P.O. Box 789
Piscataway, New Jersey 08855-0789

[b]Rutgers University
Department of Biological Sciences
P.O. Box 1059
Piscataway, New Jersey 08855-1059

[c]Department of Environmental and Community Medicine
UMDNJ-Robert Wood Johnson Medical School
Piscataway, New Jersey 08855

Endotoxemia is associated with hepatic damage and impaired functioning. The initial hepatic changes induced by endotoxin primarily involve reticuloendothelial cells. This is followed by degenerative changes in hepatocytes.[1,2] Similar damage and dysfunction have also been described following exposure of hepatocytes to endotoxin *in vitro*. However, little is known about the mechanisms underlying these effects. Hepatocytes are known to produce nitric oxide *in vitro*[3] which has been reported to alter their functioning and to inhibit protein synthesis.[4] Nitric oxide also decreases the proliferation of different cell types including lymphocytes,[5] smooth muscle cells,[6] and bone marrow leukocytes.[7]

In the present studies we examined the potential role of nitric oxide in hepatocyte injury induced by acute endotoxemia, which was characterized histologically by increased vacuolization and the appearance of mitotic figures within hepatocytes. Liver parenchymal cells were isolated from female Sprague-Dawley rats 48 hours after injection with *Escherichia coli* bacterial lipopolysaccharide (5 mg/kg intravenously). Nitric oxide was measured in hepatocyte culture medium after treatment of these cells with increasing concentrations of the inflammatory mediators lipopolysaccharide and/or gamma interferon (IFNγ). We found that hepatocytes from endotoxemic rats produced significantly more nitric oxide than did cells from control rats (TABLE 1). This was correlated with increased expression of protein and mRNA for the inducible form of nitric oxide synthase, as demonstrated by Western and Northern blot analysis, respectively. These results suggest that endotoxin primes hepatocytes for nitric oxide production. We also found that hepatocytes from endotoxemic rats displayed enhanced proliferation and protein synthesis when compared with cells from control animals (TABLE 1). Increased production of nitric oxide by hepatocytes after acute endotoxemia was associated with marked inhibition of proliferation and protein synthesis (TABLE 1) and the appearance of degraded cytoplasmic DNA (not shown). These are characteristics of injured hepatocytes. These effects were partially reversed by the addition

TABLE 1. Effects of Acute Endotoxemia on Nitric Oxide Production, Proliferation, and Protein Synthesis by Isolated Hepatocytes

Lipopolysaccharide (µg/ml)	Control Rats		Endotoxemic Rats	
	+ Media	+ IFNγ	+ Media	+ IFNγ
	Nitrite (µM/well)			
0	4.6 ± 0.8	8.3 ± 2.5	6.2 ± 0.3	73.6 ± 0.1
0.25	8.5 ± 3.0	9.0 ± 1.0	62.5 ± 0.1	89.4 ± 2.4
1.0	7.8 ± 1.6	10.5 ± 2.5	81.5 ± 1.6	94.4 ± 2.2
5.0	5.6 ± 0.2	12.4 ± 1.8	92.0 ± 2.7	103.3 ± 2.3
	(^{3}H)Thymidine Uptake (cpm/well)			
0	391 ± 42	198 ± 51	3,706 ± 345	1,420 ± 262
0.25	850 ± 50	200 ± 23	2,584 ± 303	180 ± 32
1.0	322 ± 17	266 ± 39	1,170 ± 159	175 ± 41
5.0	371 ± 22	120 ± 26	359 ± 88	214 ± 23
	(^{3}H)Leucine Uptake (cpm/well)			
0	922 ± 199	1,021 ± 56	5,938 ± 125	5,029 ± 758
0.25	845 ± 92	1,191 ± 141	1,911 ± 96	884 ± 58
1.0	595 ± 91	370 ± 44	1,948 ± 214	564 ± 62
5.0	378 ± 52	284 ± 31	1,742 ± 149	581 ± 36

of N^G-monomethyl-L-arginine (L-NMMA), an inhibitor of nitric oxide synthase, to the cultures. Taken together these results suggest that increased production of nitric oxide during endotoxemia may contribute, at least in part, to the pathogenesis of hepatic injury.

SUMMARY

Hepatocytes from control and endotoxemic rats were cultured for 40 hours in 96-well dishes in medium containing 0–5 µg/ml of lipopolysaccharide in the presence or absence of 50 U/ml IFNγ. Nitric oxide production was quantified by the accumulation of nitrite in the culture medium by the Greiss reaction. Hepatocyte proliferation and protein synthesis were measured by (^{3}H)thymidine (TdR) and (^{3}H)leucine (Leu) incorporation, respectively. Results are the mean ± standard error of triplicate wells from four experiments.

REFERENCES

1. NOLAN, J. P. 1975. Gastroenterology **69:** 1346–1356.
2. HIRATA, K., A. KANEKO, K. OGAWA, H. HAYASAKA & T. ONOE. 1980. Lab. Invest. **43:** 165–171.

3. CURRAN, R. D., T. R. BILLIAR, D. J. STUEHR, K. HOFMAN & R. L. SIMMONS. 1989. J. Exp. Med. **170:** 1769-1774.
4. CURRAN, R. D., T. R. BILLIAR, D. J. STUEHR, J. B. OCHOA, B. G. HORBRECHT, S. G. FLINT & R. L. SIMMONS. 1990. Ann. Surg. **212:** 462-471.
5. ALBINA, J. E. & W. HENRY. 1991. J. Surg. Res. **50:** 403-409.
6. SCOTT-BURDEN, T., V. B. SCHINI, E. ELIZONDO, D. C. JUNQUERO & P. M. VANHOUTTE. 1992. Circ. Res. **71:** 1088-1100.
7. PUNJABI, C. J., D. L. LASKIN, D. E. HECK & J. D. LASKIN. 1992. J. Immunol. **149:** 2179-2184.

The Role of *Streptococcus viridans* in Human Infections in Mauritius

JAGDISH RAI

Department of Health and Medical Science
Faculty of Science
University of Mauritius
Reduit, Mauritius

Streptococci whose colonies produce a greenish discoloration on blood agar (alpha hemolytic streptococci) are usually ignored or underrated as nonpathogenic viridans streptococci. Recent studies have shown a definite relation between these microorganisms and different human infections. In the present study 17,800 clinical specimens such as throat swabs, pus swabs, aspirated pus, vaginal swabs, urine, blood, and cerebrospinal fluid of patients with serious infections were processed for bacteriologic examination, resulting in isolation and identification of various species of viridans streptococci from patients with serious infections who reported to or were admitted to hospitals in Mauritius. The species of *Streptococcus viridans* isolated from clinical specimens mainly include *S. anginosus, S. sanguis, S. mutans,* and *S. mitis.* Analysis of these results indicates that various types of *S. viridans* are associated with serious human infection and that the pathogenic role of these microorganisms cannot be overlooked or underrated, making it obligatory for the Clinical Microbiological Laboratory to report on *S. viridans* isolates along with the results of their antibiotic susceptibility.

The work is continuing with special emphasis on the following aspects: (a) correlation between the presence of microorganisms (predominant) and the cellular response, that is, polymorphonuclear leukocytes in clinical material such as throat swab, pus swab, cerebrospinal fluid, other body fluids, vaginal smears/urethral smears, and urine (centrifuged deposit) as demonstrated by direct detection with the help of gram staining of the smears prepared from the clinical specimens; (b) presence of microorganisms (direct detection and isolation/identification by culture) in body cavities that are normally free from microorganisms such as cerebrospinal fluid, pleural fluid, pericardial fluid, peritoneal fluid, urine, and blood, especially with accompanying inflammatory cells (i.e., polymorphonulear leukocytes/pus cells) in the clinical specimens; (c) therapeutic response to appropriate antimicrobial drugs, that is, antibiotics (clinical improvement), eradication/significant reduction in microorganisms as seen by direct detection or culture, and decline in cellular reaction on instituting appropriate therapy after antimicrobial susceptibility testing; (d) demonstration of rising titer of specific antibodies to the suspected isolates in the patient's serum; and (e) demonstration of a cell-mediated immune response in the patient such as blast transformation and macrophage migration inhibition phenomena.

TABLE 1. Specimens Processed

Spec. No.	Type of Specimen	No. of Specimens Processed	Age (yr)/Sex Distribution									
			0–4		5–11		12–16		19–30		Over 30	
			M	F	M	F	M	F	M	F	M	F
1	Throat swab	1,553	150	125	218	214	162	150	158	148	113	115
2	Pus/wound swab	1,230	115	150	147	133	132	116	121	114	133	114
3	Vaginal swab	1,110	—	202	—	286	—	223	—	210	—	189
4	Urethral swab	148	—	—	—	—	25	38	21	25	19	20
5	Eye swab	525	48	37	57	40	68	64	66	59	45	41
6	Ear swab	157	14	12	28	14	22	14	21	16	9	7
7	Nasal swab	31	3	2	5	4	4	3	4	2	3	1
8	Blood culture	777	78	64	92	79	94	82	87	71	72	63
9	Cerebrospinal fluid	222	21	17	33	26	25	21	24	19	21	15
10	Pleural fluid	80	—	—	—	—	16	12	14	11	15	12
11	Peritoneal fluid	90	—	—	—	—	17	13	21	16	14	9
12	Urine	11,102	700	628	912	875	1,292	1,283	1,242	1,224	1,477	1,469
13	Sputum	775	—	—	111	103	112	97	106	91	33	72
	Total	17,800	1,129	1,129	1,603	1,774	1,959	2,116	1,385	2,006	2,004	2,132

TABLE 2. Viridans/Non-beta Hemolytic Streptococci (figures in parentheses are percentage)

Type of Specimen	No. of Specimens Processed	S. anginosus	S. sanguis	S. mutans	S. mitis	Any Other Type	Total
Throat swab	1,553	11 (12)	20 (23)	6 (7)	26 (30)	25 (28)	88
Pus/wound swab	1,230	5 (31)	6 (37)	1 (6)	2 (13)	2 (13)	16
Vaginal swab	1,110	—	—	—	4 (100)	—	4
Urethral swab	148	2 (17)	3 (25)	—	2 (17)	5 (41)	12
Eye swab	525	3 (12)	3 (12)	4 (16)	5 (20)	10 (40)	25
Ear swab	157	4 (31)	4 (31)	1 (8)	2 (15)	2 (15)	13
Nasal swab	31	1 (17)	2 (33)	—	1 (17)	2 (33)	6
Blood culture	777	2 (22)	3 (34)	—	2 (22)	2 (22)	9
Cerebrospinal fluid	222	1 (25)	1 (25)	—	—	2 (50)	4
Pleural fluid	80	—	—	—	—	—	—
Peritoneal fluid	90	—	1 (100)	—	—	—	1
Urine	11,102	2 (7)	1 (3)	2 (7)	10 (33)	15 (50)	30
Sputum	775	5 (20)	12 (48)	1 (4)	6 (24)	1 (4)	25
Total	17,800	36 (15)	56 (24)	15 (6)	60 (26)	66 (29)	233

REFERENCES

1. COYKENDALL, A. L. 1989. Classification and identification of the Viridans streptococci. Clin. Microbial. Rev. **2:** 315–328.
2. RUOFF, K. L., J. A. FISHERMAN, S. B. CALDERWOOD & L. J. KUNZ. 1983. Distribution and incidence of viridans streptococcal species in routine clinical specimens. Am. J. Clin. Pathol. **8:** 854–858.
3. RUOFF, K. L. 1989. *Streptococcus anginosus (S. milleri)*: The unrecognised pathogen. Clin. Microbiol. Rev. **1:** 102–108.
4. WHITLEY, R. A., H. FRASER, J. M. HARDIE & BEIGHTON. 1990. Phenotypic differentiation of streptococcus intermedius, streptococcus constellatus and streptococcus milleri group. J. Clin. Microbiol. **28:** 1497–1501.
5. WHITWORTH, J. M., P. W. ROSS & I. R. POXTON. 1992. Use of rapid carbohydrate utilization test for identifying ''*streptococcus milleri* group.'' J. Clin. Pathol. **44:** 329–333.

Effects of Acute Endotoxemia on Production of Cytokines and Nitric Oxide by Pulmonary Alveolar and Interstitial Macrophages

THERESA M. WIZEMANN AND DEBRA L. LASKIN

Department of Pharmacology and Toxicology
Rutgers University
P.O. Box 789
Piscataway, New Jersey 08855-0789

The lung is highly sensitive to damage induced by endotoxin.[1] This major component of the gram-negative bacterial cell wall is normally confined to the gastrointestinal tract and is effectively removed from the portal circulation by the Kupffer cells of the liver.[2] If this route of elimination fails or if infection occurs outside the portohepatic circulation, lung macrophages may become exposed to circulating endotoxin. Alveolar macrophages are known to be activated *in vitro* by lipopolysaccharide, the primary component of endotoxin, to release mediators such as tumor necrosis factor alpha[2] (TNFα) and nitric oxide,[3] which are involved in inflammation and have been implicated in tissue injury. The role of pulmonary interstitial macrophages in these processes is unknown.

The present studies were designed to analyze the response of interstitial and alveolar macrophages to *in vivo* exposure to lipopolysaccharide. Alveolar macrophages were obtained by lavage of perfused lungs 48 hours after treatment of rats with lipopolysaccharide (5 mg/kg iv) or control. Lung tissue was then digested with collagenase (175 U/ml) and the resulting cell population enriched for interstitial macrophages by adherence to tissue culture dishes.[4] The release of TNFα by alveolar and interstitial macrophages was quantified by measuring the ability of supernatants from cultured macrophages to lyse actinomycin D-sensitized L929 cells. Both macrophage subpopulations were found to produce TNFα (TABLE 1).

Treatment of rats with lipopolysaccharide resulted in a decrease in TNFα production by interstitial macrophages, but had no effect on alveolar macrophages. Nitric oxide was quantified by the accumulation of nitrite in the medium using a modified Greiss reagent.[5] Macrophages cultured overnight were treated with various concentrations of lipopolysaccharide and/or rat gamma interferon (IFNγ). After 48 hours of incubation supernatants were collected and analyzed for nitric oxide. Both cell types produced nitric oxide in response to IFNγ and lipopolysaccharide. Alveolar macrophages produced more of this mediator than did interstitial macrophages. Production of nitric oxide was dependent on L-arginine and inhibited by the nitric oxide synthase inhibitor N-monomethyl-L-arginine. Although treatment of rats with lipopolysaccharide had no effect on nitrite accumulation by either alveolar or interstitial macrophages, Western blot analysis revealed increased inducible nitric oxide synthase in these

TABLE 1. Effects of Acute Endotoxemia on Production of TNFα by Alveolar and Interstitial Macrophages[a]

	Alveolar Macrophages		Interstitial Macrophages	
Time (h)	Untreated Rats	Endotoxemic Rats	Untreated Rats	Endotoxemic Rats
4	53.6 ± 3.6	65.9 ± 8.1	59.6 ± 6.5	33.4 ± 9.6
8	56.1 ± 2.7	68.0 ± 8.1	61.0 ± 2.9	36.3 ± 7.5[a]
18	43.4 ± 7.5	41.0 ± 14.3	50.9 ± 5.9	25.5 ± 4.8[a]
24	28.8 ± 3.7	36.4 ± 19.3	38.7 ± 9.0	10.9 ± 4.9[a]

[a] Conditioned medium was collected from alveolar and interstitial macrophages cultured for 4, 8, 18, and 24 hours and analyzed for tumor necrosis factor activity. Data are represented as the percentage of cytotoxicity. Each value is the average ± SE from three experiments.

[a] Significantly different from untreated rats ($p \leq 0.05$, Student's t test).

cells. Together our data suggest that acute endotoxemia is associated with alterations in TNFα and nitric oxide production by lung macrophages.

REFERENCES

1. WELBOURN, C. R. B. & Y. YOUNG. 1992. Br. J. Surg. **79:** 998–1003.
2. CALLERY, M. P., T. KAMEI, M. J. MANGINO & M. W. FLYE. 1991. Arch. Surg. **126:** 28–32.
3. LAVNIKOVA, N., J.-C. DRAPIER & D. L. LASKIN. 1993. J. Leukocyte Biol., in press.
4. LAVNIKOVA, N., S. PROKHOROVA, L. HELYAR & D. L. LASKIN. 1993. Am. J. Respir. Cell Mol. Biol. **8:** 384–392.
5. GREEN, L. C., D. A. WAGNER, J. GLOGOWSKI, P. L. SKIPPER, J. S. WISHNOK & S. R. TANNENBAUM. 1982. Anal. Biochem. **126:** 131–138.

Invariant Chain Dissociation from Class II MHC Is a Catalyst for Foreign Peptide Binding[a]

V. E. REYES,[b,d] M. DAIBATA,[c] R. ESPEJO,[b] AND
R. E. HUMPHREYS [c]

[b]University of Texas Medical Branch
Galveston, Texas 77555

[c]University of Massachusetts Medical School
Worcester, Massachusetts 01655

The class II MHC-associated invariant chain (li) acts as a chaperone in facilitating the transport and assembly of class II MHC molecules in the endoplasmic reticulum and their sorting to compartments containing endocytosed antigens. As a result of their association with li, class II MHC αβ chains do not bind self, endogenous peptides resident in the ER.[1] Class II MHC-li complexes move through the Golgi apparatus and eventually enter the endocytic pathway. Class II MHC-li complexes reside in endosomal compartments for 2–3 hours prior to the exit of class II MHC to the cell surface. While in endosomes, class II MHC become free of li through the action of cathepsin B on li.[2] This dissociation event permits class II MHC to bind peptides, become stable, and egress to the plasma membrane.[3] Our studies demonstrate that the binding of T-cell–presented peptides to class II MHC occurs as a concurrent process with the release of li by cathepsin B. Another endosomal protease, cathepsin D, which cleaved but did not release li, did not enhance peptide binding. However, trace levels of cathepsin D in the presence of cathepsin B further enhanced peptide binding by class II MHC.

Because peptide binding to affinity-purified class II MHC is very slow, relative to the time required for peptide binding by living cells, we decided to examine whether a class II conformational intermediate formed during the release of li is more efficient in binding peptides than is either class II MHC-li complexes or li-freed class II MHC. We incubated solubilized microsomal membranes from an HLA-DR-1⁺ cell line (JESTHOM) with a radiolabeled, HLA-DR-1–restricted influenza virus MA(18-29) peptide which was coupled to a heterobifunctional cross-linker (HSAB). Incubations were done at pH 5 for various time periods in the presence of varying concentrations of cathepsin B, which cleaves and releases li from class II

[a]This work was supported by grants IM-582 and JFRA-374 from the American Cancer Society, grant AHA-91013560 from the American Heart Association, and grant AI 34043 from the National Institutes of Health.

[d]Address for correspondence: Victor E. Reyes, PhD, University of Texas Medical Center, 301 University Boulevard, Route C-66, Galveston, Texas 77555-0366.

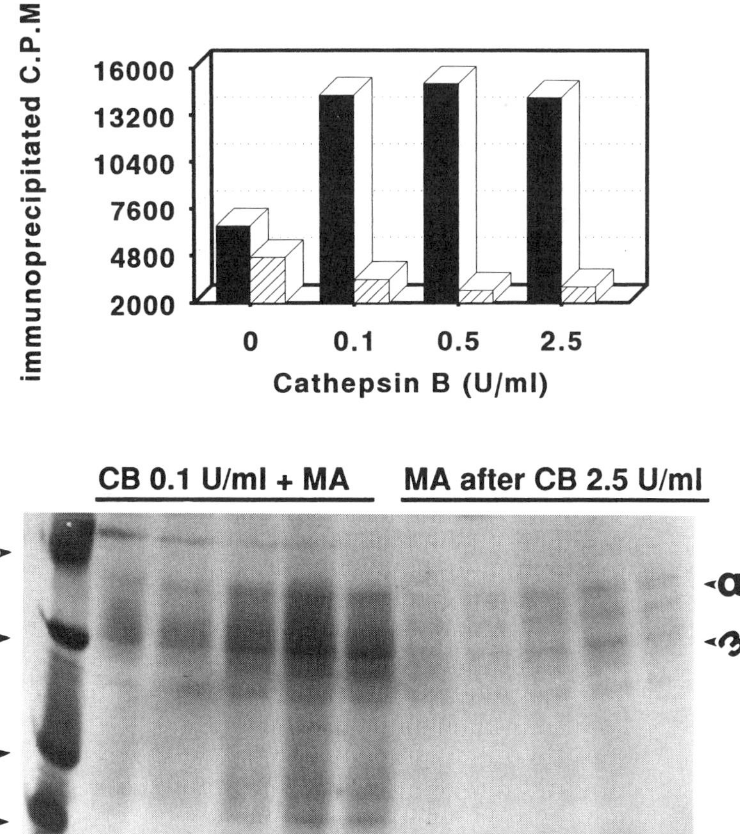

FIGURE 1. Binding of photoactivated, *N*-hydroxysuccinimidyl-4-azidobenzoate (HSAB) derivative of influenza virus MA(18-29) to MHC class II α,β chains as a function of time of digestion with varying concentrations of cathepsin B (CB). The iodinated peptide was added to the solubilized microsomal membrane proteins from JESTHOM cells (HLA-DR-1⁺) with CB, which cleaved li for varying periods of time at room temperature, pH 5.0. After each incubation, the enzyme was inactivated by 1 : 1 dilution with 2 mM PMSF, 10 mM *N*-ethylmaleimide acid, and 1 mM iodoacetamide in 10 mM Tris, pH 9.0, and the peptides were cross-linked to the α,β chains after ultraviolet light activation of the azido group. (**A**) These samples were immunoprecipitated with anti-class II monoclonal antibody (IVA12, ATCC) and coprecipitated radioactive peptide was measured. Maximal peptide coprecipitation was detected with as little as 0.1 U/ml CB. In all experiments, the concentration of MA(18-29) is 100 nM.

(*continued*)

MHC. At the end of each incubation, cathepsin B was neutralized with leupeptin. Samples were then exposed to ultraviolet light to induce cross-linking of the peptides to class II MHC α and β chains. Cross-linked complexes were immunoprecipitated with anti-HLA-DR monoclonal antibody (IVA12) and analyzed by SDS-PAGE and autoradiography. By this method, peptides cross-linked to either α or β chains of class II MHC were detected as early as 5 minutes after treatment, with a gradual increase in peptide bound as a function of time and cathepsin B concentration (FIG. 1A). Negligible levels of peptide binding occurred without cathepsin B. Peptide binding to class II MHC was more efficient (three to fourfold) if the peptide was present during li dissociation than if added afterwards (FIG. 1B).

Another endosomal protease, cathepsin D, which we and others have shown to cleave li without inducing its dissociation from class II MHC,[2,4] did not have any effects on peptide binding by class II MHC molecules. However, when the lowest dose of cathepsin D (0.1 U/ml) shown to cleave li was added to our assay in the presence of multiple concentrations of cathepsin B, there was an apparent synergy in inducing peptide binding to class II MHC (FIG. 2). These results were reproduced in three independent experiments. The specificity of [^{125}I]MA(18-29) binding to its restricting allele, HLA-DR-1, was confirmed by competition with either cold, homologous peptide or a heterologous HLA-DR-1-restricted peptide, influenza HA(306-318). Both peptides were able to compete with labeled MA(18-29) for binding. An HLA-DP-restricted dengue virus NS3(251-265) peptide and an HLA-B37-restricted influenza NP(336-356) were unable to compete.

In summary, the endosomal proteases cathepsins B and D, in addition to playing a role in generating peptides of a suitable size for binding to class II MHC, have also been shown by us and others to cleave li while leaving class II MHC α and β chains intact. Complete removal of li is mediated by cathepsin B. The occurrence of this event in endosomal/lysosomal compartments containing processed, endocytosed peptides appears to lead to the formation of a class II conformational intermediate which is receptive to peptides. Peptide binding to class II MHC complexes freed of li is not an efficient process, which in part explains the slow rates of peptide association to affinity-purified, class II MHC which were previously reported. The demonstration that cathepsin D, which alone does not affect peptide binding, can magnify the

---

FIGURE 1. (*continued*)
(**B**) Enhancement of peptide binding during CB digestion of li. Detergent-solubilized microsomal membranes containing MHC class II α,β,li trimer were incubated at room temperature at pH 5.0 with varying amounts of CB for 30 minutes in the presence of ^{125}I-labeled HSAB-MA(18-29) peptide, cross-linked, and processed as for **A**. Alternatively, after incubation with microsomal membranes for 30 minutes in the absence of MA(18-29) peptide, the enzyme was inactivated by 1 : 1 dilution with pH 5.0 buffer containing 2 mM PMSF, 10 mM *N*-ethylmaleimide, and 1 mM iodoacetamide. ^{125}I-labeled HSAB-MA(18-29) was added to the assay for 30 minutes and the samples were returned to pH 7.0 with 10 mM tris, pH 9.5, followed by photoactivation for peptide cross-linkage. Immunoprecipitates subjected to SDS-PAGE and the gels were autoradiographed. Much greater amounts of peptide are bound when the peptide is present during li proteolysis.

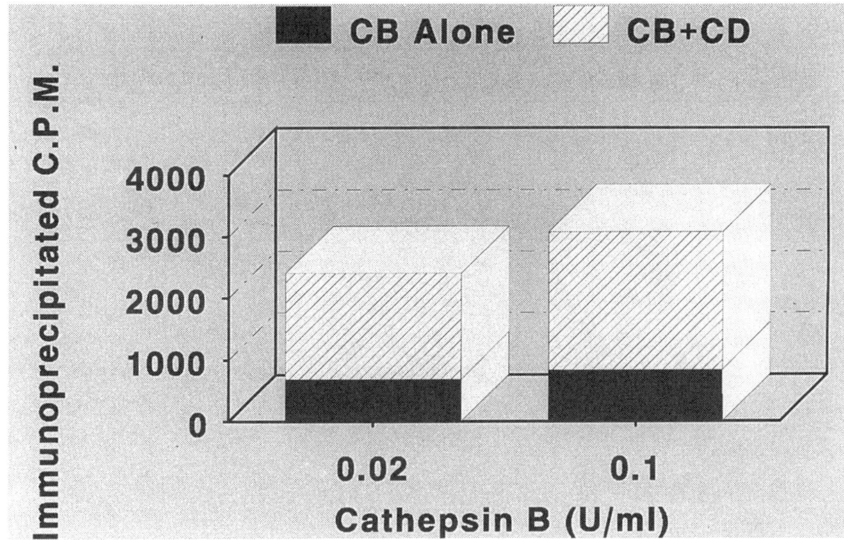

FIGURE 2. Cathepsin D (CD) enhancement of peptide binding in the presence of cathepsin B. Iodinated HSAB-MA(18-29) peptide and nonradiolabeled microsomal membranes were incubated at room temperature with or without 0.1 U/ml CD for 10 or 30 minutes in the presence of varying amounts of cathepsin B (CB). After subsequent photoactivation and immunoprecipitation with anti-class II monoclonal antibody, the samples were counted and subjected to SDS-PAGE and autoradiography.

cathepsin B-mediated enhancement of peptide loading by class II MHC possibly reflects the creation of a more cathepsin B-sensitive li intermediate. Thus, the concerted action of both enzymes on li in the presence of foreign, endocytosed peptides leads to the removal of li and the simultaneous ($\approx$5 minutes) binding by class II MHC of available peptides.

REFERENCES

1. NEWCOMB, J. R. & P. CRESSWELL. 1993. J. Immunol. **150:** 499–507.
2. REYES, V. R., S. LU & R. E. HUMPHREYS. 1991. J. Immunol. **146:** 3877–3880.
3. ROCHE, P. A., C. L. TELETSKI, D. R. KARP, V. PINET, O. BAKKE & E. O. LONG. 1992. EMBO J. **11:** 2841–2847.
4. MEHRINGER, J. H., M. R. HARRIS, C. S. KINDLE, D. W. McCOURT & S. E. CULLEN. 1991. J. Immunol. **146:** 920–927.

Nitric Oxide Has an Immunoregulatory Role Other Than Antimicrobial Activity in *Legionella pneumophila* Infected Macrophages

YOSHIMASA YAMAMOTO, HERMAN FRIEDMAN,
AND THOMAS W. KLEIN

Department of Medical Microbiology and Immunology
University of South Florida College of Medicine
Tampa, Florida 33612

Legionella pneumophila is a facultative intracellular bacterium that causes legionellosis in humans and is inhibited by cell-mediated mechanisms. Recently our studies showed that the fate of *L. pneumophila* in macrophages, which is modulated by cytokines such as gamma interferon (IFNγ),[1] is critical for the course of infection.[2] Therefore, how the macrophages respond to *Legionella* infection is important in the final outcome of that infection. Nitric oxide (NO) was recently discovered as an important effector molecule for macrophage functions inasmuch as this molecule has direct toxicity not only for microorganisms but also for tumor cells.[3] However, the essential role of NO in infection, especially its immunologic role, is poorly understood. In the present study, the possible role of NO in *Legionella* infection, especially in *Legionella*-macrophage interaction, was examined. Thioglycolate-elicited mouse peritoneal macrophages obtained from *Legionella*-susceptible A/J mice[4] were used in this study. When macrophage monolayers were treated with murine recombinant IFNγ (20 U/ml) for 24 hours, *Legionella* growth in the otherwise permissive macrophages was significantly inhibited. *Legionella* growth inhibition was approximately 99.4% in the IFNγ-treated macrophages. Nitric oxide production in *Legionella*-infected macrophages primed with IFNγ was measured as nitrite production using Griess reagent.[5] IFNγ treatment alone induced only a small amount of NO (268 ± 39 nmol of nitrite/mg of macrophage protein). However, IFNγ plus infection induced 628 ± 93 nmol of nitrite/mg of protein at 48 hours after infection.

Induction of inducible macrophage NO synthase (M-NOS) mRNA in *Legionella*-infected macrophages primed with IFNγ was also examined by a polymerase chain reaction following reverse transcription of mRNA (RT-PCR). *Legionella* infection induced an increased steady-state level of M-NOS mRNA. These results clearly showed that *Legionella* infection of IFNγ-primed macrophages generates NO. Nitric oxide inhibitors such as *N*-monomethyl-L-arginine (L-NMMA) or aminoguanidine, as well as culture of the macrophages in arginine-free medium, completely inhibited

[a] This work was supported by grant AI 16618 from the National Institute of Allergy and Infectious Diseases.

TABLE 1. Effect of NMMA on the Production of Interleukin-6 (IL-6) and Nitric Oxide (NO) in *Legionella*-Infected Macrophages[a]

Treatment	Control		*Legionella* Infection	
	IL-6[b]	NO[c]	IL-6	NO
None	1.6 ± 0.09[d]	34.2 ± 3.4	4.6 ± 0.7	55.2 ± 3.1
L-NMMA	1.6 ± 0.08	<1.2*	15.3 ± 2.1**	1.5 ± 0.3*
D-NMMA	1.6 ± 0.12	35.8 ± 1.5	4.6 ± 0.5	45.8 ± 5.6

[a] Macrophage monolayers (1×10^6 cells/culture) were treated with 20 U/ml of IFNγ for 24 hours and then infected with *Legionella* for 30 minutes. After infection, macrophage monolayers were washed to remove nonphagocytized bacteria and incubated in the presence or absence of 2.5 mM *N*-monomethyl-L-arginine (L-NMMA) or *N*-monomethyl-D-arginine (D-NMMA) for 24 hours.

[b] Amount of IL-6 (ng/culture) in culture supernatants measured by ELISA.

[c] Amount of NO (μM/culture) in culture supernatants measured as nitrite using Griess reagent.

[d] Data represent the mean ± SD of triplicate cultures. Representative experiment from three different experiments.

*$p < 0.001$; **$p < 0.003$ compared with group receiving no treatment.

NO production in the *Legionella*-infected macrophages. However, anti-*Legionella* activity was not diminished in NO inhibitor-treated macrophages that produced little NO. That is, NO does not correlate with anti-*Legionella* activity in macrophage cultures.

It is widely recognized that macrophages are important cytokine-producing cells and such cytokines serve a pivotal role in immunity to infection. *Legionella* infection in macrophages induces cytokines such as interleukin-1 (IL-1) and tumor necrosis factor (TNF),[6,7] whereas IL-6 production is minimal. However, when *Legionella*-infected macrophages were treated with L-NMMA, IL-6 production in culture supernatants of the macrophages increased more than three times as compared with non-L-NMMA-treated macrophages infected with *Legionella*. Nitric oxide production in L-NMMA-treated macrophages was completely inhibited. By contrast, the chemical isomer of L-NMMA, *N*-monomethyl-D-arginine (D-NMMA), did not induce any change in IL-6 production and no inhibition of NO production (TABLE 1). Reconstitution of NO by the addition of nitroprusside, which generates NO in aerobic conditions, reduced IL-6 production to normal levels (data not shown). These results strongly indicate that NO may modulate the production of IL-6 induced by *Legionella* infection in macrophages primed with IFNγ. Thus, the study of *Legionella* growth in macrophages treated with No inhibitors and analysis of IL-6 production in *Legionella*-infected macrophages suggest that NO may have an immunoregulatory role in *Legionella*-infected macrophages rather than merely a direct antimicrobial effect.

REFERENCES

1. KLEIN, T. W., Y. YAMAMOTO, H. K. BROWN & H. FRIEDMAN. 1991. J. Leuk. Biol. **49:** 98–103.

2. YAMAMOTO, Y., T. W. KLEIN, C. NEWTON & H. FRIEDMAN. 1992. J. Immunol. **148:** 584–589.
3. MONCADA, S., R. M. J. PALMER & E. A. HIGGS. 1991. Pharmacol. Rev. **43:** 109–142.
4. YAMAMOTO, Y., T. W. KLEIN, C. A. NEWTON, R. WIDEN & H. FRIEDMAN. 1988. Infect. Immun. **56:** 370–375.
5. MIGLIORINI, P., G. CORRADIN & S. B. CORRADIN. 1991. J. Immunol. Methods **139:** 107–114.
6. WIDEN, R., T. W. KLEIN, C. A. NEWTON & H. FRIEDMAN. 1989. Proc. Soc. Exp. Biol. Med. **191:** 304–308.
7. ARATA, S., C. NEWTON, T. W. KLEIN, Y. YAMAMOTO & H. FRIEDMAN. 1993. Proc. Soc. Exp. Biol. Med. **203:** 26–29.

Identification and Sequencing of a Plasmid (pYV96)-Encoded Gene Product of *Yersinia enterocolitica* Recognized by Antibodies in Sera of Patients with Autoimmune Thyroid Disease[a]

N. S. BARTENEVA, A. G. EVSTAFIEVA,
V. N. GORELOV, AND B. E. WENZEL

Cell- and Immunobiological Laboratory
Department of Internal Medicine
Lübeck Medical University
Ratzeburger allee 160
23562 Lübeck, Germany

Certain bacterial infections may play a role in the pathogenesis of several autoimmune disorders including autoimmune thyroid disease (AITD). Patients with AITD more frequently show serum antibodies against *Yersinia enterocolitica* (YE) than do healthy controls.[1] Moreover, immunoglobulins of patients recovering from YE infections react with one of the principal thyroid autoantigens, the thyroid-stimulating hormone receptor (TSHR).[2] These and other findings support an association between AITD and enteropathogenic *Yersinia.* Target antigens for antibodies from AITD patients which react with *Yersinia* microbes may be *Yersinia* outer membrane proteins (Yops), which comprise important virulence factors encoded by the pYV plasmid of YE and are target antigens for antibodies in AITD.[3]

We demonstrated several prevailing bands of *Yersinia* preparations in the range of 36–37 and 47–49 kD which react with sera from AITD patients. To further study the potential relation between YE infection and AITD, we attempted to identify *Yersinia* antigens that would react with IgG and IgA antibodies from patients' sera. The *Clu*I gene library of pYV (0:9 serogroup, strain 96 of YE) was constructed using the pBluescript-SK⁺ vector and *Escherichia coli* XL-Blue as the host. Recombinant clones were screened by Western blotting with anti-Yops sera and human sera from AITD patients. The expressed protein from clone 75 had similar differential mobility on SDS-PAGE analysis as YOP 37 of YE (FIG. 1). Furthermore, using Southern blotting and deletion mutagenesis, we identified a gene which encoded this protein, as part of car-operone of YE.[4] This operon contains a set of genes that encode proteins

[a]These studies were supported by Deutsche Forschunggemeinschaft/SFB 367/B6. A.E. and V.G. are the recipients of a grant from the Medical University of Lübeck, Lübeck, Germany.

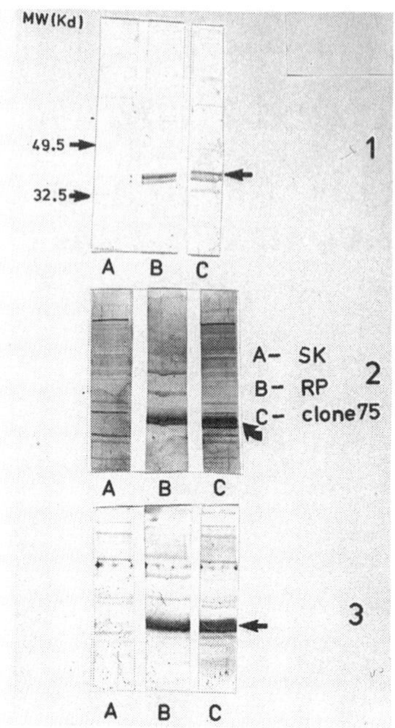

FIGURE 1. Western blotting analysis of clone 75 (*lane* C) in comparison with Yops from YE of serogroup 9 (*lane* B) and the *E. coli* strain XL1-Blue, containing pBluescript-SK⁺ (*lane* A). Sera from AITD patients (1–3) were used in a 1 : 100 dilution. *Arrows* point to the Yop37 band.

```
pYVe96    MTINIKTDSPIITTGSQIDAITTETVGQSGEVKKTEDTRHEAQAIKSSEASLSRSQVPEL   60
pYVe227   ----------------L------------------------------------------
pIB1      ----------------L--------K----I-----------------------------

pYVe96    IKPSQGINVALLSKSQGDLNGTLSILLLLLELARKAREMGLQQRDIENKAAITAQKEQVA  120
pYVe227   --------------------------------------------------T-S-------
pIB1      --------------------------------------------------T-T-------

pYVe96    EMVSGAKLMIAMAVVSGIMAATSTVASAFSIAKEVKIVKQEQILNSNIAGRDQLIDTKLQ  180
pYVe227   ---------------------------------------------------------M-
pIB1      ----------------------------------------------------E------M-

pYVe96    QMSNTSDKAVSREDIGRIWKPEQVADQNKLALLDKEFRMTDSKANAFNAATQPLGQMANS  240
pYVe227   ----AG-----------------------------------------------------
pIB1      --G-IG-----------------------------------------------------

pYVe96    AIQVHQGYSQAEVKEKEVNASIAANEKQKAEEAMNYNDNFMKDVLRLIEQYVSSHTHAMK  300
pYVe227   -----------------------------------------------------------
pIB1      -----------------------------------------------------------

pYVe96    AAFGVV      306
pYVe227   ------
pIB1      ------
```

FIGURE 2. Deduced amino acid sequences of the Yop37 protein from plasmid of YE strain 96 (serogroup 0:9) in comparison with Yop37 proteins from YE strain W227 (0:9) and YP strain IB1. *Dashes* denote sequence identity. Amino acids from pYVe227 and pIB1 are indicated where the sequences differ. Sequence was set up according to the dideoxy-chain termination method of Sanger *et al.* using direct blotting electrophoresis DNA sequencer (''GATC GmbH'', Germany), and it also was repeated by the usual radioactive method with ³⁵S-dATP.

of similar molecular weight (range 37-44 kD). We sequenced the cloned gene to eliminate the possibility that the recombinant product of clone 37 is a truncated form of Yop44 or Yop41. The deduced sequences of the Yop37 proteins were obtained from the cloned gene of YE strain 96 (sequenced by us) and were compared with pYV227 of YE and pIB1 of *Y. pseudotuberculosis* (YP) (both sequenced by Häkansson *et al.*[5]) (FIG. 2). Our results indicate that quantitatively there is a similar degree of difference in the amino acid sequence between different species (YP and YE; 97.4% identity) and between different strains of the same serogroup (0:9; W22709 strain and 96 strain; 97.7% identity). Yop37 proteins from YE and YP, however, show a molecular weight difference in SDS-PAGE (37 and 34 kD), which suggests a different three-dimensional configuration as a result of just a few amino acid alterations. A computer search of homologies between amino acid sequences of Yop37 and an important thyroid autoantigen, TSHR, did not reveal any significant level of homology when compared to randomly scrambled sequences. However, we cannot rule out cross-reactivity between secondary or tertiary structures of Yop37 and the TSHR or other thyroid autoantigens.

In conclusion, we identified and sequenced one *Yersinia* antigen, which is frequently recognized by antibody in sera from patients with AITD. We are currently investigating the role that Yop37 may play in AITD.

REFERENCES

1. WENZEL, B. E., T. F. FRANKE, A. E. HEUFELDER & J. HEESEMANN. 1990. Autoimmune thyroid diseases and enteropathogenic *Yersinia enterocolitica*. Autoimmunity **7:** 295-303.
2. WOLF, M. W., T. MISAKI, K. BECH, M. TVEDE, J. E. SILVA & S. H. INGBAR. 1991. Immunoglobulins of patients recovering from *Yersinia enterocolitica* infections exhibit Graves' disease-like activity in human thyroid membranes. Thyroid **1:** 315-320.
3. WENZEL, B. E., J. HEESEMANN, K. W. WENZEL & P. C. SCRIBA. 1988. Antibodies to plasmid-encoded proteins of enteropathogenic *Yersinia* in patients with autoimmune thyroid disease. Lancet **1:** 56.
4. BARTENEVA, N. S., V. GORELOV, A. EVSTAFIEVA, I. ZUBASHEV, O. NOVIKOVA & B. E. WENZEL. 1993. Molecular characterization of bacterial antigens from entheropathogenic *Y. enterocolitica* 0:9 recognized by specific antibodies in sera from patients with autoimmune thyroid disease. In preparation.
5. HÄKANSSON, S., T. BERGMAN, J.-C. VANOOTEGHEM, G. CORNELIS & H. WOLF-WATZ. 1993. YopB and YopD constitute a novel class of Yersinia Yop proteins. Inf. Immunity **61:** 71-80.

Active Immunization against *Salmonella typhi* by Oral Administration of Fast Neutron Irradiated Cells

F. V. DIMA, D. IVANOV, AND S. V. DIMA

Department of Experimental Pathology and Microbiology
Cantacuzino Institute and Institute of Atomic Physics
Splaiul Independentei 103
Bucharest 70.100, Romania

Typhoid fever continues to be a major health problem in developing countries where high morbidity and mortality values have been reported. The worldwide index for typhoid fever is estimated to exceed 30 million cases per year with 500,000 deaths annually.[1] In the last two decades several attenuated *Salmonella typhi* strains have been suggested.[2-4]

In this study we investigated the protective capacity of the new typhoid vaccine inactivated with fast neutron radiation (FNIV) compared with acetone-killed and dried vaccine (AKD). The protective capacity was estimated by the following parameters: (1) survival rate; (2) shedding the challenge strain; (3) antibodies to *S. typhi* antigens measured in serum and jejunal fluids by the ELISA method; (4) mitogenic response in spleen cells from rats immunized with FNIV or AKD vaccines; and (5) SEM observations.

Experimental results indicated that the protective capacity of FNIV against infection with *S. typhi* Ty2-6A strain is characterized by: (1) survival rate of 78.4% in rats immunized with FNIV, 54.8% in rats given AKD vaccine, and 23.2% in control animals; (2) shedding of the virulent strain for 3-5 days in 11.5% of rats immunized with five FNIV doses, 5- 9 days in animals given AKD vaccine, and 15-22 days in control rats; (3) development of antibodies in serum and jejunal fluids in rats after feedings with FNIV, with lower antibody levels in animals that received AKD vaccine (TABLE 1); and (4) splenic lymphocytes from rats given FNIV responded to higher uptake of (^{3}H)TdR when stimulated with *S. typhi* extract or phytohemagglutinin in contrast to lower values in rats given AKD vaccine and control animals (TABLE 2). Examination with the scanning electron microscope confirmed the results obtained by other methods. The better protective capacity of the FNIV compared with acetone-killed *S. typhi* vaccine is possibly due to the harmless action of the inactivation method. In connection with this, we suggest two mechanisms of action: (1) irradiation with fast neutrons destroys both plasmid and chromosomal DNA without altering the integrity of bacterial cells, and (2) ionizing radiation produces the selective removal of the toxic properties of endotoxin while retaining the immunologic character.[5,6]

In summary, fast neutron irradiated typhoidic vaccine demonstrated marked protective capacity against infection with the *S. typhi* Ty2-6A virulent strain.

TABLE 1. Evaluation of Immune Response

	Antibodies to *S. typhi* Antigens								
	Serum						Jejunal Fluids (sIgA)		
	LPS		H		Vi				
Vaccine	IgG	IgA	IgG	IgA	IgG	IgA	LPS	H	Vi
AKD	3/12	2/12[a]	3/12	1/12	0/12	0/12	2/12	0/12	0/12
FNIV	6/14	8/14	5/14	2/14	4/14	2/14	9/14	3/14	1/14

ABBREVIATIONS: AKD = acetone-killed vaccine; FNIV = fast neutron irradiated vaccine; sIgA = secretory IgA.

[a] No. positive/no. tested. Fourfold rise in titer from prechallenge to postchallenge was considered significant.

TABLE 2. (^{3}H)Thymidine Incorporation by Splenic Lymphocytes from Rats Immunized with *S. typhi* Vaccines

| | | (^{3}H)TdR Uptake (cpm × 10^{-3}) by Cultured Cells | | |
Vaccine	Experiment	No Mitogen	PHA (10 μg/ml)	Ty2 (25 μl/ml)
AKD	1	3.65 ± 0.05[a]	28.57 ± 1.03	15.29 ± 0.92
	2	2.93 ± 0.17	25.88 ± 0.71	18.62 ± 0.83
FNIV	1	1.86 ± 0.09	37.55 ± 1.65	21.38 ± 1.47
	2	3.22 ± 0.55	33.14 ± 1.06	25.74 ± 2.19

ABBREVIATIONS: AKD = acetone-killed vaccine; FNIV = fast neutron-irradiated vaccine.
[a] Mean ± SE of triplicate.

REFERENCES

1. CRYZ, J. S., E. FURER, L. S. BARON, K. F. NOON, F. A. RUBIN & D. J. KOPECKO. 1989. Infect. Immun. **57:** 3863–3868.
2. GERMANIER, R. & E. FURER. 1975. J. Infect. Dis. **118:** 293–306.
3. DIMA, F. V. 1983. Arch. Roum. Path. Exp. Microbiol. **42:** 191–198.
4. TACKET, O. C., D. H. HONE, H. CURTIS III, S. M. KELLY, O. LOSONKY, L. GUERS, A. M. HARRIS, R. EDELMAN & M. M. LEVINE. 1992. Infect. Immun. **60:** 536–541.
5. EVANS, G. D., D. J. EVANS, JR., A. R. OPEKUN & D. Y. GRAHAM. 1986. Ann. Sclavo No. 1–2: 155–156. Proc. Sclavo Int. Conf. Siena, Italy.
6. CSAKO, G., E. A. SUBA, A. AHLGREN, C. M. TSAI & R. J. ELIN. 1986. J. Infect. Dis. **153:** 98–108.

Role of Porins from *Salmonella typhi* in the Induction of Protective Immunity

A. ISIBASI,[a,b] J. PANIAGUA,[a] M. P. ROJO,[a]
N. MARTÍN,[a] G. RAMÍREZ,[a] C. R. GONZÁLEZ,
C. LÓPEZ-MACÍAS,[a] J. SÁNCHEZ,[c] J. KUMATE,[a] AND
V. ORTIZ-NAVARRETE [a]

[a]*Unidad de Investigación Médica en Inmunoquímica*
CMN Siglo XXI
IMSS. Mexico City, Mexico

[c]*Patología Experimental*
CISEI
INSP
Cuernavaca, Mor. Mexico

We previously demonstrated the ability of outer membrane proteins (OMPs) to induce protection against challenge with *Salmonella typhi* in mice; it was also possible to transfer this protective effect with immune sera against OMPs.[1] The antigens responsible for this protective status are two different porins.[2] Both cellular and humoral mechanisms of immunity might be involved in the protection achieved. The presence of cellular immunity is evidenced by the ability of these proteins to activate T lymphocytes from mice immunized with OMPs or with porins isolated from *S. typhi*.[3] A similar lymphocytic proliferative response is also observed in individuals vaccinated against typhoid fever or in patients in the convalescent phase of typhoid fever.[4] Nevertheless, the specific role that each porin plays in protection is unknown. Recently, the gene encoding Omp C was cloned[5]; therefore, we decided to assess its capacity to induce active protection against *S. typhi* in mice. We also identified hypothetical B-cell epitopes in this protein and demonstrated immunoreactivity for two of those proposed sequences.

MATERIALS AND METHODS

Isolation of Omp C Recombinant Porin. Omp C recombinant porin (rOmp C) was isolated, according to a method described previously,[2] from *Escherichia coli* UH302 transformed with the plasmid pST13.[5]

Evaluation of Active Protection. For active protection assays, groups of 10 BALB/ c mice, each weighing 18-20 g, were twice immunized intraperitoneally with a 2-

[b] Address for correspondence: P. O. Box 73-032, México, D.F., C.P. 03020, México.

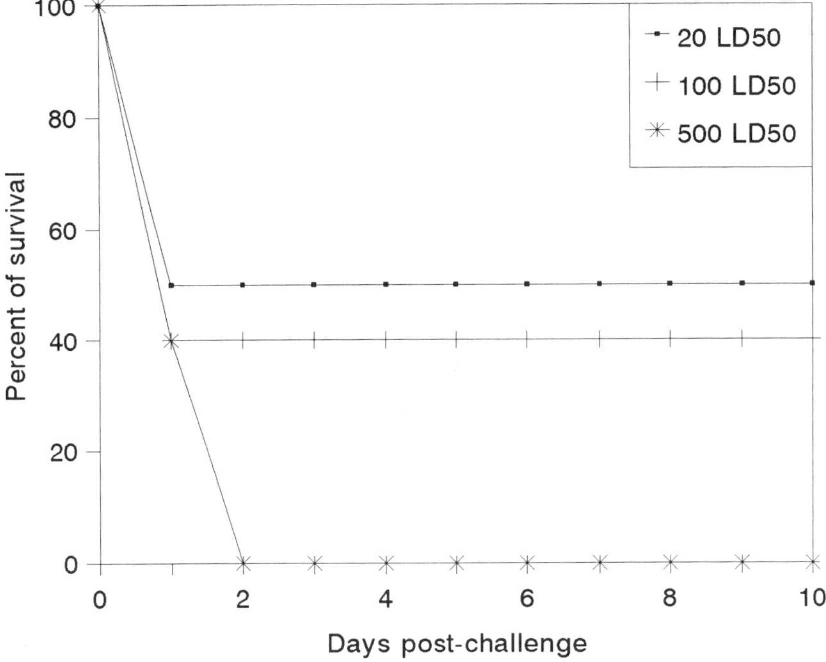

FIGURE 1. Protection induced by *S. typhi* Omp C porin.

week interval between immunizations with 10 μg of rOmp C. Ten days after the last injection, mice were challenged intraperitoneally with 20, 100, and 500 50% lethal doses (LD_{50}) of *S. typhi* strain suspended in 5% mucin. Protection was evaluated as the percentage of survival during the 10 days following the challenge.

B-Cell Epitopes of Omp C Porin. Potential antigenic residues of the native protein were identified by the prediction algorithms of Karplus and McCammon[6] (from PCGENE® software).

RESULTS AND DISCUSSION

Protection Induced by Salmonella typhi *Omp C Porin.* The *S. typhi* Omp C porin was expressed in the porin-deficient *E. coli* UH302 strain. The recombinant porin was isolated from the outer membrane of *E. coli* and purified by gel filtration chromatography. The rOmp C eluted in the same chromatography fraction as did the native Omp C,[2] which shows that the rOmp C is assembled as a trimmer. A partially protective effect was observed with the immunization of rOmp C; 50% of the mice survived against a challenge of 20 LD_{50} and 40% of survival was obtained with a challenge of 100 LD_{50} (FIG. 1). These results suggest that Omp C indeed plays a role in the induction of protection against *S. typhi* in the experimental model used; however, to get the protective status, a second porin is required.[2]

TABLE 1. Predicted B-Lymphocyte Epitopes from *S. typhi* Omp C

Region	Sequence	B Value
5–11	NKDGNKL	1.084
26–32	DKGSDGD	1.109
64–70	QETGSND	1.121
122–128	QQRGNGY	1.088
150–156	QGKNGSV	1.098
157–163	SGEQTQG	1.105
167–173	LNQNGDG	1.092
198–234	TADQNNT	1.106
247–254	TSNGSNPS	1.333
286–292	QSKGKDI	1.105

B-Cell Epitopes of Omp C Porin. Ten potential antigenic regions were identified in the protein sequence (TABLE 1). One of these epitopes is not shared with *E. coli* Omp C, so it could be involved in the specific immune response against *S. typhi.* Two of the 10 predicted epitopes, the epitope formed by amino acid 246-255 as a fusion protein and the epitope comprising residues 285-303 as a synthetic peptide, were synthesized. Antibodies against these two sequences recognized the trimmer of native porin as well as rOmp C. These results suggest that the two selected epitopes are exposed segments on the surface of the porin; therefore, they could be the major antigenic determinants involved in the production of antibodies against *S. typhi.*

REFERENCES

1. ISIBASI, A., V. ORTIZ, M. VARGAS, J. PANIAGUA, C. GONZÁLEZ, J. MORENO & J. KUMATE. 1988. Infect Immun. **56:** 2953-2959.
2. ISIBASI, A., V. ORTIZ-NAVARRETE, J. PANIAGUA, R. PELAYO, C. GONZÁLEZ, J. A. GARCÍA & J. KUMATE. 1992. Vaccine **10:** 811-813.
3. GONZÁLEZ, C. R., A. ISIBASI, V. ORTIZ-NAVARRETE, J. PANIAGUA, J. A. GARCÍA, F. BLANCO & J. KUMATE. 1993. Microbiol. Immunol. **37:** 793-799.
4. BLANCO, F., A. ISIBASI, C. R. GONZÁLEZ, V. ORTIZ, J. PANIAGUA, C. ARREGUÍN & J. KUMATE. 1993. Scand. J. Infect. Dis. **25:** 73-80.
5. AGUERO, J., G. MORA, M. J. MROCZENSKI-WILDEY, M. E. FERNÁNDEZ-BEROS, L. ARON & F. C. CABELLO. 1987. Microb. Pathog. **3:** 399-407.
6. KARPLUS, M. & A. MCCAMMON. 1983. Ann. Rev. Biochem. **53:** 263-300.

Effective Stimulation of the Mucosal Immune Response by Parenteral Vaccination with Weak Antigen Associated with a Nucleoprotein Vehicle

V. J. LEVENSON AND T. P. EGOROVA

Walter Reed Army Institute of Research
Washington, DC 20307-5100

Gabrichevsky Institute of Microbiology
Moscow, Russia

Efficiency of vaccines depends on the proper choice of an epitope-bearing component and on the use of an appropriate vector or delivery system. With a powerful delivery system, even very weak antigens (devoid of a built-in amplifier component) could be used in a vaccine design. In this study, the nucleoprotein particles (NP) were found to be an efficient delivery system for the weakly immunogenic O-polysaccharide (OP). This natural complex seems to be a promising candidate vaccine against *Shigella* infection.

Avirulent, form I *Shigella sonnei* strain 9090 cells were disrupted by sonication and fractionated by ultracentrifugation or by polyethylene glycol precipitation. The OP-NP preparation has a UV-absorption maximum at 260 nm. As shown by chemical analyses, it is composed mainly of RNA and proteins. Sedimentation profile and ultrastructural patterns are typical for ribosomes and their subunits.[1]

The O-specific component was detected in trace amounts by serologic tests and isolated by affinity chromatography.[2] This component is a lipid-free polysaccharide similar to "native hapten."[3] It has extremely low immunogenic activity when injected alone into animals.[4] The complex of O-polysaccharide and NP could be dissociated by EDTA treatment which is indicative of noncovalent bonds between the two components. OP-NP complexes were nontoxic in mice, rats, rabbits, guinea pigs, and monkeys. For example, doses up to 5,000 μg caused no deaths in mice.

Subcutaneous immunization with OP-NP complexes without any adjuvant elicited highly significant ($p < 0.001$) local protection of guinea pigs against *S. sonnei* (FIG. 1). No protection against *S. sonnei* was seen with OP-NP complexes from *Escherichia coli*, *S. minnesota*, and *S. flexneri*.[1]

Rhesus monkeys were protected from dysentery caused by oral challenge with virulent *Shigella* in five experiments (74 monkeys total). The overall efficiency of vaccination ($EV = [1\text{-}V/C] \times 100$, where V and C are the disease frequency in control and vaccinated monkeys) was 89%. Vaccine did not prevent pathogen excretion after challenge, but it reduced the length of excretion.

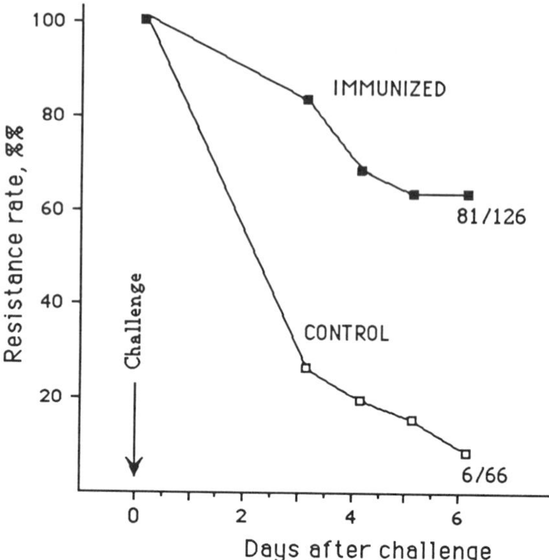

FIGURE 1. Mucosal protection in guinea pigs after parenteral vaccination with OP-NP complexes. Summarized data of six independent experiments. Animals were challenged with virulent *S. sonnei* strain 1041 2 weeks after subcutaneous injection of 200 μg OP-NP. The ratio of resistant eyes to total challenged eyes is shown for vaccinated and control (nonimmunized) group. The difference between two groups is highly statistically significant ($p < 0.001$).

Parenteral immunization with OP-NP complexes induced not only systemic responses but also secretory IgA O-antibody response in saliva of monkeys (TABLE 1), in tears of guinea pigs, in bile (rats and monkeys), and in intestinal secretions (mice and monkeys). Injection of OP-NP to pregnant guinea pigs led to the appearance of IgA antibody in milk.[5] This could be used in the context of lactogenic immunity to shigellosis.

CONCLUSIONS

1. The nucleoprotein particles (ribosomes) can serve as an extremely potent delivery system, providing amplification of immunogenicity by several orders of magnitude.

2. Nucleoprotein particle-amplified antigen is capable of inducing mucosal immunity and protection when given parenterally.

3. The natural complex of nucleoprotein particles with haptenic O-polysaccharide from *S. sonnei* is a promising candidate vaccine against shigellosis.

4. A similar approach can be fruitful in developing other vaccines of medical or veterinary importance.

TABLE 1. Secretory IgA Response to OP-NP Vaccine in Monkeys

Group of Monkeys[a]	Animals (n)	Salivary IgA O-Antibody Level[b]	
		Titer^{-1}	Log$_2$ (mean ± SE)
Immunized once	12	23	4.5 ± 0.6
Immunized twice	8	69	6.1 ± 0.9
Infected	4	104	6.7 ± 0.5
Normal	4	2	1.0 ± 0.7

[a] Monkeys were injected subcutaneously with one or two 600-μg doses of OP-NP vaccine. The interval between injections in case of twofold immunization was 2 weeks. The nonimmunized animals were studied before challenge (normal monkeys) or after oral challenge with 10^{10} cells of virulent *S. sonnei* strain (infected monkeys).

[b] IgA O-antibody titers were determined on the 14th day after vaccination or challenge in ELISA. The difference between the control group and the vaccinated or challenged monkeys is statistically significant ($p < 0.01$). The difference in the antibody level induced by infection and twofold immunization is not statistically significant.

REFERENCES

1. LEVENSON, V. J., T. P. EGOROVA, Z. P. BELKIN, V. G. FEDOSOVA, Ju. L. SUBBOTINA, E. Z. RUKHADZE, E. K. DZHIKIDZE & Z. K. STASSILEVICH, 1991. Infect. Immun. **59:** 3610–3618.
2. LEVENSON, V. J. & T. P. EGOROVA. 1990. Res. Microbiol. **141:** 707–720.
3. ANACKER, R., R. FINKELSTEIN, W. HASKINS, M. LANDY, K. MILNER, E. RIBI & P. STASHAK. 1964. J. Bacteriol. **88:** 1705–1720.
4. LEVENSON, V. J., Z. P. BELKIN, T. P. EGOROVA, M. M. LYUBINSKAYA & S. Yu. SASYKINA. 1991. Zh. Microbiol. (Moscow) **7:** 25–29.
5. CHERNOKHVOSTOVA, E. V., M. M. LYUBINSKAYA, Z. P. BELKIN & V. J. LEVENSON. 1990. Int. Arch. Allergy Appl. Immunol. **92:** 265–267.

Protection against Invasion of the Mouse Pulmonary Epithelium by a Monoclonal IgA Directed against *Shigella flexneri* Lipopolysaccharide

A. PHALIPON,[a] P. MICHETTI,[b] M. KAUFMANN,[b]
J. M. CAVAILLON,[c] M. HUERRE,[d]
J. P. KRAEHENBUHL,[b] AND P. J. SANSONETTI [a]

*Unité de [a]Pathogénie Microbienne Moléculaire, [c]d'Immuno-
allergie, et [d]d'Histopathologie
Institut Pasteur
28 rue du Dr Roux
75015 Paris, France*

*[b]Institut de Biochimie
ISREC
1066 Epalinges, Switzerland*

Bacteria belonging to the genus *Shigella* cause a dysenteric syndrome in humans by invading the colonic mucosa.[1] Systemic as well as mucosal immune responses elicited in infected hosts after natural or experimental infections are directed mainly against the lipopolysaccharide and against a set of proteins associated with invasion and encoded by a 220-kb virulence plasmid.[2] Despite many studies, the respective role of systemic and mucosal responses in the protection against shigellosis remains to be determined.

To study the role of the mucosal immune response directed against the lipopolysaccharide, we generated a hybridoma producing a monoclonal immunoglobulin A (mIgA) antibody directed against a specific determinant of the *S. flexneri* serotype 5 lipopolysaccharide. This hybridoma was obtained by oral immunization of BALB/ c mice with virulent live bacteria and subsequently fusing Peyer's patch lymphoblasts with mouse myeloma cells. The correlation between the presence of mIgAC5 and protection was studied by using the "backpack" model.[3] Subcutaneous hybridoma tumors were obtained by injecting mIgAC5 hybridoma cells in the upper back of mice. These tumor-bearing mice were secreting mIgAC5 at the mucosal level. In the absence of a mouse model of intestinal infection by *S. flexneri,* a model of invasion of the pulmonary epithelium was used.[4] Tumor-bearing mice secreting mIgAC5 into their respiratory tract were challenged intranasally with *S. flexneri* strains. The level of secretion of interleukin-6 (IL-6), a key member of the cytokine network involved in the host defense against infection, and the intensity of histopathologic damage of lung tissues were measured to evaluate the severity of the infection process in the presence and the absence of mIgAC5. After *S. flexneri* 5-intranasal challenge, but not *S. flexneri* 2-challenge, levels of IL-6 were significantly lower in mice secreting

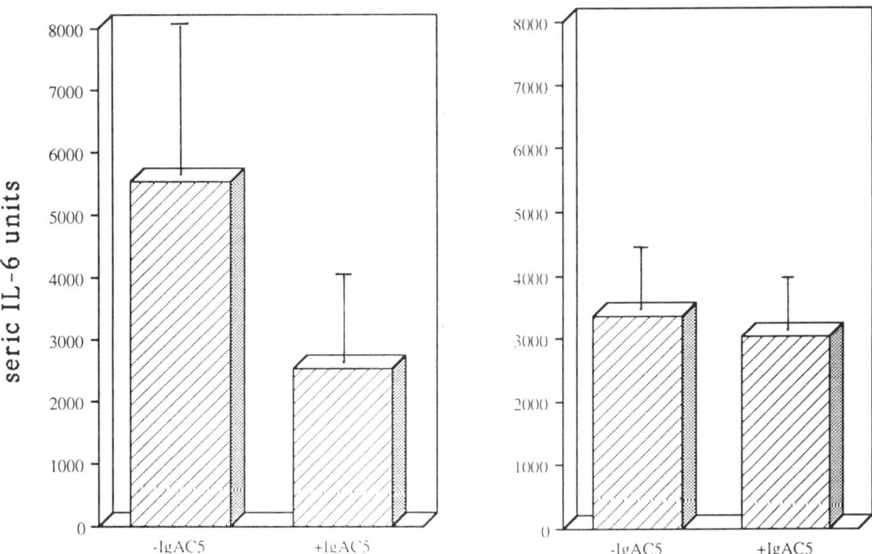

FIGURE 1. IL-6 response in mice after intranasal challenge with *S. flexneri* strains. Naive (−mIgAC5) or mIgAC5-secreting mice (+mIgAC5) were challenged with *S. flexneri* 5a (**A**) or *S. flexneri* 2a (**B**). Each seric IL-6 value corresponds to the mean of seric IL-6 values of 10 mice. Standard deviations are indicated.

mIgAC5 than in the control group (FIG. 1). In addition, mice secreting an irrelevant mIgA had an IL-6 response similar to that of naive mice after being challenged with *S. flexneri* 5 strain (data not shown). In mice secreting mIgAC5, no destruction of the pulmonary epithelium was observed by lung histopathologic studies after *S. flexneri* 5-challenge. By contrast, substantial destruction of the epithelium was observed in the presence of mIgAC5 after *S. flexneri* 2-challenge which was similar to that observed in infected naive mice. mIgAC5 specifically prevents the polymorphonuclear cell infiltrate observed in naive mice after intranasal challenge.

Together these results demonstrate that mIgAC5 protects mice from invasion of the pulmonary epithelium by bacteria. Moreover, this protection correlates with the amount of locally secreted mIgAC5. This study represents the first direct demonstration that the mucosal immune response constituted by secretory IgAs directed against lipopolysaccharide is the major component of the protection against *Shigella* infection.

REFERENCES

1. SANSONETTI, P. J. 1991. Genetic and molecular basis of epithelial cell invasion by *Shigella* species. Rev. Infect. Dis. **13:** S285-292.
2. OBERHELMANN, R. A., D. J. KOPECKO, E. SALAZAR-LINDO, E. GOTUZZO, J. M. BUYSSE, M. M. VENKATESAN, A. YI, C. FERNANDEZ-PRADA, M. GUZMAN, R. LEON-BARUA & R. B.

SACK. 1991. Prospective study of systemic and mucosal immune responses in dysenteric patients to specific *Shigella* invasion plasmid antigens and lipopolysaccharides. Infect. Immun. **59:** 2341–2350.

3. WINNER, L. S., III, R. A. WELZTIN, J. J. MEKALANOS, J. P. KRAHENBUHL & M. R. NEUTRA. 1991. New model for analysis of mucosal immunity: Intestinal secretion of specific monoclonal immunoglobulin A from hybridoma tumors protects against *Vibrio cholerae* infection. Infect. Immun. **59:** 977–982.

4. MALLETT, C. P., L. VAN DE VERG, H. H. COLLINS & T. L. HALE. 1993. Evaluation of *Shigella* vaccine safety and efficacy in an intranasally challenged mouse model. Vaccine **11:** 190–196.

Immunogenicity of Two Types of *Shigella flexneri* 2a O-Specific Polysaccharide-Tetanus Toxoid Conjugates

VSEVOLOD Y. POLOTSKY, RACHEL SCHNEERSON,
DOLORES BRYLA, AND JOHN B. ROBBINS

National Institute of Child Health and Human Development
National Institutes of Health
Bethesda, Maryland 20892

A fully expressed lipopolysaccharide (LPS) is essential for the virulence of *Shigella* and is capable of inducing protective immunity proposed to be conferred by serum IgG.[1,2] Two known methods of LPS detoxification are: (1) 1% acetic acid hydrolysis which cleaves 2-keto-3-deoxy-D-manno-octonate (KDO)-α-D-Glc*p*NAc-(1->3) bonds and yields O-specific polysaccharide attached to the residual "core" oligosaccharide (O-SP); and (2) hydrolysis with hydrazine which hydrolyzes ester bonds on lipid A and releases partially deacylated LPS (DeALPS).[3]

The unsatisfactory immunogenicity of the O-specific polysaccharide led to the development of conjugate vaccines for shigellosis. Conjugates composed of *S. dysenteriae* type 1 O-SP bound to the tetanus toxoid (TT) and *S. flexneri* 2a O-SP or *S. sonnei* O-SP bound to the recombinant exoprotein A of *P. aeruginosa* were synthesized.[4] Here we compare biochemical properties and immunogenicity of *S. flexneri* 2a LPS detoxified by acid or base hydrolysis and bound to TT.

The LPS of *S. flexneri* type 2a was treated with acetic acid (O-SP) or hydrazine (DeALPS). O-SP was eluted from a Sepharose CL-6B column as one peak with molecular weight of ~17,000 Da. DeALPS was more heterogeneous and formed two peaks with molecular weights of ~10,000 Da and ~30,000 Da. The LPS, O-SP, and DeALPS of *S. flexneri* 2a yielded an identity reaction with *S. flexneri* 2a hyperimmune serum by double immunodiffusion. SDS-PAGE detected 120 ng of LPS. By this assay, LPS in O-SP and DeALPS was reduced > 620-fold and ~40-fold respectively. *Limulus* amebocyte lysate assay (LAL) could detect 0.125 ng/mL of LPS. By this assay, a 5-10 × 10^3-fold reduction of LPS activity in the O-SP and 2-4 × 10^3-fold reduction in the DeALPS were detected.

The O-SP and DeALPS were conjugated to TT. O-SP-TT and DeALPS-TT eluted in the void volume of a CL-6B Sepharose column, whereas O-SP, DeALPS, and TT were retarded by this column. TT and LPS antisera formed a line of identity with both conjugates by double immunodiffusion. The saccharide/protein (weight/weight) ratios in the conjugates were 1 : 4.5 and 1 : 2, respectively.

The immunogenicity of these conjugates was evaluated in 4-week-old outbred mice injected subcutaneously, with 2.5 μg of O-SP or DeALPS alone or as a conjugate, three times 2 weeks apart and bled 2 weeks after the first injection and 1 week after the second and third injections. LPS antibodies were not detected after any injection of 2.5 μg of O-SP alone. DeALPS elicited low levels of IgM antibodies after the third injection. Two of three O-SP-TT conjugates induced significant rises of IgM antibodies after three injections: 3.1 (0.5–22) (25th–75th centiles in parentheses) ELISA units *vs* <1 after one injection, $p < 0.05$. All O-SP-TT conjugates enhanced IgG antibody production after the third injection: 2.7 (0.3–71.8), 1.5 (0.3–8.0), and 12.9 (3.5–40.3) units *vs* <0.2 after one injection, $p < 0.001$. DeALPS-TT conjugates did not induce IgM antibodies after three injections but did elicit IgG after two injections. DeALPS-TT$_1$ raised IgG antibodies after three injections and DeALPS-TT$_2$ did not. Three injections of O-SP-TT conjugates elicited higher levels of both IgM and IgG antibodies than those of DeALPS-TT (3.73 *vs* 0.4, $p < 0.001$).

The different immunogenicity of the two conjugates may be related to the higher protein/saccharide ratios of the O-SP-TT conjugates than those of the DeALPS-TT. Seemingly, this higher protein/saccharide ratio of the O-SP-TT conjugates was more critical for immunogenicity of *S. flexneri* type 2a conjugates than the higher molecular weight of the DeALPS.

REFERENCES

1. COHEN, D., M. S. GREEN, C. BLOCK, R. SLEPON & I. OFEK. 1991. J. Clin. Microbiol. **29:** 386–389.
2. ROBBINS, J. B., C. CHU & R. SCHNEERSON. 1992. Clin. Infect. Dis. **15:** 346–361.
3. GUPTA, R. K., S. C. SZU, R. A. FINKELSTAIN & J. B. ROBBINS. 1992. Infect. Immun. **60:** 3201–3208.
4. TAYLOR, D. N., A. C. TROFA, J. SADOFF, C. CHU, D. BRYLA, J, SHILOACH, D. COHEN, S. ASHKENAZI, Y. LERMAN, W. EGAN, R. SCHNEERSON & J. B. ROBBINS. 1993. Infect. Immun. **61:** 3678–3687.

Cross-Reactive Protection Eliciting Epitopes of Pneumococcal Surface Protein A

BETH A. RALPH, DAVID E. BRILES, AND
LARRY S. McDANIEL

The University of Alabama at Birmingham
Birmingham, Alabama 35294

In the developing world, respiratory infections with *Streptococcus pneumoniae* are one of the major causes of death among children less than 5 years of age.[1,2] The pneumococcal polysaccharide capsule is an important virulence determinant that is also able to elicit protective, type-specific antibodies.[3,4] Unfortunately, children generally do not make protective responses to the isolated capsular polysaccharides comprising the present pneumococcal vaccine.[5-8] Efforts are underway worldwide to prepare multivalent polysaccharide-protein conjugate vaccines that could be used to elicit protective responses in children. Although the chemical conjugate vaccines being developed will probably be efficacious in young children, the technical sophistication and costs associated with their production will likely prevent their widespread use in developing countries. Thus, candidate pneumococcal proteins are being examined in the hope that they will be able to form the basis of a less expensive and more widely available pneumococcal vaccine.

One such protein is pneumococcal surface protein A (PspA). PspA is a serologically variable molecule present on all pneumococci.[9] It is required for full virulence of the pneumococcus and can elicit antibody protection against pneumococcal challenge.[10-13] PspA consists of four distinct domains: a coiled-coil α-helical region, a proline-rich domain, a stretch of 10 highly conserved 20 amino acid repeats, and a hydrophobic region at the COOH-terminus. It is linked to the cell surface at its COOH-terminal end via the ten 20 amino acid repeats, with the NH_2-terminal half of the molecule extending beyond the cell wall. The repeat region is slightly hydrophobic in nature. This hydrophobicity suggests that this region may have interactions with the cell membrane. The proline-rich domain may act to strengthen PspA's attachment to the cell wall.[12,14]

In previous studies, epitopes on PspA reactive with monoclonal antibodies were mapped using truncated fragments of PspA with intact native NH_2-termini or intact native COOH-termini. The protective epitopes were mapped to either the NH_2-terminal 115 amino acids or to amino acids 192 to 260 of PspA. It was found that the monoclonal antibodies (mAbs) that recognized epitopes within the 192-260 amino acid region were more cross-reactive than were those that recognized the NH_2-terminal 115 amino acids. Five of the nine mAbs used in the study were shown to be protective against otherwise fatal pneumococcal infection in mice. Of the five protective mAbs, four of them mapped to the 192-260 amino acid region.[15] A PspA fragment extending from amino acid 192 to amino acid 588 (the COOH-terminus) has been made. Immunization of mice with this fragment of PspA is able to elicit protection against fatal pneumococcal infection. These data indicate that the region of PspA from amino acids 192-260 contains protection-eliciting epitopes and may have potential for use in a pneumococcal protein vaccine.

REFERENCES

1. SPIKA, J. S., M. H. MUNSHI, B. WOJTYANIAK, D. A. SACK, A. HOSSAIN, M. RAHMAN & S. K. SAHA. 1989. Acute lower respiratory infections: A major cause of death in children in Bangladesh. Ann. Trop. Pediatr. **9:** 33.

2. GREENWOOD, B. M., A. M. GREENWOOD, A. K. BRADLEY, S. TULLOCH, R. HAYES & F. S. J. OLDFIELD. 1987. Deaths in infancy and early childhood in a well vaccinated, rural, West African population. Ann. Trop. Pediatr. **7:** 91.

3. AUSTRIAN, R. 1979. Pneumococcal vaccine: Development and prospects. Am. J. Med. **67:** 547.

4. MACLEOD, C. M., R. G. HODGES, M. HEIDELBERGER & W. G. BERNHARD. 1945. Prevention of pneumococcal pneumonia byu immunization with specific capsular polysaccharides. J. Exp. Med. **82:** 445.

5. KLEIN, J. O., D. W. TEELE, J. L. SLOYER, JR., J. H. PLOUSSARD, V. HOWIE, P. H. MAKELA & P. KARMA. 1982. Use of pneumococcal vaccine for prevention of recurrent episodes of otitis media. *In* Bacterial Vaccine. Sadoffs, Eds.: 305-310. Thieme-Stratton Inc. New York.

6. GRAY, B. M., H. C. DILLION & D. E. BRILES. 1983. Epidemiological studies of *Streptococcus pneumoniae* in infants: Development of antibody to phosphocholine. J. Clin. Microbiol. **18:** 1102.

7. GOTSCHLICH, E. C., I. GOLDSCHNEIDER, M. L. LEPOW & R. GOLD. 1977. The Immune Response to Bacterial Polysaccharides in Man.: 391. Raven. New York.

8. COWAN, M. J., A. J. AMMANN, D. W. WARA, V. M. HOWIE, L. SCHULTZ, N. DOYLE & M. KAPLAN. 1978. Pneumococcal polysaccharide immunization in infants and children. Pediatrics **62:** 721-727.

9. CRAIN, M. J., W. D. WALTMAN, J. S. TURNER, J. YOTHER, D. F. TALKINGTON, L. S. MCDANIEL, B. M. GRAY & D. E. BRILES. 1990. Pneumococcal surface protein A (PspA) is serologically highly variable and is expressed by all clinically important capsular serotypes of *Streptococcus pneumoniae*. Infect. Immun. **58:** 3293-3299.

10. MCDANIEL, L. S., J. S. SHEFFIELD, P. DELUCCHI & D. E. BRILES. 1991. PspA, a surface protein of *Streptococcus pneumoniae,* is capable of eliciting protection against pneumococci of more than one capsular type. Infect. Immun. **59:** 222-228.

11. MCDANIEL, L. S., J. YOTHER, M. VIJAYAKUMAR, L. MCGARRY, W. R. GUILD & D. E. BRILES. 1987. Use of insertional inactivation to facilitate studies of biological properties of pneumococcal surface protein A (PspA). J. Exp. Med. **165:** 381-394.

12. TALKINGTON, D. F., D. L. CRIMMINS, D. C. VOELLINGER, J. YOTHER & D. E. BRILES. 1991. A 43-kilodalton pneumococcal surface protein, PspA: Isolation, protective abilities, and structural analysis of the amino-terminal sequence. Infect. Immun. **59:** 1285-1289.

13. BRILES, D. E., J. YOTHER & L. S. MCDANIEL. 1988. Role of pneumococcal surface protein A in the virulence of *Streptococcus pneumoniae*. Rev. Infect. Dis. **10:** S372.

14. YOTHER, J. & D. E. BRILES. 1992. Structural properties and evolutionary relationships of PspA, a surface protein of *Streptococcus pneumoniae*, as revealed by sequence analysis. J. Bacteriol. **174:** 601–609.
15. MCDANIEL, L. S., B. A. RALPH, D. O. MCDANIEL, J. YOTHER, C. K. STOVER & D. E. BRILES. Localization of protection eliciting epitopes on PspA (pneumococcal surface protein A) of *Streptococcus pneumoniae*. In press.

CD4[+] Th$_2$ T Cells Elicited by Immunization Confer Protective Immunity to Experimental *Borrelia burgdorferi* Infection[a]

T. DHARMA RAO, ARYEH FISCHER, AND
ALAN B. FREY

Department of Cell Biology and Kaplan Cancer Center
New York University School of Medicine
550 First Avenue
New York, New York 10016

The nature of the immune response to immunization with inactivated *Borrelia burgdorferi* was investigated. A CD4[+] population of anti-spirochete T cells was elicited in mice injected with *B. burgdorferi* extracts (B-31) and was established as a cell line, termed RBN2.1. RBN2.1 was able to transfer resistance to infection (by N-40) to naive recipients.[1] Assay of antigen-specific cytokine production demonstrates that the RBN2.1 line was of the Th$_2$ subclass. These data suggest that T-cell–mediated protective immunity to infection by *B. burgdorferi* can be elicited by active immunization. Active immunization or transfer of anti-spirochete RBN2.1 T cells into uninfected mice fails to induce symptoms of Lyme arthritis or carditis, implying that the presence of spirochete is required for development of the pathophysiologic consequences of Lyme disease.[1]

Although several possible mechanisms can be hypothesized, the basis for the anti-spirochete phenotype of RBN2-1 T cells *in vivo* is currently unknown. Preliminary data suggest that mice receiving RBN2.1 cells that are challenged with infectious spirochete produce anti-spirochete Ig with increased kinetics compared with control mice (T. D. Rao, unpublished data). The humoral anti-spirochete immune response may in turn impact upon resistance to infection.

It may be seen that anti-*B. burgdorferi* T cells that are elicited in immune mice recognize an antigenic epitope(s) different from the epitope(s) that elicits T cells in infection.[2] Comparison of *B. burgdorferi* antigens that elicit T-cell reactivity in infected mice with those that are reactive with T-cell line RBN2-1 will resolve this point. Why the pattern of T-cell reactivity is different in immune versus infected mice is not known, but it may be related to differences in antigen processing of live spirochete and soluble spirochetal proteins. In this regard we note that purified peritoneal macrophages produce Transforming Growth Factor β-$_1$ in response to

[a]This research was supported by a grant from DARPA (N00014-90-J-2032). A.B.F. was the recipient of a Whitehead Presidential Fellowship and a Research Career Development Award from the Irma T. Hirschl Charitable Trust.

364

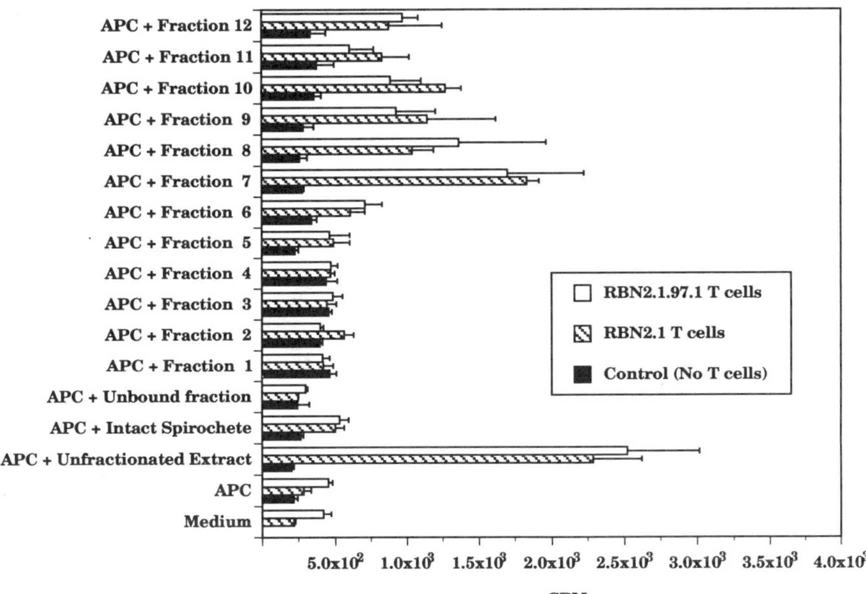

FIGURE 1. Spirochete-reactive T cells were derived from lymph nodes by nylon wool purification and then coculture in 24-well dishes in the presence of *B. burgdorferi* extract (10 μg/ml) as described.[1] Immune cells were tested for spirochete reactivity by the standard (^{3}H) thymidine uptake assay. Anti-spirochete T-cell line RBN2.1 was tested for expression of cell surface CD4 or CD8 markers by antibody staining and FACS analysis. This cell line, like the freshly isolated anti-spirochete lymph node cells, was CD4[+] CD8[−1]. RBN2.1 cells were also tested for cytokine production to characterize the functional subtype. Conditioned media from cultures of antigen-stimulated or nonstimulated RBN2.1 cells were tested for production of interleukin-2 (IL-2) and IL-4 by bioassay using CTLL-2 cells. RBN2.1 was determined by this assay to secrete IL-4 exclusively.[1] A clone was derived by limit dilution (97.1) which was determined to be phenotypically identical to the parental RBN2.1 cell line (T. D. Rao, unpublished results).

Anti-spirochete T cells were used as the basis of an antigen-presenting assay as follows. *B. burgdorferi* extract was subjected to FPLC (Mono Q) and fractions were eluted by an NaCl gradient. Individual fractions were analyzed by SDS-PAGE (FIG. 2) and also tested for the ability to stimulate proliferation of RBN2.1 cell line or clone 97.1 using freshly isolated syngeneic spleen cells as antigen-presenting cells (FIG. 1). Fractions 7–12 contain the antigenic proteins that are reactive with the anti-spirochete T cells.

coculture with *B. burgdorferi in vitro* which may be speculated to impact upon the nature of the resultant immune response. This observation is being pursued further.

In experiments designed to identify antigens reactive with RBN2.1 T cells, soluble spirochetal extracts were subjected to chromatography by FPLC, and fractions were analyzed by SDS-PAGE and also tested for the ability to stimulate anti-spirochete RBN2.1 T cells (FIGS. 1 and 2). The antigen purification data which used RBN2.1 cells as the basis of *in vitro* antigen presentation showed that the reactive antigen(s) has apparent molecular weight greater than 50 kD, indicating that major *B. burgdorferi*

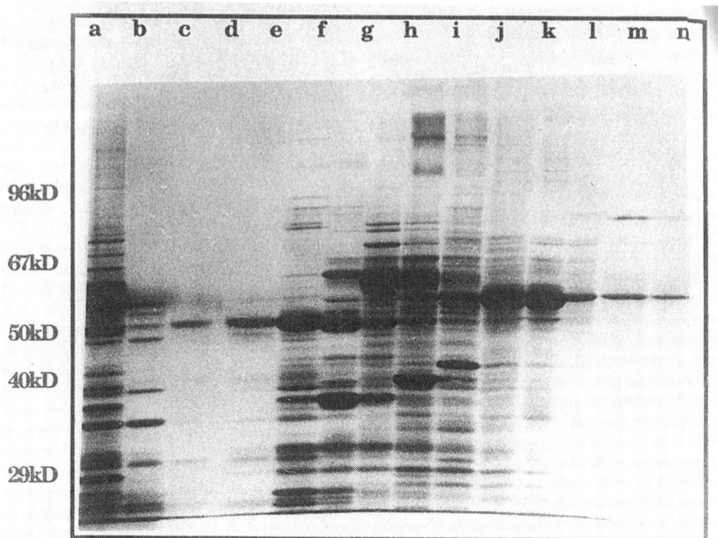

FIGURE 2. FPLC fractions were assayed for protein concentration, and 7 μg of each fraction were analyzed by SDS-PAGE that was developed by a silver stain procedure. The following are assignments of SDS-PAGE lanes and FPLC fractions; *lane a,* material loaded onto the FPLC column (''unfractionated extract''); *lane b,* the material not adsorbing to the column (''unbound''); *lane c,* fraction 2; *lane d,* fraction 3; *lane e,* fraction 4; *lane f,* fraction 5; *lane g,* fraction 6; *lane h,* fraction 7; *lane i,* fraction 8; *lane j,* fraction 9; *lane k,* fraction 10; *lane l,* fraction 11; *lane m,* fraction 12; and *lane n,* fraction 13.

surface antigens OspA, OspB, or flagellin are not the target. Identification of *B. burgdorferi* antigens that are recognized by anti-spirochete T cells able to confer protective immunity to infection will guide the rational design of recombinant anti-*B. burgdorferi* candidate vaccines.

REFERENCES

1. T. D. RAO, D. JACOBS & A. B. FREY. 1994. Murine CD4$^+$ Th$_2$ T cells can be elicited by immunization which confer protective immunity to experimental *Borrelia burgdorferi* infection. Submitted.

2. DESOUZA, M., A. SMITH, D. BECK, G. TERWILLIGER, E. FIKRIG & S. BARTHOLD. 1993. Long-term study of cell-mediated responses to *Borrelia burgdorferi* in the laboratory mouse. Infect. Immunity **61:** 1814–1822.

Immunopotentiating Ability of Neisserial Major Outer Membrane Proteins

Use As an Adjuvant for Poorly Immunogenic Substances and Potential Use in Vaccines

LEE M. WETZLER

The Maxwell Finland Laboratory for Infectious Diseases
Boston City Hospital
Boston University School of Medicine
Boston, Massachusetts 02118

Neisserial porins, a group of major outer membrane proteins (OMP) of pathogenic Neisseria, have been demonstrated to have potential adjuvant activity by various investigators. For example, (1) meningococcal outer membrane vesicles were used successfully to improve the immune response to the *Hemophilus influenzae* type B capsule, and this vaccine, manufactured by Merck, was recently licensed by the FDA[1]; (2) gonococcal porins have augmented the immune response in animals to malaria-derived peptides;[2] (3) neisserial porins have augmented the immune response to human gangliosides in melanoma patients and their tumors decreased in size after immunization (personal communication, Dr. P. Livingston); and (4) neisserial porins, when formed into proteosomes and immunized into animals without additional adjuvants, induced significant immune responses.[3] The experiments to be described were performed to investigate this phenomenon.

Purified meningococcal group C capsular polysaccharide (CPS) was used as a test antigen to measure the potential adjuvant properties of the neisserial OMP. CPS was used successfully in antimeningococcal vaccines, but the response is relatively short-lived and not adequate in infants.[4] Murine immunizations were performed using purified CPS cross-linked with lipid and formed into non-covalent complexes (proteosomes) with each of four purified neisserial OMP class 1 (C1) or class 3 (C3) proteins from *Neisseria meningitidis* or protein IA (PIA) or protein IB (PIB) proteins from *N. gonorrhoeae*. The OMP were chromatographically purified[5] from mutants lacking the other major outer membrane proteins (respectively, C4/C3 or C4/C1 minus meningococci and protein III minus gonococci[6]) to insure that the response measured was solely due to the specific proteins being tested. Groups of eight lipopolysaccharide-resistant mice (strain C3H/HeJ) were immunized with 25 μg of CPS associated with 25 μg of each OMP formed into proteosomes. The mice were immunized three times, 2 weeks apart, and pooled sera were collected prior to each immunization and 2 weeks after the third immunization. Anti-CPS IgG and IgM was measured by ELISA.

Levels of anti-CPS IgG were higher in mice immunized with CPS associated with C1, C3, PIA, or PIB proteosomes than in mice immunized with plain CPS or

"

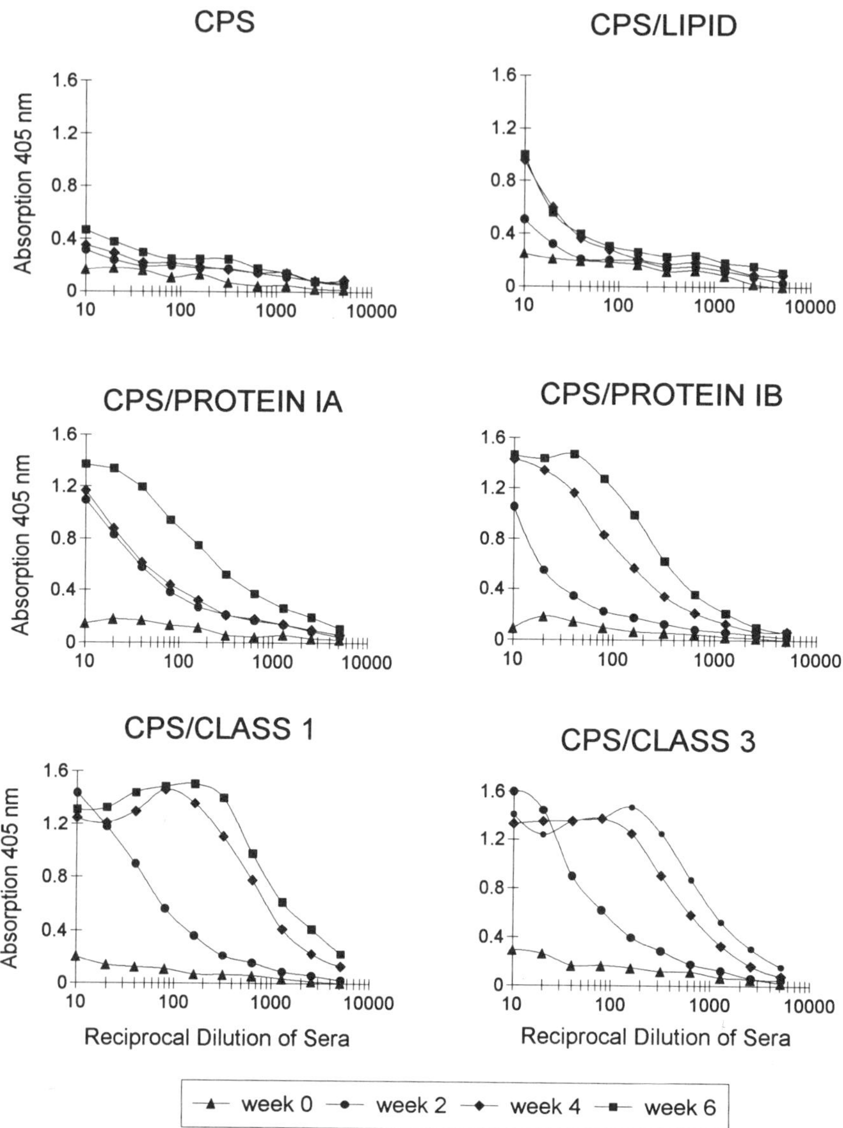

FIGURE 1. ELISA curves of pooled sera from each separate group of mice immunized with meningococcal group C capsular polysaccharide (CPS). ELISA measures the anti-CPS IgG response. The reciprocal dilution of the sera is on the abscissa, and ELISA optical density at 405 nm is on the ordinate. The six groups were immunized with (1) CPS, (2) CPS cross-linked with lipid (CPS/ lipid), (3) CPS/protein IA proteosomes (CPS/PIA), (4) CPS/protein IB proteosomes (CPS/PIB), (5) CPS/class 1 proteosomes (CPS/class 1), or (6) CPS/class 3 proteosomes (CPS/class 3). The data shown are for the sera collected 2 weeks after the third immunization. The anti-CPS IgG level was greater when the immunizing preparations included the neisserial outer membrane proteins.

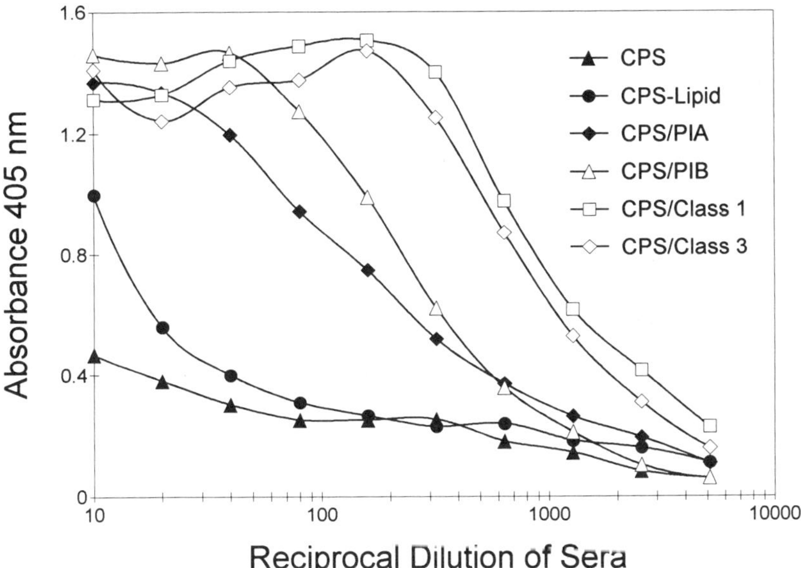

FIGURE 2. ELISA curves of pooled sera from the same six groups of mice in Figure 1. ELISA measures the anti-CPS IgG response. Mice were immunized at week 0, 2, and 4 and sera collected before each immunization and 2 weeks after the third immunization. The data are shown for the last sera collection to demonstrate the relative immunopotentiating ability of the neisserial porins.

CPS/lipid (FIG. 1). This demonstrates that the increased antibody response to CPS was due to the use of the neisserial porins and not to cross-linking alone. Mice immunized with CPS associated with C1 or C3 had the greatest increase in anti-CPS IgG over CPS/PIB or CPS/PIA immunized mice. In addition, a booster effect was seen after each immunization when the porins were used (FIG 2), suggesting that the response was T-cell dependent *versus* the usual T-cell-independent immune response seen with polysaccharides. In addition, the anti-CPS IgM response was greater when the porins were not present in the complexes, also implying that a T-cell-dependent response was induced when CPS was immunized with the porins.

CPS was cross-linked with lipid to allow insertion in the porin proteosomes without covalent bonds. Protein carriers, when covalently linked to haptens have long been known to help induce antibodies to these haptens. With the use of non-covalent complexes, the immune augmentation seen with neisserial OMP could be due to mechanisms distinct from the classical hapten-carrier model. B lymphocytes, when incubated with purified PIA or PIB, can costimulate CD3 cross-linked CD4 T lymphocytes (data not shown) Costimulation (second signal activity) is an important step in specific T-lymphocyte activation[7] and could be a possible mechanism for the porins' immunopotentiating ability.

REFERENCES

1. DONNELLY, J. J., R. R. DECK & M. A. LIU. 1990. J. Immunol. **145:** 3071–3079.
2. LOWELL, G. H., W. R. BALLOU, L. F. SMITH, R. A. WIRTZ, W. D. ZOLLINGER & W. T. HOCKMEYER. 1988. Science **240:** 800–802.
3. WETZLER, L. M., M. S. BLAKE, K. BARRY & E. C. GOTSCHLICH. 1992. J. Infect. Dis. **166:** 551–555.
4. GOTSCHLICH, E. C. 1984. Meningococcal meningitis. *In* Bacterial Vaccines. R. Germanier, Ed.: 237–255. Academic Press. New York.
5. WETZLER, L. M., M. S. BLAKE & E. C. GOTSCHLICH. 1988. J. Exp. Med. **168:** 1883–1897.
6. WETZLER, L. M., E. C. GOTSCHLICH, M. S. BLAKE & J. M. KOOMEY. 1989. J. Exp. Med. **169:** 2199–2209.
7. SCHWARTZ, R. H. 1992. Cell **71:** 1065–1068.

Microbial Pathogenesis and Immunity: A Perspective

FREDERICK A. MURPHY[a] AND STEPHEN A. MORSE[b]

[a]School of Veterinary Medicine
University of California, Davis
Davis, California 95616

[b]Division of Sexually Transmitted Diseases Laboratory Research
National Center for Infectious Diseases
Centers for Disease Control and Prevention
Atlanta, Georgia 30333

At a conference like this, the organizers can only go so far in organizing the subtopics into a logical sequence, which adds up to a complete story—in this case, the complete story of microbial pathogenesis and the immune response to infection. More organization is expected of a book. In a book, it is easy to see how all the parts fit together, what's missing, where opportunities for further research lie, where we go from here. Perhaps this last contribution to this conference is meant to be more like a book or at least its table of contents.

Of the many choices available for organizing this "table of contents" on the subject of pathogenesis and the immune response to infection, the approach chosen by Cedric Mims appears to be the most useful. Mims[1] cuts across the many disciplines of experimental pathology, microbiology, and immunology and favors consideration of the effects of infection on the whole host organism. His approach emphasizes common mechanistic principles and allows broad comparisons of pathophysiologic effects of different kinds of infections in different organs and tissues. This is of particular value when we extrapolate from laboratory models to infections of humans, where we are limited in how we can manipulate variables. We need all the help we can get when we jump from inbred to outbred subjects and when we cross the wide gulf dividing experimental science and the "clinical trial."

The Mims scheme of organization first centers on the strategies used by etiologic agents to gain entrance to the body, to extend from the entry site to key target sites, including those responsible for morbidity and mortality, and then to extend to those sites responsible for transmission to the next host. This is the realm of pathobiology, that is, what the pathogen does when unfettered by human intervention. Although little time in this conference was spent on this theme overall, there have been some very exciting new concepts concerning entry. However, even when discussing entry, the diversity is overwhelming; nothing would appear to be more different than the entry of HIV via sexual transmission and the entry of *Shigella flexneri* into gut epithelium. Nevertheless, some aspects of this process are shared by vastly different pathogens.

Perhaps this is the place to comment on viral pathogenesis versus bacterial pathogenesis. As the fields of virology and bacteriology have drifted apart, some

371

people have said that there is still common ground, the basis for getting together to share insights—pathogenesis has been mentioned as part of the common ground; after all, it is the same immune system that these pathogens are dealing with. But, based on this meeting, this may not be true. The realm of viral pathogenesis has become very different from the realm of pathogenesis covered at this meeting. For example, considerable emphasis was placed on nonspecific factors affecting the invasion and spread of microorganisms. The importance of physical barriers (mucosal, epithelial, etc.), nonimmune aspects of acute inflammation, and antibiotics (magainin, defensins) was discussed; however, there was little discussion of receptors and the very specific bases for viral entry and tropism. There are other examples which suggest that with the growth of these fields, the pathogenesis of viral and microbial diseases will drift apart further. Perhaps a future meeting can bring these fields back together.

Within the realm of the pathogenesis of the unfettered infection process, concepts relating to target cell damage in relation to the generation of the progeny microorganisms and viruses required for each succeeding step in the infection process and for their ultimate perpetuation in nature are introduced by Mims.[1] This is followed by concepts relating to host immune response and inflammatory response and to host immunopathologic response, again organized with respect to their effects on the completion of the infection cycle and the perpetuation of the microorganism or virus in nature. The result is a holistic view, leading to means of intervention in the course of infection and intervention for disease prevention and control. For example, the theme cited several times during the conference, that the successful microorganism or virus must not kill its host too quickly for fear of being buried with its host, is certainly a universal truth.

The first session topic of this conference focused on how microorganisms evade host defense mechanisms. This presumed that we knew enough about how these pathogens attack and that the host would fight back effectively. Spectacular illustrations presented during this session demonstrated that microorganisms were incredibly diverse in their evasion tactics. It would be naive to try to simplify the differences in the tactics used by *Toxoplasma gondii, Neisseria gonorrhoeae, Listeria monocytogenes,* and *Mycobacterium tuberculosis* to evade host defenses, yet this very successful group of pathogens employs only a small fraction of the variety of evasive tactics used by microorganisms and viruses taken as a whole. After hearing how *T. gondii* hides out in its vacuole, it would be interesting to know if the parasite proteins, which inserted into the vacuolar membrane, could be developed as a potential vaccine.

In the same session, it was pointed out that physical sequestration, controlled microenvironments, nutritional flux, antibodies (and complement), blocking antibodies, actin polymerization propulsion, protected cell-to-cell spread, inhibition of phagosome fusion, escape from the phagosome, life in the cytoplasm, and many specific microbial enzyme and toxin actions were all used selectively in the evasion of host defenses. Nevertheless, it's interesting how quickly we turn to tactics used to evade the *immune response* per se rather than to more primitive physiologic host defenses. One might also ask about late events. Are we so focused on studying early events in the pathogenesis of infection, in the interaction between microbe and host, that we have stopped thinking about the importance of late events, especially in regard to the pathologic consequences of infection.

The Mims scheme is based on the premise that the major physiochemical distinctions in chemical composition, mode of replication, etc., of the many different microorganisms do not necessarily predict distinctions in host-parasite interactions. Rather, his approach focuses on those holistic characteristics that most likely relate to target specificity (tropism), transmissibility, growth kinetics, and host cell and tissue damage and/or dysfunction, those characteristics that are more important pathogenetically and to the end users of pathogenetic information, the pathologist, the clinician, the epidemiologist, and the researcher working on prophylaxis and therapeutics.

In the second session, the conference turned to antigenic variation and T-cell interactions. We faced one of the great enigmas of pathogenesis: how can microorganisms, especially certain viruses, maintain phenotypic stability while exhibiting such incredible genotypic variation? As pathogens "change their coats" via mutational drift and recombinational shift, discarding old antigenic profiles and presenting new ones, how can the host's immune response ever keep up? As in the case of HIV, the host does not keep up and neutralization escape mutants eventually dominate and disease progresses. There is a sense that in such cases we have explored the limits of the host's antiviral armamentarium, whereas the virus is just toying with the first few of its many tricks. Will it not always be true that microorganisms will be quicker to find ways to change and evade the host, while the host will always have to compromise, adapting ancient mechanisms to specific changes as best it can?

The Mims concept serves well in organizing discussions of the pathogenesis of individual diseases. However, it also extends well from the individual to the population as a whole. In fact, understanding the pathogenesis of a disease in the individual host provides important insight and explanation of the behavior of the disease in the host population and, conversely, a lack of understanding of pathogenetic mechanisms in the individual reduces many epidemiologic and disease control concepts to empirical observations.

In the third and fourth sessions, the area of host response to microbial infection and the specific area of cytokines were examined. The presentations represented an expansive perspective–from thymic hormone response, to natural killer cell response, to comprehensive coverage of the cytokine array of these and all other cells responding to infection. We heard quite a bit about the Th1 and Th2 T-cell dichotomy of response, affected by the nature of antigens, the anatomic location of the response, and many other variables. In the end, the more we know about this important dichotomy, the more intrigued we become about what we do not know about its regulation and other effectors. In this case, there is a sense that many important answers are imminent. As Th1 and Th2 T cells are studied further, especially in regard to the exquisitely regulated cytokine induction cascade, it is easy to imagine many "accelerator," "adjuvant," or "modulator" activities being added to vaccine constructs; the cytokines that act on epithelial and parenchymal cells (IL-8, IL-1, and IL-12) and those that act on the immune system (IL-2, IL-4, IFN-γ etc.) will all need comprehensive testing. Surely DHEA, vitamin D, and other approaches for eliciting mucosal immunity and immunity in older people will have to be tried as well. And certainly, minigenes and DNA per se and idiotypes, which offer great promise for novel vaccine development, especially where very complex "cocktails" of antigens are called for, will need clinical trials. An important point in this regard is that despite the predictive value of models, we will not know the real value of these vaccine strategies until they are tried in humans.

In the fifth session of the conference, discussion turned to bacterial attachment, adherence, host receptors, and mechanisms of cell and tissue injury in microbial infection. For bacterial diseases, this is the realm of adhesion and adhesins, invasion and invasins, colonization, mucosal inflammation, cell invasion, and cell killing. Considering that there is no animal model that mimics all aspects of gonococcal disease, it is amazing how many lessons are being taught in these areas by studies of *Neisseria gonorrhoeae*. But if gonococcal pathogenesis is too subtle, just think about *Shigella flexneri*—as violent in its very specific way of invading the colon as turpentine injection.

In the sixth and last session of the conference, the agenda centered on vaccination and immunoprophylaxis, the ultimate attempt of humans to interfere with the infection, progression, and transmission of microbial and viral pathogens. This was a fitting conclusion to the program as we must study pathogenesis not just because it is fascinating, but because it is crucial if we are to press on with the development of more rational means of intervention in the course of microbial and viral infections.

REFERENCE

1. MIMS, C. A. 1987. The Pathogenesis of Infectious Disease, 3rd Ed. Academic Press. London.

Subject Index

Index of Contributors